D1563563

THE CITADEL OF THE SENSES
AND OTHER ESSAYS

The Citadel of the Senses
and Other Essays

Macdonald Critchley

C.B.E., M.D., F.R.C.P., Hon. F.A.C.P.

The National Hospital
Queen Square
London, England

Raven Press ■ New York

Raven Press, 1140 Avenue of the Americas, New York, New York 10036

Made in the United States of America

Library of Congress Cataloging in Publication Data

Critchley, Macdonald.
  The citadel of the senses.

  Includes bibliographies and index.
    1. Neurology—Addresses, essays, lectures.
I. Title.   [DNLM: 1. Neurology—essays.   WL 9 C934c]
RC244.C75   1985   612.8   85-2365
ISBN 0-88167-105-3

The material contained in this volume was submitted as previously unpublished material, except in the instances in which credit has been given to the source from which some of the illustrative material was derived.

for Eileen

Preface

Somerset Maugham regarded old age as the time to undertake those tasks shirked in youth because they would have taken too long. This second collection of jottings is thus explained.

My previous volume *The Divine Banquet of the Brain* was largely prompted by sentiments of nostalgia. This symptom, I find, is still active, motivating me to share memories of personalities and events of an earlier, prescientific age of neurology. It was a time of adventure, excitement and promise. My initial contact with clinical medicine even transcended the expectations of my boyhood. Hence I pay tribute to my first chief Newman Neild, to whom I served as Clerk and then House Physician. Though an anachronism and an eccentric, a cat that walked alone, he was tireless in his encouragement during an impressionable period.

Something like reverence applies to my attitude towards such neurological giants as Jackson and Gowers. I had never met either of them—both died before I had left school—but when at the age of 23 I stepped over the threshold of The National Hospital, Queen Square, I became aware of an uncanny feeling that they were still there, haunting the wards and quizzing me closely. They were not alone, for Horsley, Ferrier, and Bastian, too, were lurking around, watching me, breathing down my neck. But they were benevolent, inspiring ghosts, all of them.

At Queen Square I came under the spell of not one guru but several, all of whom had worked cheek by jowl with those legendary pioneers that still, spook-like, waited around the corner. I learned to know them at secondhand but intimately nonetheless.

The wards were cosy, with their caged birds and blazing coal-fires; the ward sisters autocratic, imperious, Junoesque. Like Agag, one had to tread warily. "Sir William Gowers would never approve," they would mutter to me, or "Dr. Jackson never said anything like that."

In those days, after passing through the swing doors into the entrance hall, one was assailed by a strong and evocative aroma made up of a blending of biological ammonia with stale coarse-cut tobacco. This smell of tobacco has vanished, but in the Twenties it was very much there, piquant and compelling. Today it is no more than a memory, but a vivid one, full of associations.

I can conjure up the mosaic of the ground floor which was like a Roman villa. When the war came, maintenance men were no longer available and protective floorboards were laid down. There they remain, and today no one but myself seems aware of the artwork that lies beneath.

Similar feelings of magic followed me whenever I visited Paris. Babinski—as far as I can recall, I never met personally—was there, still an important though remote figure, stalking in silence down the Rue de Seine on his way to the Société de Neurologie. I knew his associates very well indeed. Alajouanine, friend of Ravel, equally conversant with the literature of both France and England. It was he who first acquainted me with la paralysie des amoureux. Then there was Mondor, surgeon, member of the Académie française and author of *A propos du faune*. Jean Delay I knew in those days, biographer and disciple of André Gide; René Leriche, that philosopher-surgeon and crony of Matisse; de Clérambault, crazy as a coot but brilliant; the polymath Lhermitte, a veritable Dr. Casaubon; the lovable André Thomas, who, in his late nineties, took up the study of the newborn; Crouzon, the epicure; and Marcel Pétiot, psychiatrist and mass murderer. No wonder that Paris, like London, was heady wine, though of quite a different vintage.

Such youthful sentiments of awe—that "white light of wonder" to use G. K. Chesterton's words—linger and, I suppose, provoke an inadequate expression in this present volume. As Lord Bacon put it, "to write treatises requireth leisure in the worker and leisure in the reader...which is the cause which hath made me choose to write certain brief notes set down rather significantly than curiously."

Nether Stowey,   *Macdonald Critchley*
Somerset   1985

Contents

The Citadel of the Senses: The Nose as Its Sentinel

Among the attributes of the brain which the elder Pliny assigned were "the crowning pinnacle," "the Seat of Government of the Mind," "the Regulator of the Understanding," and in particular "the Citadel of Sense-perception." What are conventionally termed special senses are five in number, though others might well exist of which we have little understanding. To some degree they are endowments of the entire animal species, but as subjective experiences they are best comprehended in *Homo sapiens*.

The sense of smell, subserved by the first cranial nerve, does not merit its relative neglect by scientists, for to a student of neurology it offers an unprecedented medley of problems and observations. Some of the latter are factual, others speculative, but all are exciting. Although smell contributes considerably to the sense of taste, this sense modality is not considered in detail. Rather, we shall linger at what Bunyan called the nose-gate to the city of Mansoul, to the exclusion of the other four portals. Let us then emulate McKenzie, who, in his *Aromatics and the Soul* proclaimed "I sing of smells, perfumes, odours, whiffs and sniffs, of aromas, bouquets, fragrances, and also, though temperately and restrainedly I promise you, of effluvia, reeks, foetors, stenches and stinks."

In cookery, Brillat-Savarin taught that the nose is the sentinel that proclaims "Halt! who goes there?"

Incidentally, how does one define a smell? Dictionaries are at a loss and either resort to listing synonyms or else beg the question by referring to the act of smelling. The *O.E.D.* fares no better than Dr. Samuel Johnson. Brain morphology or comparative anatomy is the logical introduction of osmics, that is, the science of smell. Certain insects, such as butterflies and moths, have uncanny powers of detecting others of their species more than a mile away. Such a feat has been equated with a Londoner sniffing out a female in Siberia. Whether this process of communication depends upon olfaction as we know it is uncertain, and some other, little understood form of transmission may be at work.

Fish are also sensitive to "osmyls," or odoriferous substances, within their aqueous environment. Here the perceptive organ may not be confined to the region of the jaw but extend to large areas of skin over the flanks or underbelly. McCartney (1972) declared that some migratory fish such as the salmon can detect traces of toxic substances, and that the eel can perceive 1 cm^3 of phenyl ethyl alcohol in a volume of water equal to that of Lake Constance. It is believed that the salmon smolt finds and returns to its parent river by means of its sense of smell.

In most lowly mammals smell warns about predators or prey in the vicinity. It is also a powerful agent in the breeding impulse. In short, olfaction is vital for survival. Wood-Jones described a process in comparative anatomy which he named "the rise of the smell-brain." Superior to the sensorimotor neurons as existing in fish, reptiles, and birds, a layer of cortical cells develops. This new structure is also "superior" in function and lies over the older cellular masses like a pallium, or mantle. Its role is mainly that of olfaction. Except for a shallow hippocampal groove, it is smooth, or "lissencephalic." Later, a superficial furrow appears which represents the beginnings of a rhinal fissure separating the rhinencephalon from a more caudal neopallium concerned with mobility and with tactile, auditory, and visual perception. In man, the rhinencephalon includes the olfactory bulbs, peduncles, anterior perforated substance, piriform area, and amygdaloid nucleus. The septum, hippocampus, fornix, gyrus fornicatus, mammillary bodies, and anterior nuclei of the thalamus are possibly also olfactory in function. In subhominid mammals the brain is macrosomatic, being principally concerned with the sense of smell.

Later, other fissures appear, indicating a considerable expansion of the gray matter of the brain corresponding with an elaboration of function within the neopallium.

The mammal steadily evolves new biological characteristics. Its world of smell is also enriched by specialized tactile stimuli arising in the most forward region of the body. The entire shape of the body changes; its skull is now conspicuous for its prominent muzzle or snout, at the tip of which is a pigmented and highly sensitive cap of mucous membrane kept continuously moist. Not only is it receptive to an abundance of olfactory stimuli, or osmyls—most too faint for human detection—it is also highly sensitive to touch. Behind and alongside this wet-nosed muzzle is a complicated arrangement of vibrissae or feelers. Thus the creature "noses its way" around, rooting out food, all the time on the alert for alarm signals indicating the proximity of foes. A specialization has taken place in the maxillary area, something which Edinger called the "oral sense." Centrally it is associated with the appearance in the thalamus of a nucleus rotundus, and in a cortex a region which represents the beginnings of a somaesthetic or parietal lobe.

The mammalian osmophoric or olfactory-receptive area is characterized by its structure and its extensity. There is a greater vomerine development in animals than in man, and the conchae within the nose are more numerous. Whereas the human olfactory area measures 5 to 10 mm^2, it is as much as 150 mm^2 in a dog. The sensitive area is ciliated and pigmented. In humans it is yellowish in colour, while in macrosomatic animals it is dark brown or black. Pigment is believed to be important, for unduly pale specimens of herbivores are thought to be poorly protected against the ingestion of poisonous plants. Albinism in humans is often associated with total or partial anosmia.

At this point one must consider those imposing offshoots from the main vertebrate tree, namely the *proboscidae*. Because of their heavy tusks a counterbalance is required in the way of a short, stout neck. Were it not for an elaboration of the snout and upper lip to form an elongated, mobile, sensitive, and prehensile trunk, these animals would not be able to drink. This structure enables them to suck water and gather food which they convey to the mouth. The elephant's trunk is actually a tool of incredible delicacy as well as strength. Whether its perceptual efficiency is accompanied by an olfactory potential that puts the elephant within the category of a macrosomatic is uncertain, though without doubt it surpasses *Homo sapiens* in that respect. Not surprisingly, the elephant's brain is large, especially in its transverse diameter, and the cortex is highly convoluted.

Morphology indicates that olfaction is, or was, the principal guardian of the gateways to the citadel of the senses, even though it is the one least understood. But in *Homo sapiens* there is a decline in the smell-brain, with an enhancement in vision, hearing, and the dexterity of the forelimbs, now freed from locomotory duties.

The dog, especially the trained tracker or sniffer, is certainly the most familiar if not the supreme exponent of smell and one in which olfaction has been studied most convincingly. A dog can be conditioned to smell out 1 mg of butyric acid in 100 million cubic metres of air and, to quote McCartney again, "can follow fresh and old human scent-tracks on various kinds of surfaces under various weather conditions, can distinguish between such tracks when they are not less than a few months old, and when following a particular track, can ignore cross and diversionary tracks."

These bald, factual details are impressive, but they do not unravel or explain the nature of the canine world of smell. How does a dog learn not only to perceive but also to identify the myriad osmic stimuli that constantly bombard and excite his rhinencephalon? Smell constitutes a matter of compelling interest or curiosity. Like a sleuth, the dog trots along the highway, nose down, proceeding from one minilandmark to another, periodically pausing to ascertain which other dogs have preceded him. Not content with this pleasurable quest, he contributes, for some obscure reason, his personal quota of information. Suppositions there are, it is true, but none is convincing. Staking out of territory is plausible but too artless to be wholly acceptable. The dog's visual milieu seems of minor importance. Auditory perception, although surpassing our own, does not compete with the fascination of his world of smell. The dog's aesthetic standards are not ours; indeed, what for us is fragrant and delectable does not by any means apply to him. Stenches, mephitic and nauseous, often hold a curious attraction. Here lies an uncharted territory which invites scientific study.

It took the genius of Virginia Woolf to venture into this arena. Concerning Elizabeth Barrett Browning's spaniel Flush, who was Browning's companion on her sojourn in Italy, Woolf wrote:

> Flush wandered off into the streets of Florence to enjoy the rapture of smell. He threaded his path through main streets and back streets, through squares and alleys by smell. He nosed his way from smell to smell; the rough, the smooth, the dark, the golden. He went in and out, up and down, where they beat brass, where they bake bread, where the women

sit combing their hair, where the birdcages are piled high on the causeway, where the wine spills itself in dark red stains on the pavement, where leather smells and harness and garlic, where cloth is beaten, where vine leaves tremble, where men sit and drink and spit and dice—he ran in and out, always with his nose to the ground, drinking in the essence; or with his nose in the air vibrating with the aroma. He slept in this hot patch of sun—how sun made the stone reek! He sought that tunnel of shade—how acid the shade made the stone smell! He devoured whole bunches of ripe grapes, largely because of their purple smell; he chewed and spat out whatever tough relic of goat or macaroni the Italian housewife had thrown from the balcony—goat and macaroni were raucous smells, crimson smells. He followed the swooning sweetness of incense into the violet intricacies of dark cathedrals; and, sniffing, tried to lap the gold on the window-stained tomb.*

When we turn to the question of olfactory perception in man, we revert to a relatively humbler category, nevertheless a highly complex one. A sense of smell is a general endowment, but not to an identical degree in all. Individual differences exist as regards acuity of smell. To some, these are innate variations, but some are the product of environmental circumstances. The detection of a smell does not necessarily imply its identification. If it be true, as has been alleged, that the average person can detect 2,000 to 4,000 odours—and some, with practice, as many as 10,000—then it is obvious that our vocabulary would not be able to keep pace with this multitude of stimuli. Most persons have experienced the predicament of being unable to name an odour which seems quite familiar. Aesthetic judgement is yet another gift, one which is bestowed with less liberality.

It is a common occurrence that a perfume, whether it is identified or not, is a potent agent in evoking memories of events in the remote past. Hughlings Jackson asserted that although smell occupies in man a lowly rank as a "digestive sensation," in another way its rank is high. It has been called, he said, the most suggestive of all the senses; and smells have a remarkable power in that they call up remembrances of past scenes or happenings. This has important neurological implications.

The evocative property of smell is, of course, well known and naturally has not escaped the notice of writers. It is an occurrence shared by taste as well as smell. For example, Marcel Proust, in his introspective way, was well-nigh obsessed with the smell of things. In one passage he set out at length how his aunt would offer him madeleines after she had dipped them in her teacup. Immediately the flavour would cull up the memory of an old gray house as vividly as in a theatrical set. The sight or the feel of the madeleine had no such effect. For Emile Zola, olives would, without fail, conjure up scenes of Provence where he had lived many years before.

Another property of olfaction is even more interesting. Although refinement in odorous appreciation is largely inborn, it can also be trained, just as a tracker dog can be conditioned to root out drugs. We here again witness the intimate alliance

*From *Flush* by Virginia Woolf. Reprinted with permission by Harcourt Brace Jovanovich, Inc. and Hogarth Press as well as the estate of Virginia Woolf.

of smell and taste. In the ability to judge and evaluate haute cuisine or vintage wines, the two senses cooperate. Those whose epicurean gifts are delicate find their vocation as wine importers or tea tasters. Indeed the combined action of smell and taste may obliterate memories that are more down to earth. Was it not Hilaire Belloc who, reminiscing in his club, confessed he could not remember the village or even the name of the girl, but the wine they drank had been Chateau Grillet 1906?

To another climate belongs the stockpile of body odours, and these are far more offensive to others than to the one from whom they emanate. This was expressed in the classic era in the phrase *stercus cuique suum bene olet* (everyone's dunghill smells all right to himself). Certain odours are peculiar to a given ethnic group, who are unaware of them, although they are all too evident to those of a different race. Thus while blacks are said by whites to be characterised by a distinctive smell, this observation is reciprocal (the Fee-Fi-Fo-Fum syndrome). This is not a matter of prejudice but is a product of anatomical vagaries. Body smells proceed from specialized apocrine glands. They vary in number, size, and distribution according to race and sex. Even in a homogeneous Caucasian stock, distinctive odours may be emitted by individual members. The smell itself is the product of the chemical composition of the secretion, modified perhaps by the bacterial action dependent on personal hygiene.

Apocrine glands are present in hairy parts of the body such as the mons veneris, anus, and particularly the armpits (Fig. 1). Chemically the secretion belongs to the caprylic group of iron-containing fatty acids. A sensitive nose, it is claimed, can detect an odour peculiar to red-headed subjects. Even more, it has been asserted that members of a family group sometimes share a specific and detectable odour that may even permeate their clothing.

The acuity of the sense of smell varies from person to person. A sensitive nose does not necessarily accompany high discrimination among other sense modalities, e.g., art, music, literature. The skilled wine taster does not necessarily also possess a sense of absolute pitch. Sensitivity to smell depends largely, though not entirely, upon the physical state of the nasal mucous membrane. It is temporarily reduced if the cell layer is too moist or too dry, or if it is inflamed or congested. The young are said to have a keener sense of smell than adults, though not necessarily as sophisticated. It takes time to develop olfactory finesse, and the peak is not reached until adolescence. Without doubt nonsmokers are at an advantage. General fatigue, hunger, and malaise reduce the keenness of smell, as do such environmental influences as the temperature and the degree of movement of the air, and especially the presence of tobacco smoke.

Olfactory perception fatigues readily, so that the recipient quite quickly becomes unaware of the presence of an odour which would immediately assail a newcomer. This action is not an all-or-none phenomenon, for adaptation to one odour does not prevent the recognition of another smell appearing a little later.

Another osmophoric property is that of "masking," whereby one smell may obliterate another so as to produce a neutral or odour-free state. An example in point is balsam of Tolu, which abolishes the smells of wax and of rubber.

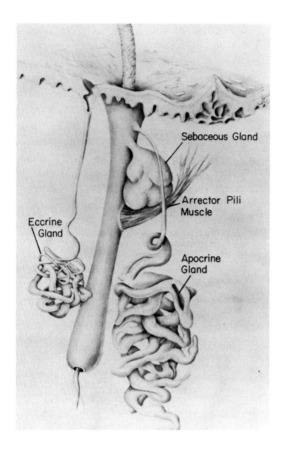

Sebaceous Gland

Arrector Pili
Muscle

Eccrine
Gland

Apocrine
Gland

FIG. 1. An apocrine gland. (From Monligna, W., and Parakkal, P. F.: *The Structure and Function of the Skin*, p. 332. Academic Press, New York, 1974, with permission.)

The potency of some odours is shown by the minute amounts which are perceptible. For example, the threshold for vanillin is 1 two-millionth of a milligram in a cubic metre of air. Such an amount is referred to as an MIO, or minimum identifiable odour.

In some cases the quality of the smell alters dramatically as the concentration decreases or increases. Jasmine, for example, we think of as fragrant and pleasurable; Dickens regarding it as "the *Omphalos* of the floral world, the Isis of flowers; and in a civil war among the gardens, it would be crowned Empress and Queen of all." However, in quantity, it changes to a grossly obnoxious stink because of its component indole. Minute amounts of such foetid animal products as musk, civet, or ambergris are important in the preparation of synthetic perfumes.

The Role of Smell in Medical Diagnosis

Diagnosticians during the last century who relied heavily on the appearance of the tongue, the feel of the pulse, and the physical state of the motions often claimed that certain diseases imparted a distinctive odour to the sickroom. Typhoid, typhus, diphtheria, rheumatic fever, nephritis, and the plague have all been associated with distinctive smells. Usually the patient is oblivious of this, doubtless being thoroughly adapted to the smell. Measles may be an exception, for a mild but nauseous aroma is sometimes detected by the patient as well as the doctor.

As if the world were not sufficiently rich in olfactory contacts, man—and more especially woman—has felt the need to seek additional osmic stimuli of which there is a considerable variety. The practice of perfumery can be traced back thousands of years, but undoubtedly over the past half century there has appeared a plethora of cosmetics, including odoriferous compounds. During this period the male sex has not remained wholly detached.

For as long as written languages have been in use, perfumes have been mentioned. The ancient Egyptian embalmers utilized them. Perfume figures repeatedly in the Song of Solomon. From time to time perfumes were referred to by Omar Khayyám (AD 130), and one suspects that an even greater sensitivity would have been shown had the poet not been such a "dram-drinking, drivelling, droning dotard" as Dr. Hastie alleged. We also find Horace (65–8 BC) deploring the sacrifice of rich farmlands to the building trade, erecting villas for the rich " . . . violet beds, all kinds of rare blossoms tickling the sense of smell, perfumes to drown those olive orchards mentioned in the past for a farmer's livelihood" (*Carmina*, Bk. II, XV). As an example of sensuous and sophisticated verse dating from the first century AD we find among Martial's epigrams the following odorous gallimaufry:

> Breath of a young maid as she bites an apple, effluence that comes from Coryeian saffron; perfume such as when the blossoming vine hangs with early clusters; the scent of grass which a sheep has just cropped; the odour of myrtle; of the Arab spice-gatherer; of rubbed amber; of a fire made pallid with eastern frankincense; of the earth when highly sprinkled with summer rain; of a chaplet that has felt locks dewy with spikenard; with all these, Diadumenus, cruel boy, thy kisses are fragrent.
>
> III. LXV.

Perfumes participate in the rituals of various religions throughout the world. In the Christian church today incense is used, particularly in the Roman Catholic and the Byzantine Orthodox services, a practice which dates from the fifth century. In Judaism, the practice of animal sacrifice, which had been universal during the second exile, gradually ceased, and the sprinkling of the altar with blood gave way to the burning of incense. Mohammedans, too, have a keen awareness of odours, though their liking for spikenard is not shared by most Europeans. The Koran contains a prayer "Oh God, make me to smell the odours of Paradise, and bless me with its delights, and make me not to smell of the fires of Hell."

What is the motive that underlies the wearing of scent? One object, of course, is to counteract offensive odours, whatever their source. During the Middle Ages the fragrance of flowers, especially rosemary and rue, was believed to protect the wearer against the plague. When men discarded wigs as an adornment, they kept their hair tidy by the local application of oily dressings. Later hair oil was artificially scented so that odorous pomades became popular mainly among men. Then arose a vogue for deodorants to ablate the body odours offensive to others.

Most important of all inducements for perfumery is its reputed aphrodisiac attribute affecting not so much the wearer as the recipient of the opposite sex. The evolution of synthetic compounds with an agreeable flavour, coupled with cunning and persuasive sales promotion, has made the cosmetic–perfumery industry big business today. Advertising has surpassed itself. One perfume ("scent" is now an unfashionable word) is claimed to be retailed only on the production of a marriage certificate! To what extent are these costly products really and truly alluring? In all probability, far less than is claimed. Could it be that the principal action of perfumery is narcissistic, rather than seductive?

The laboratory has not yet entirely ousted the traditional methods of concentrating and extracting the odour of certain blossoms and gums, using a process of *enfleurage*. One ton of rose petals is still needed to produce 1 pound of attar of roses. Musk, castor, ambergris, and especially civet are still utilized in minute quantities as fixatives.

Apothecaries for a considerable period were responsible for the manufacture of perfumes. Those who specialized in this art or mystery usually occupied premises in Bucklesbury in the City of London, their trademark being a civet cat. In the *Merry Wives of Windsor* we find Falstaff referring to Mistress Ford with a "smell like Bucklesbury." The Great Fire of 1666 raged with exceptional ferocity throughout Bucklesbury because of the highly combustible material stored within the warehouses.

Refined and delicately perfumed substances are often added to foods and beverages to combine with the "gusts" or primary units of taste in order to impart an attractive flavour. Those who have lost the sense of smell lose, almost entirely, their ability to taste; dishes are recognisable by their appearance and by the feel in the mouth of the texture of what is being eaten.

There are some who carry to extremes the pleasures of the table and the cellar. Their skill at detection and appraisal seems uncanny. At the risk of taxing the patience of those who have read my essay on "Man's Attitude to his Nose," may I quote once again my concluding paragraph?

> Now watch this gourmet. His face becomes vacant. His eyelids close and his gaze becomes lost in some far off mist. The nose alone remains alive. And what a nose! A nose with nostrils spread, diabolically voluptuous and mobile. A nose full of curiosity delicate as amber. A nose dainty with aromas. A great virtuoso of their gamut of a thousand scents. A lucid, cultured nose which evaluates, classifies and compares. A wise, translucent nose. A nose which knows! In fact, a nose!
>   Poulain & Jacqueline, *Vins et Vignes de France*

Oenophilists now and then smack of pretentiousness in their claims to recognise from the bouquet a wine's year of growth. Some allege they can detect whether the grapes had been gathered by a man or a woman, and if by the latter, whether she was married or a maid. Besides their skills in discernment, real or avowed, viniculturists and wine-bibbers tend to adopt a jargon rich in astonishing metaphors and similes, with synaesthetic loans from the language of other sense modalities. Some of these phrases are direct translations from the French tongue. Thus wines have been described as "robust," "fat," "supple," "full of stuffing," "velvety," "flabby," "vigorous," even "nervous." Wine merchants may go further. One of them has described "a naïve little domestic burgundy with no breeding, but amusing by virtue of its presumptuousness."

As one might expect, such oenological expertise has not gone unchallenged, particularly in the case of Scotch whisky. It is commonly asserted that when blindfolded one not only can distinguish malt liquors from blends but also that individual malts can be readily recognised and named, and for that matter blends also. Recently two surgical sceptics, Chadwell and Dudley, devised an experiment to test such claims (see *British Medical Journal*, 23 December 1983). Eight volunteers, four of whom were regular whisky drinkers, were blindfolded and then given a glass of three malts and three blends. Each testee was then asked (a) whether it was a malt or a blend; (b) if he could identify the distillery; and (c) if he enjoyed it. Of 72 tests, the four experienced whisky drinkers correctly recognised malts as malts in 36 instances (50%), and blends as blends 48 times (67%). Three subjects would hazard no guess. Among the inexperienced testees the results were as follows: malts were recognised as such 32 times (44%); and blends as blends 40 times (56%). Only one subject could identify the distillery of a particular malt, and on one occasion only. The researchers concluded that malts could not be singled out from blends, and that powers of discrimination did not relate to experience.

Not surprisingly, both the setup of the experiment and the conclusions therefrom did not go unchallenged. Professor Howie criticized the choice of the whiskies used as test substances, and the statistician Altman regarded the blueprint of the enquiry as not beyond reproach.

Even earlier, the claims made by reputedly accomplished wine tasters had been frowned upon as ignoring personal and environmental factors. Suggestion, too, is all important. Rabelais described how his troupe drank from the Princess Bacbuc's fountain of the purest water. By Panurge it was confidently praised as a *Beaune* of the highest quality. To Friar John it was a gallant sparkling Greek wine, while Pantagreul identified the water as the wine of *Mirevaux*, though overchilled.

Physicians are familiar with patients who complain of anosmia. Rarely is one born without a sense of smell, though it has been said that the chief scavenger of Leipzig was found at autopsy to have had no olfactory nerves. Anosmia is almost always a symptom that is acquired. In some cases it results from a viral infection; at other times it is a consequence of a long-standing septic infection within the nose. More often, anosmia is a sequela of a head injury. A fracture of the ethmoidal plate of the frontal bone may tear the olfactory nerves, causing a permanent loss of smell and great detriment to the sense of taste. The trauma may not necessarily comprise a fracture of the skull. In such cases there may be a gradual recovery of function. During the early days of convalescence it is difficult to foretell whether the anosmia will be permanent. Radiology rarely helps. Those versed in medicolegal practice usually state that if no improvement has occurred by the end of 2 years the anosmia is likely to be permanent.

Loss of taste and of smell is an unfortunate situation but not calamitous. If smell is lost, one is at least spared noisesome, putrid stenches, and it can be argued that this immunity outweighs the unfortunate failure to enjoy pleasurable fragrances. Loss of taste is a greater hardship, but oddly enough the victim retains some enjoyment at mealtimes. He learns to discriminate foodstuffs by way of their texture, and appetite certainly does not suffer. This fact is not generally known, and medical witnesses may consider that the law takes too serious a view of impaired smell and taste and so awards excessive amounts in the way of compensation. Perhaps learned judges are unduly mindful of the pleasures of a vintage claret, a Havana cigar, and a well-cooked dinner.

To one of those rare masters of olfaction engaged in the manufacture of scents, an acquired anosmia would be serious indeed. But experts whose profession it is to devise new products for the cosmetic trade are indeed few in number, being far rarer than wine tasters. The nature of their skill is enigmatic. E. P. Meunier's *Psychologie du parfumeur* (1965) is a notable contribution to this arcane subject. According to the author, such exponents are a dying breed; the necessary climate of serenity accords little with the contemporary pace. Olfactory sensibility becomes apparent at an early age, the endowment being a product of environment as well as birth. Maurice Barrès maintained that there are places which *souffle l'esprit*, and Grasse is unquestionably the locality which *souffle le parfum*. The great exponents share certain personality traits. One is enjoyment in the act of smelling, something which becomes more and more refined over the years. Another is an urge to identify, compare, and classify. Slowly there is built up a considerable olfactory memory. One can say "not only have I smelled that before, but the circumstances were such and such." Whereas anyone else might bite into an apple with enjoyment, an expert might well proclaim "Oh! This smacks of cinnamic aldehyde."

A young man embarking upon a career in perfumery will find no textbooks and no colleges of instruction. Only the experience of older colleagues is there to help him. The apprentice soon realises that he is studying a tightly locked art form. He will discover that what he learns is highly personal. Unless he has a knowledgeable parent or grandparent he can consult, he will have to endure years of groping in a certain moral and intellectual vacuum. Gradually he attains enormous patience while remaining ever receptive to inspiration, the product of his phenomenal memory for odours. This may come to him in the night, as the composer Debussy found. Plainly something mysterious is at work, beyond explanation. The end result is profit for the manufacturer, and for the inventor anonymity.

Hallucinations of smell coupled perhaps with taste are well-known neurological symptoms. Hughlings Jackson was the first to draw attention to what he termed "uncinate attacks," an expression nowadays replaced by "temporal epilepsy." They are often complicated by a peculiar mental state of forced memory or an odd feeling of familiarity with the surroundings (*déjà vu, déjà vecu*). Jackson called them "dreamy attacks," while Oppenheim used the term "crepuscular."

During such uncinate attacks the patient may unwittingly make smacking movements of the lips as well as chew, lick, and occasionally spit. Such a performance lasts only a minute or two and gives the impression that the subject is undergoing some gustatory experience that flouts the canons of accepted behaviour but of which he is not aware.

Hallucinations of taste and smell in the context of epilepsy usually baffle the patient's power of identification or even description. But almost always they are disagreeable.

Can Smells be Classified?

On the analogy of taste, where it is usual to identify four basic gustatory experiences (bitter, sweet, salty, sour), attempts have been made to establish certain primary odours. Over the years many have tried, but there has been no consensus. Four to 18 basic smells have at various hands been suggested, but the matter still awaits decision.

One of the most bizarre contributions to such endeavours has been the work of W. Septimus Piesse (1820–1882) coupled with that of his son Dr. Charles Piesse. The former was an analytical chemist who, in partnership with Lubin, opened a shop in Bond Street, London, where he sold various scents of his own manufacture, including "Trump Card," "Frangipani," and "Kiss-Me-Quick." He must have been invested with a vivid and unusual variety of synaesthetic imagery. In his opinion, there was an octave in odours as in music. Certain perfumes, he believed, harmonize like keys of an instrument. Thus almond, heliotrope, vanilla, and clematis blend. Citron, lemon, orange peel, and verbena do the same, but an octave higher. "Semi-odours," such as rose and rose geranium, are analogues of the semi-tones. He regarded the seven primary odours as camphor, lemon, jasmine, rose, almond, clove, and santal. The manner in which he associated smells with musical notes is illustrated in his tabulated "gamut of odours" (Figs. 2 and 3).

His son Charles qualified in medicine and in 1891 edited the fifth edition of his father's work *The Art of Perfumery*, which had originally been published in 1855. Dr. Piesse apparently abandoned his medical career to end his days as British Consul to Monaco.

The Nature of the Olfactory Stimulus

The smell receptors are unique, being ciliated bipolar cells, with their neurons conducting the stimulus directly to the brain. This statement seems unquestionable, but there is still doubt as to the nature of the stimulus itself assailing the sensitive mucous membrane. The many ideas that have been advanced fall into two principal categories. One hypothesis is that actual particles of some particular odour come into contact with the receptive mucous membrane. The opposing idea is that the stimulus is vibratory in character, as in the case of hearing and vision.

Those who have studied the subject support one or other of these notions in approximately equal number. One argument that has been put forward against the

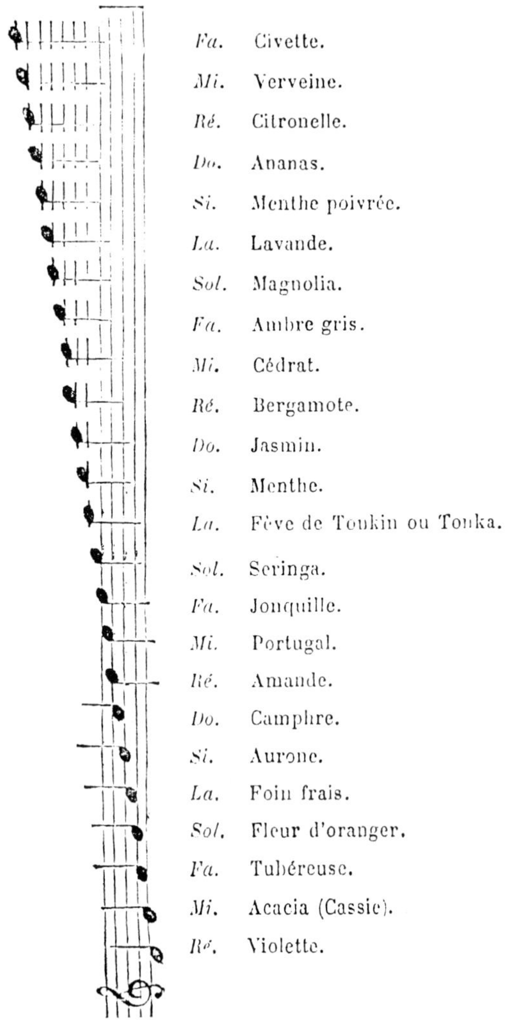

FIG. 2. Association of smells with musical notes according to Piesse: treble clef.

Fa.	Civette.
Mi.	Verveine.
Ré.	Citronelle.
Do.	Ananas.
Si.	Menthe poivrée.
La.	Lavande.
Sol.	Magnolia.
Fa.	Ambre gris.
Mi.	Cédrat.
Ré.	Bergamote.
Do.	Jasmin.
Si.	Menthe.
La.	Fève de Tonkin ou Tonka.
Sol.	Seringa.
Fa.	Jonquille.
Mi.	Portugal.
Ré.	Amande.
Do.	Camphre.
Si.	Aurone.
La.	Foin frais.
Sol.	Fleur d'oranger.
Fa.	Tubéreuse.
Mi.	Acacia (Cassie).
Ré.	Violette.

theory of chemical contact is the fact that strong-smelling substances do not lose weight however long they have been exposed to the air. This observation was made by Robert Boyle as long ago as 1673 in his *Essay on the Great Efficacy of Effluviums* and has not been contradicted.

Abuse of the Olfactory Organ

Certain volatile substances endowed with odorific properties not necessarily pleasurable in nature have been used as media for drug addiction. The practice began over a century ago with a vogue for inhaling ether and, later, chloroform in order to attain an euphoriant effect. Nitrous oxide and trilene (trichlorethylene)

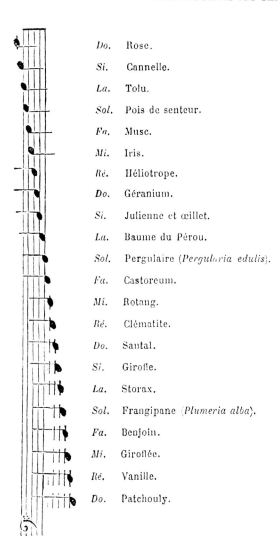

Do.	Rose.
Si.	Cannelle.
La.	Tolu.
Sol.	Pois de senteur.
Fa.	Musc.
Mi.	Iris.
Ré.	Héliotrope.
Do.	Géranium.
Si.	Julienne et œillet.
La.	Baume du Pérou.
Sol.	Pergulaire (*Pergularia edulis*).
Fa.	Castoreum.
Mi.	Rotang.
Ré.	Clématite.
Do.	Santal.
Si.	Girofle.
La.	Storax.
Sol.	Frangipane (*Plumeria alba*).
Fa.	Benjoin.
Mi.	Giroflée.
Ré.	Vanille.
Do.	Patchouly.

FIG. 3. Association of smells with musical notes according to Piesse: bass clef.

also became liable to abuse and were sources of stimulation leading to addiction. More recently a number of industrial solvents are being inhaled, such as paint thinners, paint and lacquer removers, shoepolish (turpentine), antifreeze, petrol, nailpolish (acetone), glue, and dry-cleaning material (trichlorethylene).

So we find one of the principal watchdogs of the citadel in flagrant neglect of his duty and, as it were, allowing admission to illegal and irresponsible immigrants.

Other drugs of addiction, both soft and hard, usually taken by mouth or intra-venously are also operative when ignited and the fumes inhaled. Examples are "pot" (cannabis indica) and heroin (diamorphine). The former may be rolled into a homemade cigarette; the latter is sprinkled onto a silver paper, ignited at one end, and the smoke breathed in. This is what is known as "chasing the dragon."

In all such cases, olfaction plays a very minor role. Inhalation as a portal to the nervous system has been discovered and utilized as a highly potent and very easy means for attaining hallucinatory or euphoriant experiences.

Summary

Three steps are observable in the detection of an odour. First, the perceptual organ of smell is stimulated. Second, the impulse is rapidly transmitted to the brain. Third, something takes place centrally which results in that indefinable sensation of smell.

As Moncrieff well said, "It is this third stage that is practically a closed book." Those who are intimately concerned with the workings and the aberrations of the brain should be writing that volume.

Hughlings Jackson, The Sage of Manchester Square

Just beyond the fashionable enclave where London's principal physicians and surgeons once lived and practised is the small and rather sombre Manchester Square. The northern flank is occupied by Hertford House with its famous Wallace collection. Although the private houses are elegant and spacious, they are, we must confess, grim-visaged and gloomy. Within the dark southeast corner stands No. 3, a veritable Bleak House. This is where John Hughlings Jackson, the Plato of neurology, spent most of his lonely life and where in 1911 he died at the age of 76 years. His wife, who had also been his cousin, had died 35 years previously after 11 years of a childless but happy marriage. By one of those cruel tricks that Destiny so often plays, it happened that his wife's terminal illness was characterized by countless epileptiform seizures of a focal character, the significance of which was all too evident to her husband.

Jackson never remarried, and not being gregarious or a man with intellectual interests he latterly became more and more of a recluse. He was cared for by a woman known simply as "Mead," who had originally come to the house as a parlour maid and stayed on as a factotum. At the dinner table a place was always laid for his long dead wife. His cronies were few in number, though he was widely acclaimed, respected, and held in awe by his colleagues.

His relatives, though numerous, were widely scattered, and few lived in or near London. His three brothers had long ago settled in New Zealand. Other relatives remained in Yorkshire. One branch of his family had early emigrated to Oakland, California. Closest to him was a loyal cousin, Charles Jackson, mathematics coach at "The Shop," the Military Academy at Woolwich, and known affectionately as "Slide-Rule Jackson." Living in Blackheath, "Slide-Rule" was able to visit Hughlings Jackson every week, usually taking with him his young daughter Evelyn.

It is my privilege not only to have often corresponded with this lady, now a widow of 85 living in Cheshire, but to have had opportunities of talking with her. Just a few weeks ago I visited her and was entranced by her clear recollections of "cousin John" in his latter years. She had also carried out the laborious task of constructing an elaborate pedigree, especially relating to the distaff side. Twenty-three years ago, I too, quite independently, had drawn up Jackson's family tree largely on the basis of data from New Zealand. These two pedigrees usefully interdigitate.

Jackson's solitary way of life not unnaturally conduced to a certain forgetfulness, not for remote events but for day-to-day trivia. To his absentmindedness was added increasing deafness and vertigo, so that his environment, never expansive, closed in upon him more and more. To some extent he became a benevolent eccentric. As is well known, Hughlings Jackson had always been an academic paradox. Despite his intellectual stature, his philosophical endowment, and his perspicacity, he had not been well educated. Nor was he in any respect an *arbiter elegentiae*. The visual arts, poetry, music, drama, architecture—all these meant nothing to him. He was sadly aware of his educational mediocrity, and he often commented bitterly on his inadequate schooling which, incidentally, came to an end when he was 15 years of age.

He never learned Latin, German, or Greek, but he knew French. His literary habits were odd. That is to say, in his solitude he read much, especially the works of Jane Austen, Dickens, Trollope, and Thackeray. Books, as such, meant nothing to him, and he indulged in "Tit-Bits" and, with even greater eagerness, rubbishy thrillers. These he promptly discarded, throwing page after page into the street or out of the railway carriage window on a train journey. He never amassed a library. If he needed to look up a neurological reference, he would borrow the book from a colleague. Rarely did he return the volume unprompted. After repeated requests the book might be returned, but the owner would often be dismayed to find the relevant pages torn out.

What were the origins of this father figure of neurology? Sometimes he is described as being of quite a humble background. That is not really the case. He was born in the hamlet of Green Hammerton, Yorkshire, midway between Harrogate and York. The paternal side of the family comprised respected and prosperous self-employed farmers and maltsters. The ancestry can be traced directly to a William Jackson born in 1707 in Brent Burnt, Harewood Bridge, York; more remote ancestors included women in the fifteenth and sixteenth centuries who married such worthies as the mayors of York and of Hull; there was also a Sir Richard Bowes, Bt.

It is not generally known that a cousin of Hughlings Jackson, a Miss Margaret Hardcastle Jackson, became governess to Queen Victoria's second daughter, Alice. Known in the royal household as Madgie, she remained with Princess Alice until her early marriage to Prince Louis, the Duke of Hesse-Darmstadt. Princess Alice was unfortunately a carrier of the gene for haemophilia, which she transmitted to the most attractive of her six children, "Alicky." Only three weeks after Alicky's marriage to the Crown Prince Nicholas of Russia, the Czar died, and she found herself the empress of Russia. Madgie, who had accompanied Princess Alice to Germany, was later sent for to go to St. Petersburg to look after the children, all of whom were murdered in 1918. On Madgie's return to England, she was granted a Grace & Favour residence in Regent's Park.*

---

*There are several references to Madgie in the Baroness Sophie Buxhoereden's *Life and Tragedy of Alexandra Feodorovna, Empress of Russia* (Longmans, New York, 1928). From the authoress we learn that Miss Jackson was a broadminded, cultivated person who soon gained a strong influence over her pupils. She had advanced ideas on feminine education. She tried not only to impart knowledge to her pupils but to form their moral characters and to widen their views on life. A keen politician, she was always deeply interested in all important political and social questions of the day. Miss Jackson discussed

Hughlings Jackson's mother also had an interesting background. She was Sarah Hughlings born in mid-Wales in the tiny village of Llanfihangel Rhydithon on the A488 between Knighton and Llandrindod Wells. One of her ancestors was Benjamin Hewling, whose two sons were taken prisoner after the Battle of Sedgemoor in 1685, condemned by Judge Jeffreys at the Bloody Assizes, and executed. Their elder sister Hannah Hewling married Henry, a grandson of Oliver Cromwell. One can state here and now that whatever Cromwellian characteristics were transmitted to Hughlings Jackson, no traces of cruelty or inflexibility were among them.

Young Jackson learned his letters at the village school. Afterwards he attended a school at Tadcaster, some miles away. The school no longer exists, and the original building has been incorporated within the structure of the local police station.

Each day Jackson made this journey by coach. Once something happened which made an unforgettable impression upon him. The coachman took along with him his 17-year-old daughter, and the two youngsters sat on the driver's seat. Suddenly the girl was taken ill. She screamed aloud: "I can't talk." Sure enough, her speech was grossly impaired, and she was paralysed down one side. The coach was halted, then turned round, and the girl was taken home. Though she improved, she never fully recovered her speech, and she died 12 years later.

Another incident of this sort occurred when the Jackson family took rooms at the seaside for their annual holiday. They found to their astonishment that the landlady, a jolly woman who was always laughing, could not speak. She seemed to understand what was said to her, but all that she could utter was a meaningless "Watty, watty, watty" over and over again. Here was an experience that Jackson tucked away in his mind which 20 years or so later he was to retrieve, identify, and label.

Young Jackson was finally sent for a year to a Quaker school in Nailsworth, Gloucestershire, specializing in natural science, philosophy, and French. Apparently it was an advanced, experimental school. We know nothing of the circumstances that took him there, how he fared, and why he left so early. I have found, however, that there was a Quaker family living at Cirencester 10 miles away; their name was Hewlings and may well have been related to Jackson's mother.

The next step in Jackson's career was his apprenticeship to a fashionable practice in York run by Dr. William Charles Anderson and his son Dr. Temple Anderson. They lived at 23 Stonegate, a house which still stands and now forms the attractive premises of the York Medical Society. Two years later he was enrolled as a student at the York Medical School, which no longer exists, being incorporated within the University of Leeds. In 1855 he spent a few months in London walking the wards of St. Bartholomew's Hospital, where he came under the spell of James Paget. In

---

all such matters with the children, awakening their interest in intellectual questions. Gossip of any kind was not permitted.

For many years there was an affectionate and frequent correspondence between Madgie and Princess Alicky in which the latter would sign herself "PQ no. 111," which was a shortened version of "My Poppet Queen, No. 3." (See also *Nicholas & Alexandra*," by Robert K. Massie. World Books, London, 1967.)

April 1856 he qualified by attaining the diploma of the Society of Apothecaries of London. Full details of this examination, his examiners, and the marks he was awarded are preserved in the City of London Archives at the Guildhall.

Returning to Yorkshire he was appointed resident medical officer at the York Dispensary. Apparently he was outstandingly efficient, earnestly following up every fatal case to the postmortem room. He was fortunate in having among his chiefs a most exceptional man, Dr. Thomas Laycock. This farsighted physician was highly intrigued by nervous disorders and was one of the supporters of Marshall Hall and his theories of reflex activity. Laycock undoubtedly fostered Jackson's interest in neurology, and when later he was promoted to the chair of medicine at Edinburgh he likewise inspired another student, David Ferrier.

In 1859 Jackson went back to London and lodged at 4 Finsbury Circus, together with his friend and fellow graduate from Yorkshire, Jonathan Hutchinson, who was 7 years older than he was. The following year he was successful in attaining as an external student the M.D. St. Andrews, something which 2 years later became no longer possible, the Senate having at long last realised the point of Samuel Johnson's quip.*

At this period, Jackson was becoming more and more interested in pure philosophy. In particular he was attracted to the work of Herbert Spencer who, inspired by the theories of Charles Darwin, was thinking in terms of evolution as concerning mental processes. As is well known, Jackson began to think seriously of abandoning medicine in favour of a career in academic philosophy. Fortunately, Jonathan Hutchinson dissuaded him and shrewdly advised his friend that it would be wiser to continue with his medical career and to incorporate within it a philosophical way of thinking.

Meanwhile it was necessary to live. The two friends were lucky enough to secure work as reporters for the *Medical Times & Gazette*. Their job was to attend meetings of every medical society in and around London and to record their transactions. These duties brought them in touch with all the medical and surgical elite, and the clinical meetings gave them the opportunity of seeing many rare and remarkable cases. Jackson was becoming fascinated by neurology. This culminated when that brilliant eccentric Brown-Séquard intimated to him that a vacancy for an assistant physician was likely to materialize at the recently founded Hospital for the Paralysed and Epileptic in Queen Square. Jackson applied and was successful. His duties entailed paying domiciliary visits to house-bound patients living in the poorer quarters of Holborn, St. Pancras, and Bloomsbury.

The hospital had been opened in 1860, i.e., 2 years previously, the two original members of the staff being Dr. J. S. Ramskill and C. E. Brown-Séquard. Two surgeons were coopted, namely William Fergusson, surgeon to the royal family, and J. Z. Laurence, whose interests later turned towards ophthalmology.

---

*Concerning the University of St. Andrews, which was poorly endowed but prolific with its honours, Dr. Johnson said: "Let it persevere in its present plan and it may become rich *by degrees.*"

Five years later Jackson became a full physician, and he joined the staff of the Metropolitan Hospital and 2 years after that the London Hospital. At the latter, Jonathan Hutchinson was already a consulting surgeon with a special interest in dermatology. Meanwhile Jackson had left Finsbury Circus and was living in Queen Square itself, a few doors away from that popular pub "The Queen's Larder." After his marriage he moved to 38 Bedford Place in Bloomsbury.

Jackson was to continue at the National Hospital for most of his life, for when his retirement was due at 65 his colleagues invited him to continue for another 10 years.

His method of working was unique. A searching clinical examination was followed by a faithful recording of the patient's behaviour. He noted exactly what the patient did and said, his every delay, hesitancy, faulty response, and gesture. This was only the beginning. He went on to ponder, and to ask himself—why? He strove to unravel the fundamental problems which pervaded the nervous system and which resulted in that particular pattern of altered function. His thinking was speculative and far ahead of contemporary notions. He visualized levels of function within the nervous system which in disease disintegrated in inverse ratio to their order of development, like the blossoms on a tree. He did not entirely reject anatomical localization but conceived of it in only the broadest sense. The duality of the brain was realised, and he assigned considerable importance to the nondominant hemisphere.

He was no teacher and an indifferent lecturer, for his voice was soft and did not carry. He could not transmit to his students his novel and obscure ideas. How right was Hazlitt when he said that the chief disadvantage of knowing more and seeing farther than others is to be not generally understood. His colleagues, too, were out of their depth, but they were shrewd enough to realise that Jackson had a message to impart of tremendous significance. Not only did they admire him for his intellect, they revered him as a person, for he was gentle, modest, and grateful for any service his juniors afforded him, however trivial. Jackson did not attain a following by attending neurological meetings and explaining his theories in simple language. What kept him away was not shyness and certainly not unfriendliness, but sheer boredom. Like Henry James he could not abide listening to lectures or visiting theatres. If ever he was coaxed into a theatre he would slip away during the first interval.

His medium of communication was the written word. He spent his so-called leisure hours at his desk, and his contributions to journals were numerous. Unfortunately, he never published a monograph. Though he wrote much, he found it anything but easy to commit his thoughts to paper. His prose style was turgid and often obscure. One reason was his compulsive search for precision. This led him to qualify, modify, or amplify almost every one of his statements. Hence a profusion of subordinate clauses, parenthetical afterthoughts, and footnotes. He would go to extremes to acknowledge any help afforded him. For example, instead of saying that the patient had no knee jerks, he would write: "I am indebted to my house-physician [Dr. So & So] for kindly informing me that the patellar reflexes were in abeyance." Consequently his manuscripts—like those of Marcel Proust—were incredibly untidy, with afterthoughts, additions, erasures, remarks inserted vertically along the margins. Some of his papers were typed, but here again by the time they were in the hands of the printer there were manifold alterations in his barely legible handwriting.

Though his papers make difficult reading, they are full of witty turns of expression and scintillating phrases, especially in his contributions to aphasia. He spoke of "a clotted mass of spasm," "feminine oaths," "detonating commas," "stillborn prepositions," "barrel organisms," "scientific blasphemy." Carlyle's writing, he said, was like "high power swearing." After an ophthalmoscopic examination of a patient he said that the optic disk looked as though it had been trodden on.

As I said, his fellow neurologists held him in the highest esteem, a lectureship was endowed in his name, and he was invited to deliver the first Hughlings Jackson lecture. He was the recipient of the Moxon Gold Medal of the College of Physicians. His portrait was painted by Lance Calkin. The original was bequeathed to the Royal College of Physicians, and copies hang in the London and National Hospitals. At the latter a marble bust was commissioned (Fig. 1). William Gowers, that difficult and unapproachable neurologist, was invited to perform the ceremonial unveiling. Confronting the rest of the staff, Gowers flung back the covering sheet with the words: "Behold, the master!"* To employ a much abused cliché, Jackson was indeed a legend in his own lifetime.

Jackson had no hobbies but he enjoyed weekend rambles with Jonathan Hutchinson in Surrey, putting up for the night in Haslemere or Frensham Ponds. On visits to Hutchinson's country home he would sit silently in front of the fire at one end of an elongated room while his host was ensconced before another fire at the opposite end. Every year he would revisit his beloved Yorkshire, for he asserted that Green Hammerton was the original Garden of Eden. Though taking no active role in politics, Jackson was a staunch Conservative and was often heard to declare "Thank Heaven we have a House of Lords."

During his last years he would from time to time be driven in his carriage and pair to the hospital and ask to see any interesting cases there might be in the wards. The house physicians vied with each other in spotting his approach into the Square and in being the first to greet him in the front hall.

Kinnier Wilson had a carefully guarded notebook in which, like Boswell, he recorded in detail his conversations with the great man. Years later Wilson allowed me to peep occasionally at this invaluable notebook. Wilson died 45 years ago, and the present location of this volume is unknown. It was last seen in 1935 when

---

*Where is the bust today? A humiliating question. It was 60 years ago when I first crossed the threshold of Queen Square, and there the bust stood, a symbol of welcome and encouragement. Over the ensuing decades it continued to gaze at me with benignity. According to the whim of those in authority, its precise location varied. Latterly it was a lonely figure in the lobby of the Rockefeller Library. Just 3 months ago the base was found to be standing empty. Some dastardly sneak thief had filched the bust. Fumbling as well as furtive, the vandal had dropped the precious booty, as evidenced by a handful of marble chips. Will it ever be retrieved? It cannot remain hidden forever.

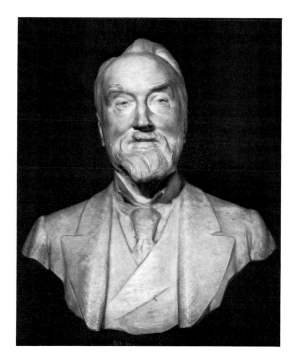

FIG. 1. Hughlings Jackson, the sage of Manchester Square.

a Jackson centenary dinner was held with Kinnier Wilson, the then president of the neurological section of the Royal Society of Medicine, in the chair. He produced this notebook and read aloud snippets from it. Amongst the neurological pundits at the dinner sat a shy young man from New Zealand, a Dr. Douglas, who was Jackson's grandnephew by marriage.

When Gordon Holmes was on duty, Jackson would often invite him to accompany him on a ride in his landau. Eagerly Holmes would take his place next to the master, and off they would go to Richmond, Kew, or Epping Forest. When they reached their destination, Jackson would tell James Brown the coachman to stop; and then, shaking his passenger by the hand, thank him warmly for his company and leave him to find his way back as best he could.

Over the course of many years Jackson kept up a correspondence with Herbert Spencer, who died in 1903. His few close friends included Thomas Buzzard, who outlived him, and Jonathan Hutchinson. His junior colleague James Taylor, whom I remember well, was also close to him. Taylor had had the incredible privilege of having served as assistant and secretary to both Jackson and Gowers, two men whose only common bond was their genius.

Latterly, Jackson was regularly visited by James Taylor and, more particularly, by cousin Charles and little Evelyn. Towards the latter, Jackson was generous and kind: He "never talked down to me," so she told me 70 years later. After tea, they would all clamber into the landau, and Jackson would take them to Mudie's bookshop. Evelyn would be gravely presented with a book, of either her choosing or his.

I have had the opportunity of reading Jackson's will, drawn up in 1911. There were gifts to those in his employ; £500 was left to James Taylor, and cousin Charles was given all the furnishings of Manchester Square, which included a large ebony bookcase empty, however, of books. Charles was given strict instructions to destroy "with his own hands" all the letters, diaries, case notes, and professional correspondence.

Its an odd paradox that Jackson's work first attained recognition in Europe when his papers had been read in German translation by such men as Pick, Freud, Sittig, and von Monakow. They conveyed their admiration to Henry Head, then working on the Continent, who on his return brought them forcibly to the attention of his British colleagues. Oscar Wilde was all too right when he said: "There are some works which wait, and which one does not understand for a long time; the reason is that they bring answers to questions that have not yet been raised."

Sir William Broadbent well said: "There are two kinds of knowledge, one consisting in the accumulation and certification of facts and their natural relation: the other of a more profound character, comprehending the underlying significance of phenomena." It is the latter of these to which Hughlings Jackson has so largely contributed.

My First Chief: Newman Neild

Every so often in the medical profession there turns up an individual to whom the term eccentric would not be unfairly applied. Recluse, antiquarian, anachronist, sorcerer's apprentice—each of these appellations could be attached to that intriguing personality, Newman Neild. Born in Manchester in 1872, he was of Quaker stock, for his father, Theodore Neild, was principal of Dalton Hall. His mother was formerly Helen Newman. He was educated at Bootham School, York, and at Owen's College, Manchester, and after qualifying held resident posts at the Manchester Royal Infirmary, the Brompton Hospital, and Great Ormond Street. At the first of these he came under the influence of Julius Dreschfeld, and at the other two he made life-long friendships with those great men who were at that time medical registrars: Robert A. Young and George F. Still, respectively. Neild settled in practice in Bristol and in 1901 was appointed assistant physician to the General Hospital, which he served until his sudden death in 1934.

Neild's principal interests lay in materia medica and therapeutics, but they were of past centuries. He did not pretend to be scientific, for he practised the healing art with enthusiastic unorthodoxy.

Simples and medicinal plants fascinated him, and he owned an important collection of herbals. He did not hesitate to utilize many of these mediaeval remedies, and when he chose he borrowed freely from folklore and from the armamentarium of homoeopathy—though employing these drugs in his own allopathic fashion. His students were privileged to witness such empirical gestures as scutellaria for debility, ignatia for depression, zinc for night sweats, bichromate of potash for premenstrual pain, cane sugar for heart failure, injections of seawater for shock, garlic (in the boots) for chest disease. Neither heroic doses nor very small ones were despised. Thus he employed steadily increasing amounts of Fowler's solution for chorea, and massive doses of calomel for mild constipation. On the other hand, patients with troublesome vomiting might be required to sip a tumbler of water to which a single drop of Lugol's iodine had been added. It is not surprising that with their therapeutic innovations of salvarsan and insulin, Neild looked askance at his colleagues, and they, in turn, at him. He was very much the cat that walked alone.

Disease of the nervous system intrigued him, though neurology was not the subject dearest to him. However, when stimulated by eager inquirers, he responded to the challenge and went to great trouble to find satisfying replies. One of his more unorthodox yet most useful activities was to devise a pantomimic mnemonic concerning the distribution of the corporeal dermatomes. His students were told to follow him in a drill whereby he would clap his hands on various parts of his anatomy, chanting meanwhile "C5, C6, C7—D3, D5, D7, D9, D11, L1 and 2, L3,

First appeared in an abbreviated form as an obituary in Munk's *Roll*, vol. 5, Royal College of Physicians, London.

L4, S1, S2, S3 and 4." This ritual served as a rapid *aide mémoire* for spinal localization. A little later, his students requested another mnemonic, this time for the autonomic supply to the viscera; after a week, Newman Neild concocted a diagrammatic schema. Though less readily recalled, it nevertheless proved useful.

He would likewise invent simple methods for remembering the principal signs of certain neurological syndromes. These mnemonics could be either recited aloud or symbolized graphically. Thus Friedreich's ataxia, according to Neild, was typified by "three signs above the waist, four below." These were: nystagmus, scanning speech, and scoliosis; absent knee jerks, pes cavus, upgoing toes, and an incoordinate gait (Fig. 1).

As with all other maladies, patients with disorders of the nervous system were treated by him with outdated remedies, reminiscent of folklore, even witchcraft.

Thus those with facial neuralgia had leeches applied to their brow. Neild believed that relief of the pain followed too quickly to be attributable to a mere local detumescent action. He wondered if the leech, when biting, might conceivably inject some unknown but potent pain-killing substance. To put this to the test he would sometimes apply the leeches to the big toe. The results, if I recall, were inconclusive. Patients with intractable and persistent headache were subjected to a seton inserted into the nape of the neck. The tape was left *in situ* for some days, and every 24 hours it would be pulled a little to one side and then to the other. The result was "laudable pus," and the victim usually protested that the headache was "much better." Epileptics were instructed to gather mistletoe in the woods and to make an infusion therefrom which was to be imbibed at least once daily. Rumour had it that Neild had even recommended mouse pie as a remedy for nocturnal enuresis in children, but I personally never saw this treatment prescribed and followed.

Rightly perhaps, Neild held the opinion that most of the female working class population of my home town suffered from chronic tea poisoning and were literally "char-ladies." He delighted in coaxing from them their precise daily intake of very strong tea, which might amount to a gallon or more. It was possible, he believed, to identify a syndrome representing an addiction to tea. The clinical picture was

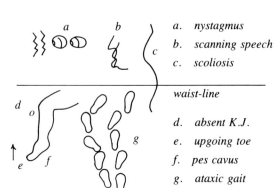

a. nystagmus
b. scanning speech
c. scoliosis

waist-line

d. absent K.J.
e. upgoing toe
f. pes cavus
g. ataxic gait

FIG. 1. Characterization of Friedreich's ataxia, according to Neild.

made up of a brown pigmentation of the skin especially under the eyes, furred tongue, bad breath, chronic dyspepsia, sour spasms, windy belches, and constipation. As far as I can recall, there were no neurological manifestations except tremor of the hands and acroparaesthesia.

At the bedside he examined his patients rapidly but in no perfunctory fashion. He took pride in the art of percussion and in cases of pleural effusion liked to demonstrate Grocco's triangle and shifting dullness by tilting the patient from one side to another. The tapping out of dull patches over swollen hilar glands was another tribute to his expertise. He paid great attention to the appearance of the tongue, the odour of the breath, and especially to the stools. Indeed a ritual visit to the sluice, where the bedpan of every patient was laid out for his inspection, was the solemn climax to his teaching round. Augury by ordure was indeed his hobby, and by observing the motions of the bowels he divined the mysteries of life and death. Obviously he loved teaching, but so torrential and so rapid was his flow of talk that students often found him difficult to follow. His quick, bird-like mind hopped from topic to topic, and his conversation was of the allusive type. Inattentive listeners or those whose wits moved at a more leisurely pace could not keep up

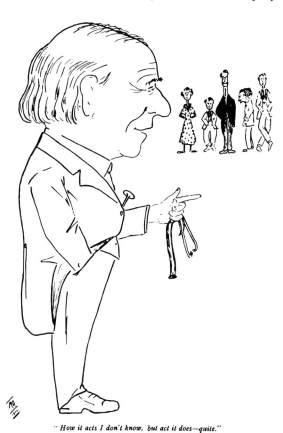

FIG. 2. Newman Neild, my first chief.

" How it acts I don't know, but act it does—quite."

with the knight's-move progression of his argument. Withal he was witty in an impish or mischievous way, and no mean mimic. Towards his pupils he was passionately loyal, and to support them and further their interests he would battle on until every imaginable obstacle was surmounted. They on their part were devoted to him, though it was obvious that "Nogs," as they called him, was out of step with most of the other chiefs.

He did not have a big practice and was not in great demand as a consultant, but his outpatient clientele was enormous. It was here that he was supreme. He conducted these clinics standing in the doorway of the waiting room and letting the patients file past. To each one he handed out some lightning-like instruction or advice, laced with a pertinent jest or a quip. He would never discharge a patient or delegate his clinic to another; nor for that matter would a single one of his flock have consented to see anybody else. Outside of medicine he had numerous interests, including botany, natural history, occultism, and the stage. He collected much: old books, flints, bric-a-brac. Porcelain was perhaps his favourite quest, and he became well known as an authority on Bristol china, especially its Delft ware.

His appearance was reminiscent of Lord Beaverbrook, for he was clean-shaven, short, and gnome-like (Fig. 2). His hair, thin on top, was worn long back and sides. His jerky movements, flitting smile, and rapid gestures mirrored his mental agility. Generous, warmhearted, but touchy, he made one think of Fluellen. Right up to the time of his death he went on with his hospital work in his usual energetic fashion, though warning notes of anginal pain had latterly been sounding. Death came suddenly on 4 July 1934.

Josef François Babinski

I suspect that the name Babinski is familiar to every medical man throughout the world, whatever his special interest, and probably to every fourth-year student as well. Can such a statement be applied to any other eponym in medicine?

Yet outside of France, Babinski remains a somewhat obscure, remote figure—little more, in fact, than a name. We feel more knowledgeable about Charcot, Pasteur, Claude Bernard, Duchenne, Dejerine, and Pierre Marie as individuals, and of course our own Hughlings Jackson, Gowers, Ferrier, and Horsley.

This is partly due to Babinski's *persona*, partly to the style of his clinical approaches, but mainly to the curious hierarchical system that used to characterize the medical establishment in France. For example, Babinski was never accorded the distinction of a departmental chair or even the title or rank of *professeur agrégé*. In France this is an invidious procedure whereby a choice is made between rival candidates, a practice where nepotism is, or was, by no means unknown. Even Charcot had been turned down at his first attempt (but was successful at his second). Babinski did not deign to submit himself to a further rebuff. Consequently he was never in charge at the Salpêtrière, although for at least 2 years he had served Charcot as his principal assistant with great distinction. Babinski had to settle for a somewhat less prestigious clinic, in the old and dilapidated La Pitié in the Faubourg St. Victor. This was in 1890. Incidentally a similar fate befell other neurological giants in France—Duchenne, Jean Lhermitte, and Charles Foix—whose intellectual status in every case was quite outstanding.

Both of Babinski's parents were Poles, the elder Babinski having lived in that part of the country under Russian rule. Having married Henryeta Weren, in 1848 when due for military service, Babinski's father, like many others, migrated to France and later took French citizenship. By profession, he was a construction engineer who eventually became successful financially. At one time his services were employed in Peru, and a plaque in Lima now commemorates his work in that country.

Josef François Babinski was born on 17 November 1857 in the Boulevard Montparnasse. With increasing prosperity the family moved to the Rue Bonaparte, and Josef and his elder brother Henri attended the Polish school in the Boulevard des Batignolles where he excelled in mathematics. Later he attended the Lycée Louis-le-Grand. In due course the older brother proceeded to the School of Mines, near the Luxembourg Gardens.

We know little of how the young Babinski reacted to the calamities among which he lived as a boy—the bombardment and siege of Paris, the triumphant march of the Prussians into the city, its occupation, the humiliating peace treaty, and then the horrors of the Commune. Perhaps the family were evacuated into the country, I cannot be sure. We do know, however, that Babinski *père* took part in erecting the fortifications of the beleaguered city.

Tranquility was restored in 1872 with the Third Republic, by which time Josef was 15 years of age. He chose medicine as a career. In 1878 he became an *interne provisoire* at the Bicêtre, and the following year he worked as *interne* to Vulpian at La Pitié, with Bucquoy and Cornil. The first of these taught him neurology, the second general medicine, and the third normal and morbid anatomy. In 1885, when he was 28 years of age, his thesis on multiple sclerosis was submitted and accepted.

Babinski's bent for clinical neurology was considerably furthered in 1887 by an unexpected death vacancy at the Salpêtrière on Charcot's service. A certain Dr. Richardière had been the first choice; Babinski was the runner-up. By a stroke of luck, Richardière became successful in winning a gold medal, a valuable international award which opened up other vistas. He withdrew his candidature, and Charcot, on the advice of Joffroy, accepted Babinski as his *chef de clinique*, without his having ever held the post of *interne*. This was in 1885, and he continued to serve as Charcot's principal assistant until 1887. He figures conspicuously in that well-known painting by Brouillet of Charcot in his clinic demonstrating a girl in an hysteroepileptic attack. Babinski was the bearded young man supporting the patient.

Owing to the intrigues of the influential Professor Charles Bouchard, Babinski's relationship with the Clinique Charcot ended at this point. In 1890 Babinski became a *médcin des hôpitaux*, and 5 years later he was elected head of the service at La Pitié, an antiquated hospital (Fig. 1) where Vulpian had worked, and Charcot too at one time. Although the Salpêtrière accepted only female patients and La Pitié males, the former was the more exalted, because Charcot, on being accorded the very first chair in clinical neurology in the world, had elected to establish his service at the Salpêtrière.

By single-minded dedication to his work, Babinski raised the status of La Pitié as a teaching hospital, and he gradually attained great popularity among postgraduates. Every morning Babinski would arrive at the hospital in a cab promptly at 9:30. Later he was driven by a chauffeur, as taciturn as himself, in a motor car his brother Henri had bought for him. After 1900 he would every so often take off a

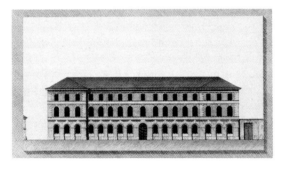

FIG. 1. Hôpital de la Pitié. (Courtesy of Wellcome Institute Library, London.)

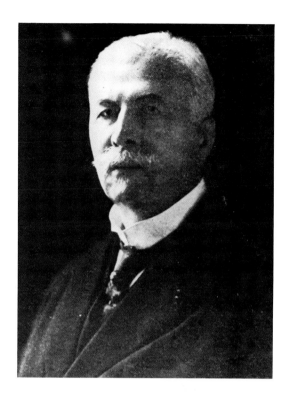

FIG. 2. Josef François Felix Babinski.

Thursday, for by that time, in company with Brissaud, Dejerine, Souques, Ballet, Meige, Pierre Marie, and some others, he had founded the Société de Neurologie de Paris. This body would meet on the first Thursday morning of each month at their premises in the Rue de Seine, not far from the hospital.

In addition to the regular daily teaching sessions, he would hold Saturday morning demonstrations throughout each May and June in an amphitheatre packed with doctors from the world over.

From the accounts left by such of his assistants as Vaquez, Chaillou, Moreau, Boisseau, Neri, and especially Clovis Vincent, de Martel, and Auguste Tournay, we can visualize something of Babinski the man, his eccentricities, and his techniques as a clinician. All writers are in agreement. First of all his appearance: He was a tall and somewhat heavily built man, impressive, dignified, and statuesque (Fig. 2). His movements were restrained, for like rich cream he moved slowly. He appeared cold and remote; perhaps he was merely shy. The beard of his days at the Charcot Clinic had been replaced by a rather full moustache. His fair hair early turned white, and in later life his features were particularized by a tiny tuft of hair in the centre of his chin, like Balzac.

All writers make special mention of his taciturnity. His arrival each morning was something of a ritual in its austere silence. Possibly he would acknowledge the presence of his chief assistant, but there was none of the compulsive handshaking all around so characteristic of French medicine, and none of the chatter of mutual greetings. Whenever he went so far as to offer his hand, it was meaningful and given with all his heart. His friends came to learn this in time.

In silence he would proceed like a high dignitary of the church to his *salle de consultations* and seat himself with his back to the window. On his right was a small table with the *impedimenta* of his discipline: percussion hammer, tuning fork, pin cushion at the ready, wisps of cotton wool, common objects for testing stereognosis, tubes for hot and cold water, and two electric batteries. On his left would sit his first assistant, and the head nurse stood at the doorway, ready to bandage the eyes of the patient during sensory testing.

Without any preamble, the door would open to admit his first patient, standing before him unclothed except perhaps for a loose gown. I am not even confident about the gown. The assistant would give a brief account of the illness and only very rarely did Babinski speak to the patient. Nothing more, perhaps, than a laconic query now and again.

If the history-taking was brief, not so the clinical examination. Still silent, Babinski with his piercing gaze would inspect the patient from top to toe before starting to test motor power, tonus, and sensibility. Often he would go back and repeat some of his tests so as to ensure their reliability. He might take as long as 5 minutes in the elicitation of a particular reflex. No comment ever fell from the master's lips, but the assistant would be taking down a detailed record of the findings.

Babinski's clinical technique was notable for its thoroughness, simplicity, and lucidity. He disdained elaborate, unorthodox bedside procedures, but if ancillary aids were needed he called upon the services of Chaillous for ophthalmology, the otologist Weil for special tests of labyrinthine function, and Delheim for electrical procedures and radiology. Attached to his service was the pathologist Nageotte, who was destined to occupy one day the chair of the Collège de France. But, as Guillain said, Babinski was not very interested in pathology, preferring to study the living rather than the dead.

Clovis Vincent held a special place in the story of Babinski. As a medical student Vincent was not attracted to neurology, saying that it was a kind of necromancy. His friend Aïtoff told him how wrong he was and that he should go and watch Babinski at work. "I did," said Clovis Vincent, "and went again and again. Eventually I became his *interne*, though even then it was a fortnight before he spoke to me." It was Babinski who later convinced Vincent of the need for neurosurgery in Paris and persuaded him, at the age of 50, to visit America and study with Cushing. In this way he became the pioneer of French neurosurgery. During the First World War Clovis Vincent was decorated on the battlefield for gallantry. In 1940, after the Germans occupied Paris, he became an active but discreet member of the resistance. Many a bailed-out British airman would be smuggled into his surgical ward. There he would remain swathed in bandages until the coast was clear and he could be sneaked across the Pyrenees. When Paris fell, the German chief military surgeon visited Clovis Vincent and directed him to continue his outpatient teaching in the ordinary way for the benefit of his army medical officers. Vincent did so and widely advertised that his first clinical presentation would deal with "war wounds of the head." The German doctors turned up in force, while Clovis Vincent demonstrated compound fractures of the skull in a dozen patients, not one of whom was over 12 years of age.

In like manner, Babinski prevailed upon another of his assistants, de Martel, to visit Victor Horsley in London and learn neurosurgery. De Martel, who was a descendant of the famous "hammer of the Saracens" and grandfather of Charlemagne, became so distressed at the French reverses that on 20 June 1940 he took a lethal dose of strychnine as the German troops marched down the Avenue des Champs Elysées.

Late in life Babinski was asked what he considered had been his greatest contribution to neurology. "When I persuaded Vincent and de Martel to take up neurosurgery" was his reply.

Earlier I spoke about Babinski's great attachment to his older brother Henri, the wealthy engineer who had studied at the School of Mines. Both were life-long bachelors. They shared an elegant apartment in the Boulevard Haussman where Henri typed all of his brother's manuscript papers. Their relationship was unusually close and cosy. They were inseparable, sharing the same interests, namely the opera, where seats were reserved for them, but in particular gastronomy. Henri was the author of a classic and monumental work, *Gastronomie Pratique*, which he wrote under the pseudonym "Ali Bab." There has been speculation as to why this *nom de plume* was chosen, and some have suggested that it implied "the *other* Babinski." Today, this large book is much sought after by collectors, and a few close colleagues were lucky enough to secure a copy. To my knowledge there are two in the United States; I know of none in Great Britain. Schaltenbrand of Würzburg has told us how Babinski, on a visit to Amsterdam in 1926, was entertained at dinner by Professor Brouwer. Schaltenbrand too was invited. All the resources of Dutch cuisine were displayed, and if I can judge by my own personal experience Brouwer probably made brief addresses explaining each course just before it was brought to the table. When Babinski got back to Paris he despatched to Myvrouw Brouwer a copy of Ali Bab's monograph on the culinary art.

This snide or at any rate ambiguous response to the hospitality of the Brouwers raises the matter of Babinski's personality. I have read widely what his contemporaries and pupils have written. I cannot escape the strong suspicion that Babinski was a cold fish. Towards his colleagues, pupils, and patients his attitude was not warm or outgoing. He seems to have had but few close friends. Neurologists respected him, although he was aloof and uncommunicative. The fact that he rarely elicited a history but relied upon exhaustive clinical examination is surely a shortcoming that put him in the category of a veterinarian of the nervous system. His words were few and often brusque. If not actually rude, they could not be regarded as couth or encouraging. Schaltenbrand, then a postgraduate student in Amsterdam, related how Babinski was invited to address the Dutch Neurological Society. The next day he made rounds at the Wilhelmina Gasthuis with Schaltenbrand. The first patient had a pupillary abnormality regarded as being of the Argyll Robertson kind. Babinski's comment was: "*that* is not an Argyll Robertson pupil." Next they showed him a patient with an upgoing toe. Babinski took the foot, scratched the sole, and proclaimed "No, he does not have *le signe d'extension des orteils*." In the laboratory the great man then asked Schaltenbrand what he was studying. The reply was "a case of Westphal-Strümpell's pseudosclerosis." Babinski's rejoinder was "a neurologist who talks of pseudosclerosis is not a neurologist, but a pseudo-neurologist."

In 1921 Babinski visited the National Hospital, Queen Square, as a guest of James Taylor. Purdon Martin, then the house physician, told me that Babinski was shown a patient with amyotrophic lateral sclerosis. Babinski remarked: "The spasticity is excessive; and what is the matter with his neck?" Sure enough the case turned out to be one of traumatic cervical spondylosis with cord compression. Those few words were virtually all that Babinski volunteered during his visit.

The interest of the Babinski brothers in haute cuisine was not merely theoretical. They certainly lived well. Egas Moniz, one time assistant to Josef, has left an account of a so-called modest and frugal lunch at the Boulevard Haussman. He and the two brothers were the sole participants. After a preliminary *vol au vent financière* came a Chateaubriand with *pommes soufflés*. This was followed by a slice of *foie gras*. For dessert there were *fraises a la Chapon fin*, that is, wood strawberries from Turenne, with kirsch and whipped cream, sprinkled with grilled almonds. Their wines included an outstanding burgundy, then a Chateau d'Yquem, and an 1815 port. Coffee in the study was accompanied by a cognac of imperial vintage.

Each August was spent by the two brothers in Deauville or Font-Roman.

When Henri developed a serious illness Josef Babinski became deeply distressed, and after Henri's death he was inconsolable. He gave up attending meetings of the Société de Neurologie and began to go downhill physically, dying 2 years later, on 20 October 1932. According to the few American obituaries available, the cause of death was Parkinson's disease, but no French appreciation has made mention of such a malady. Tournay, who was responsible for the most complete biography, stated unequivocally that it was Babinski's father Alexander who succumbed to that disease in 1899.

Neri, his loyal ex-assistant from Italy, has told us how he could not keep back his tears so shocked was he at Babinksi's appearance in June 1932. He had all the sadness of a man who was rapidly failing. "Dear friend," Babinski said, "how many years is it that we have known each other?" His voice had changed almost beyond recognition. Along with Barré of Strasbourg Neri visited him once more at the Boulevard Haussman. Calmly they chatted about what was going on in the world of neuroscience. But Babinski's features were wan and drawn; his eyes, though sunken, appeared somehow larger, and in their splendour seemed not to belong to him, but shone like beacons. In the last weeks of life he is said to have suffered moments of great pain.

On 2 June 1958 the Société de Neurologie de France organised a centennial memorial for Babinski on an international scale. From Great Britain, Sir Francis

Walshe and I attended. The ceremony synchronized with a particularly tense political crisis, and in Paris heavily armed police were ubiquitous. The principal address was by Raymond Garcin. Each national representative delivered an appreciative tribute, the outstanding contribution coming from Walshe, as might be expected. It was obvious that he entertained a particularly deep respect for the work of Babinski, even among the brilliance of the French neurological galaxy of which he had a high opinion. Other speakers included Lehoczky (Hungary), Ihsan Sükrü Aksel (Turkey), van Gehuchten (Belgium), Ott (Switzerland), Almeida Lima (Portugal), Subirana (Spain), Chorobski (Poland), Schaltenbrand (Germany), Lea Plaza (Chile), Mogens Fog (Denmark), Pearce Bailey (United States), Neri (Italy), Monrad-Krohn (Norway), Biemond (Holland), Kreindler (Romania), and Soriano (Uruguay).

At the regular meetings of the Neurological Society, Babinski spoke little, far less indeed than most of his colleagues. Occasionally he would read a short paper or present a clinical case, and woe betide the man who was rash enough to make any critical comment. When other neurologists were speaking, Babinski would seat himself in the front row of the auditorium "his handsome face tense and interested." His deep-set eyes were focused like searchlights upon the patient. Sometimes he would leave his seat and grab the patient's limb in order to satisfy himself about the state of muscle tonus. Or he would percuss with his own hammer and examine those tendon reflexes that were not well defined. Then he would resume his seat in silence.

When perusing the literature, he would make critical notes in the margin of the book. He could not tolerate confused, obscure, or imprecise writings, the product of what he called the *chieurs d'encre*, which may be translated as "ink shits." His own writing was sober, detailed, precise, and restrained. Evenings were spent at his desk. Words seemed to flow readily from his pen, but actually there had been a long period of gestation. The rough draft was always vetted by his brother, Henri, who then typed the paper. The proofs of his *Exposé des Travaux Scientifiques*, written in collaboration with Dagnan-Bouveret, were corrected again and again. After the final version had been posted to the publisher, the authors, along with Henri Babinski, relaxed over dinner at the Restaurant Laperousse.

The discovery of the renowned Babinski sign was made comparatively early in his career. During the nineteenth century neurologists had often tickled the soles of their patients' feet, noting merely whether there was a prompt or a sluggish reactionary movement of the toes. The direction of movement of the great toe must have been witnessed countless times but without registering anything in the examiners' minds. As was truly said, *"tout le monde voit, peu de personnes savent observer"* (everyone sees, but few observe). In 1895 Babinski came to the realisation that in cases of crural monoplegia or in hemiplegics a pinprick applied to the sole of the healthy limb produced a flexion movement at the hip and knee joints as well as the ankle and toes. A similar stimulus to the affected leg again would be followed by flexion at the hip, knee, and ankle, but the toes, instead of flexing, would carry out a movement of extension upon the metatarsals. This led to his classic paper in the *Comptes Rendus de la Société de Biologie* (22 February 1896).

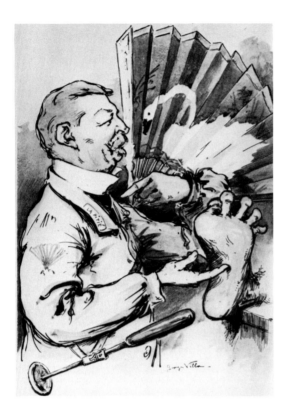

FIG. 3. The Babinski sign. (Courtesy of Wellcome Institute Library, London.)

The note was brief, merely a matter of 28 lines, and yet, as Pearce Bailey truly remarked, "the Babinski phenomenon therein described, has no equal in its combination of simplicity, diagnostic importance, and physiological implication." Here at last was a clinical shibboleth which would distinguish the organic from the hysteric, the genuine from the counterfeit. Babinski continued his clinical studies upon the effects of plantar stimulation; he observed that the toe movement was often slower on the affected than on the healthy side; that the outer side of the sole was more important in that extension might follow only when that side was stimulated, whereas the same type of provocation applied to the inner side might evoke a flexor plantar response. He observed, too, that it was an upward movement of the *great* toe that was all important. Sometimes, but certainly not always, the small toes responded by a movement of abduction, the so-called *signe de l'éventail*, or fanning of the toes (Fig. 3). He found that a tourniquet applied at calf level could sometimes cause an extensor plantar response to become a flexor, thus confirming an observation that had already been made by Ozorio de Almeida.

It is true that, strictly speaking, the Babinski sign had been described in 1893 by E. Remak. At a meeting of the Berlin Society of Neurology & Psychiatry, he demonstrated a case of transverse myelitis. He went on to say: "One is able, through stroking of the distal half of the plantar aspect of the metatarsus primus, to evoke a fairly isolated reflex of the extensor hallucis longus." Remak failed to realise the importance of this phenomenon, however, and did not pursue the matter. His remarks do not detract from Babinski's role in the discovery of this sign and its great clinical implications. As Osler once said: "In science the credit goes to the man who convinces the world, not to the man to whom the idea first occurs." Hence the accreditation rightly belongs not to Remak but to Babinski.

The most material aspect of Babinski's work was the realisation that the common factor underlying the extension of the big toe was an involvement of the pyramidal tract. Indeed in such calamitous circumstances as a transection of the spinal cord, the upgoing toe can be elicited by stimulation not only of the sole but also the dorsum of the foot, the leg, the thigh, and even the lower abdomen. Could it be that the Babinski response was merely the least common multiple of the defence reflexes described in 1912 by Marie and Foix and the mass reflex of Head and Riddoch? This idea became in time a bone of contention in which such authorities as Fulton, Pierre Marie, Foix, and Walshe among others locked horns.

Walshe, in particular, contributed much to our deeper understanding of the Babinski response. In 1914, when he was resident medical officer at the National Hospital, he wrote a detailed evaluation of the clinical importance of the extensor plantar response and its physiological significance in the light of Sherrington's researches. He kept up his interest in this subject and, working with T. R. Elliot, later showed that a permanent and irreversible lesion of the pyramidal tract was not necessarily proved by the finding of Babinski's sign. Thus it could occur as a temporary manifestation of hepatic coma, after certain drugs had been ingested, after an epileptic fit, and in the deep sleep which follows a prolonged state of induced wakefulness.

There were a few subsequent writers who ventured to express doubt as to the significance of the upgoing toe. Thus in 1956 Hoff and Breckenridge, on the basis of animal experimentation, asserted that "only convention and tradition link the Babinski plantar response with defect of pyramidal system activity." Their ideas were based upon the decerebration of over 300 dogs and more than 50 cats. In characteristic vein, the authors were castigated by Walshe, who wrote (1956): "A less adequate and informing graphic description of the findings in such a holocaust of animals it would be difficult to conceive." His wrath also descended upon Nathan and Smith, who studied the autopsy material after chordotomy and were incautious enough to say that Babinski had actually described *two* types of response depending on whether there was also fanning of the toes, and that Babinski had neglected to establish his correlation of the toe sign with lesions of the pyramidal tract. Walshe hotly criticized their paper, stating that they had based their conclusions upon an incomplete review of the literature. They had failed to mention the case described by Walshe in 1935, where surgical ablation of the leg area of the cortex was followed by a transient weakness of that limb and a permanent upgoing toe. His chief criticism was that morbid histology cannot be accepted as the final criterion by which we assess functional activity.

Babinski did not define clearly what type of mechanical excitation of the sole was needed. In his first paper he mentioned pinprick. Two years later he referred to stroking of the sole with a pin. I have the uneasy feeling that he was responsible for the ruthless, I almost said cruel, technique of a deep and painful scratching of the sole with a sharp pin. Now we know that the stimulus need not be so traumatic. A blunter implement is just as efficacious, without necessarily agreeing with Dr. Henry Miller that the ideal is the car key of a three-litre Bentley. With transection of the cord, a touch with a piece of cotton wool may suffice.

As might be expected, the success of Babinski's clinical discovery led to a multitude of lesser mortals trailing on his coat-tails as though he were the Pied Piper of neurology. These camp followers fall into two groups. First are those who contrived to bring about an extension of the great toe by other manoeuvres. Soon the lower limb became comparable to one of those pillars that adorn the kerbs of the Grands Boulevards of Paris, whereon are plastered advertisements and playbills. There were those, like Chaddock, who stroked the outer side of the dorsum. Others, like Gordon, firmly squeezed the calf. Oppenheim heavily rubbed the shinbone from above downwards. Trömers would have us press hard on the thigh muscles, and in Brazil Austregesilo was pinching the tendo Achillis. But all these were bit players in a classic drama in which Babinski was the star.

Commenting upon the inordinate number of synonyms for Babinski's index of pyramidal dysfunction, Professor Jean Lhermitte was reminded of the Spanish grandee travelling through France. Realising he would not reach his destination until late, he decided to put up for the night at a wayside inn. The proprietor asked for his identity and got the reply, "The Duke of Bejar, Marquis of Gibraleon, Count of Benalcazar y Benares, Viscount de la Puebla de Alcocer, Señor de la Villas de Copilla, Curiel y Burguillos." "Sorry," said the landlord "I haven't room for that many."

The other group who climbed upon the bandwagon are those who sought similar fame and distinction by comparable devices. Minor neurologists, especially in France, frenetically scratched, stroked, pinched, stimulated, or tickled this part of the anatomy or that—the palm, the fingers, the lips, the glabella—in search of some response which might bring them eponymous notoriety. Much of this was wasted effort.

It would bore those who are not neurologists if I were to delve more deeply into the clinical vagaries of the Babinski phenomenon, though much indeed could be said. There are ways and means of converting a flexor into an extensor and vice versa. The plantar response is not always easy to evaluate, and even neurologists of experience have at times differed vigorously in their interpretation of the findings. Perhaps it is fair to say that if the plantar response is a frank flexor on one side and equivocal on the other, the latter is probably abnormal.

In 1899 there appeared in *Brain* an important paper by James Collier, then the Junior House Physician at the National Hospital, Queen Square, to whom belongs the credit of introducing into British neurology the extensor plantar response. Collier admitted in his paper that it was Gowers who had drawn his attention to this sign.

Many other important contributions to neurology were made by Babinski. What most of us refer to as the syndrome of an occluded posterior inferior cerebellar artery is known throughout France as the Babinski–Nageotte syndrome. Early in his career Babinski studied, with Onanoff, muscle dystrophy. Like Edwin Bramwell many years later, he debated why some muscles are affected early whereas others always escape and still others occupy an intermediate position. He believed that the answer lay in the embryo, and that the first muscles to be formed were the most vulnerable. These two papers seem forgotten today.

In 1900 he described the adiposogenital syndrome, that is, a year before Fröhlich. Babinski's "rising sign," as we call it in England, was the demonstration that when a hemiplegic lying on his back with his arms folded across his chest is told to sit up the leg on the paralysed side automatically rises higher than on the other. This is a useful way of rapidly distinguishing an organic from a nonorganic case.

His principal interests were for some years focussed upon cerebellar symptomatology, describing in turn dyssynergia, adiadochokinesia, and hypermetria. In 1913 he attended the International Congress of Medicine held in London. In a session, chaired by David Ferrier, he delivered the principal lecture of the day on the topic of cerebellar lesions. The success of the paper was shown by what has been described as the "vibrant explosion of prolonged applause" and by that most un-English of reactions, a standing ovation. Babinski was visibly shaken by the reception.

In 1914 he was elected to the Académie de Médecine. Since 1905 plans were in train for rebuilding the decrepit Pitié hospital, but by August France was at war. Babinski's work load became enormously increased. The reason was that for some years before he had been turning his attention to the question of hysteria. This is not surprising in one who had been the respectful disciple of Charcot. Cases were always there in profusion, and the numbers increased dramatically among shell-shocked soldiers and civilians. Babinski at first followed Charcot's doctrine, but gradually he came to differ somewhat from his master's views upon the nature of hysteria. For one thing he preferred to employ the term "pithiatism," implying that the symptoms were evoked by suggestion and curable by persuasion. He emphasized that an hysteric never showed physical signs which could not be voluntarily reproduced. In hysterical palsies the reflexes remained unaltered. The role of hypnosis as a means of treatment was pursued, and during the war years he resorted to what his unfortunate military patients called "electrocution."

Babinski's work on hysteria, one must admit, forms a disappointing chapter in his curriculum vitae. According to Osler, "He who knows hysteria knows medicine." I doubt if Babinski ever did understand hysteria. He would have been astonished had he been spared to live through the Second World War, to observe that battle stress no longer evoked such phenomena as palsies, deafness, blindness, seizures, and amnesia. Conversion hysteria was replaced by subjective symptoms: dyspepsia, anxiety, phobias.

No one who has paid tribute to Babinski has bothered to mention two papers of his which were in quite a different vein, and, I submit, much more important and far more profound than his previous work. In 1914 he collected a series of hemiplegics not one of whom seemed to realise the fact that paralysis was present, although their minds were clear. Each patient had been a right-hander and in each one the hemiplegia was left-sided. This phenomenon he called "anosognosia," meaning unawareness of disease. That same year, he followed up this article by drawing attention to a light-hearted, noncaring attitude towards the existence of a hemiplegia. This phenomenon he termed "anosodiaphoria," or lack of concern over the presence of a lesion.

Unfortunately, Babinski did not follow up these two perspicacious articles. It was as though he had scaled a high mountain and had been permitted a glimpse of a wider vista which at that time was a *terra incognita* but into which he feared to venture. It was left to others to show that he had stumbled upon a principle which pervades the manifold disorders of higher nervous activity. To Goldstein the phenomenon exemplified a commonplace tenet in cases of cerebral lesions, that of "organic repression." Others speak of the "denial syndrome." We know that this applies not only to paralysis but also to blindness, hemianopia, deafness, and mental impairment provided they are of central origin. Twenty years previously Anton had noted how cortically blind persons did not realise they were blind or else projected their failure to see upon environmental factors such as poor illumination. Seneca had found the same phenomenon 2,000 years before. Thus unawareness, ignoral, projection, denial, and wild confabulation are now realised to be commonplace in cases of high-level brain damage.

Babinski never realised that in medicine close investigation and accurate reporting are not enough, important though they be. Simple descriptive accounts take one only part of the way. Always it is necessary to proceed further and to enquire "why? how?" and to seek out the underlying permeating precept. In this way Babinski just failed to attain supremacy.

In 1922 Babinski regretfully retired. However, on the Continent they are civilized in their attitude to the wisdom of age. Vaquez, his successor, put at his disposal accommodation where Babinski could continue to see patients and to teach whenever he chose. Babinski gratefully availed himself of this courtesy over the next 8 years—until the death of his brother shattered his initiative.

A final word about Babinski as a Pole. True, he was born a Frenchman, but his heart was in Poland. Although his colleagues pronounced his name *à la française*, Babinski never did. He attended a Polish school and presumably spoke the language. I imagine he must have been well acquainted with the Curies. At a victory parade in 1918 he cancelled his hospital work so as to watch the march-by of the Polish contingent. Emotion overcame him. When he died he was buried in the Polish cemetery at Montmorency on a hill overlooking the city of Paris.

At his christening two fairies attended: one good, the other not so good. Babinski was therefore destined throughout his life to be dogged by extremes of good luck and bad. He was unlucky in not achieving entry, as he deserved, into the citadel, the holy of holies of Parisian neurology, and dominate the Charcot Clinic at the Salpêtrière. He was unlucky, too, in that he was cheated out of professorial rank.

On the other hand, he was lucky in that early in his career, without years of toil or research (from his armchair in fact), he chanced upon the simplest and yet most momentous clinical phenomenon which brought him international fame overnight. *Venit, vidit, vicit.*

He was fortunate too in his self-sufficiency. In his close if somewhat abnormal relationship with his brother, he shared a snug and comfortable existence. Alas, like those who put all their eggs into one basket, he was irretrievably destroyed when he lost his alter ego.

Within the Pantheon of the neurosciences where does he belong? Certainly on a lofty pedestal. Can we compare him with any of the medical men familiar to us? His silence reminds us of Farquhar Buzzard, who, defying the laws of nature, rose to great heights by reason of his gravity. In his uncanny skill in coaxing physical signs Babinski came close to Gordon Holmes. His shortcoming was his failure to communicate with his patients. No one who does not probe deeply will succeed in his search for truth.

It was said of another French physician, Lasègue, that when taking a history from a patient, he would be "urging, begging, ironical, good-natured, even endearing, permitting the patient to express himself freely, or on other occasions asking him innumerable questions, but never tiring until he was sure to have obtained all possible information." If to Babinski's skill as an observer one could have added the warmth of Lasègue, supplemented by the wisdom of a Hughlings Jackson, you would have had a genius.

Let us end by quoting the words with which Auguste Tournay finished his appreciation of Babinski: *"il était beau, il fut bon, il reste vrai."*

John Addington Symonds, Primus *et* Secundus

To that hackneyed anonym "the man in the street" the name John Addington Symonds probably means nothing. Even the pronunciation is a matter of uncertainty. A classicist or an art historian would remember that there was a minor poet, a *fin de siècle* aesthete and authority on the Italian renaissance, of that name. To a medical librarian, this name might conceivably evoke the picture of an early Victorian provincial physician, an austere, highly cultivated and widely respected gentleman with perhaps the largest practice in the West of England.

Both images are correct, for there were two individuals who bore this name, related of course—the doctor being Symonds *père*, and the writer, his son.

Unwarranted neglect surrounds these two very different figures of nineteenth century England. They were vastly dissimilar in their physical and psychological constitutions, although they shared certain attributes, namely superior intellect, learning, and artistic refinement. To a philosopher of medicine, both these individuals present themselves as endowed with qualities and weaknesses that merit retelling.

Ancestry

The two who bore the name of John Addington Symonds could trace their origins to ninth century France. In 1066 an Adam Fitzsimon accompanied William the Conqueror and received grants of land in the Midlands and East Anglia. "Simon" is actually a distorted variant of "Sigmund," and for that reason the "y" in "Symonds" is pronounced as a short "i" and the "d" is sounded. The first generations in England were wealthy property owners; and although none was enobled by royalty, the distant forebears include a knight templar, a crusader, a founder companion of the Most Noble Order of the Garter, settlers in Ireland and colonists in North America,* a soldier at Agincourt, a regicide, and many distinguished ministers of religion. With the Reformation they became strict dissenters, or Puritans, and during the parliamentary civil wars (1642–1645, 1647–1649) many were active supporters of Oliver Cromwell. An ancestor became a surgeon in Atherstone, Warwickshire. It was in the city of Oxford, however, where the profession of medicine descended from one generation to another. The father of Dr. John Addington Symonds was actually the seventh in direct succession who practised

---

*In 1637 a Samuel Symonds settled in New England and held the office of deputy governor.

medicine in that city. This choice of profession was due to the exclusion of non-conformists from Oxford and Cambridge.

Over the centuries the Symonds family made important marriages, and as a result it includes many notables. In his article in *The Eugenics Review* on Further Studies in Hereditary Genius (1925), W. T. J. Gunn referred to the descendants of Dr. John Symonds of Worcestershire. These included Sir Morell Mackenzie, the laryngologist who operated upon Emperor Frederick III of Germany; Sir Stephen Mackenzie; Henry Compton, the comedian; Sir Rowland Hill, the originator of the penny postal system; George Birkbeck Hill, educationalist and Johnsonian; Lord Strachie; St. Loe Strachey, editor of the *Spectator*; Maurice Hill, a high court judge; Sir Leslie Scott, a lord justice of appeal as well as a privy councillor; Dame Katherine Furse; Sir Compton Mackenzie, author and mnemonist, and Fay Compton, his actress sister. To this galaxy should also be added many admirals in the Royal Navy; a provost of Eton; the Regius Professor of Hebrew at Oxford; the inspector general of Chinese customs; the Right Honourable John Strachey; Lord Byron; Dame Janet Vaughan, doctor of medicine and principal of Somerville College; a sheriff of London; and Lord Sidmouth, Speaker of the House of Commons and a none too successful prime minister.

Dr. John Addington Symonds

It was on the advice of an influential great-uncle, Dr. Addington of Ashley Court in Bristol, that in 1831 Dr. John Addington Symonds (b. 1808), having qualified in medicine at Edinburgh in 1828, set up in practice in the city and county of Bristol, then second only to London in size and importance.

At first he practised from No. 7 Berkeley Square. In 1834 he married Harriet Sykes. She lived only 10 years, having given birth to seven children, of whom three died early, one of the boys being hydrocephalic.

Thus at the age of 37 the doctor was left a widower with three girls and a boy to care for. His late wife's sister came to live in the family *in loco parentis*. Dr. Symonds's mother-in-law was a handsome but overpowering woman living close by in Clifton. She was a fanatical Plymouth Sister and a martinet, and to her son-in-law more of a burden than a help.

Arriving in Bristol, Dr. Symonds found himself caught up with an epidemic of cholera, and in 1832 he collaborated with an older colleague in the city, Dr. Andrew Carrick, in a paper entitled "Medical Topography of Bristol." This was a pioneer work in community medicine. A year previously, Dr. Symonds had been instrumental in founding the Bristol General Hospital, for the resources of the Royal Infirmary—probably the oldest hospital in England—were not sufficient to meet the pressure of the sick population of the expanding city.

His practice grew rapidly, and he became in great demand for consultations throughout the West Country. In 1848 he retired from the hospital staff in order to devote himself to his clientele and to allow himself more time for his studies of

English, Latin, and Greek verse; for a collection of prints and engravings; and for the reading of history, philosophy, and Egyptology.

Each day he rose at 6:00 a.m. and dedicated 2 hours to serious literature. Thereafter the whole day was assigned to his patients. On his desk in the consulting room there was always at hand a volume of classical poetry to peruse in intervals between patients and to render into English verse. He dined late, and if there were no postprandial country consultations, he would read aloud to his family for an hour or so. His usual choice was Milton or Tennyson, for he had strong likes and dislikes. Hobbies and nonacademic diversions were alien to him, but he enjoyed the company of others with comparable cultural and intellectual tastes. At the Sterling Club or in his own home, he conversed with such eminent and kindred souls as Jowett, the Master of Balliol; Dean Elliot; Dr. Carpenter; Hallam the historian; Lady Dufferin; and many others. Dr. and Mrs. Symonds were also warm friends of Mrs. Goldschmidt, better known as Jenny Lind, "the Swedish nightingale."

He wrote a good deal on paramedical subjects. In the posthumous volume *Miscellanies* (1871) were essays on the Principles of Beauty; Sleep and Dreams; Apparitions; the Relation between Mind and Muscle; Habit; and the Criminal Responsibility of the Insane. A particularly touching contribution was a lengthy tribute to his great friend that scientific polymath Dr. James Cowles Prichard, physician to the Bristol Royal Infirmary.

Although kindly and sympathetic towards the sick, he was in many ways aloof and reserved, humourless, and without any sense of fun (Fig. 1). As a strict churchgoer, Dr. Symonds was far more broad-minded than his Oxford forebears, having discarded most of their sectarian rigidity.

His professional reputation spread to the metropolis. Indeed, had he elected to live in London, he probably would have attained high office in the Royal College of Physicians. As it was, being the youngest elected Fellow, he was awarded the distinction of the Goulstonian lectureship in 1858. The topic he selected was Headache. So detailed was his dissertation, its publication required six consecutive issues of the *Lancet*. It is of interest that Symonds was familiar with the "ice-cream headache" of today. This work and other writings of his were well known to and quoted by such authorities as Hughlings Jackson, William Gowers, and Edward Liveing.

In 1851 he moved from his rather gloomy residence, having bought a beautiful and commodious mansion known as Clifton Hill House (Fig. 2), built in 1747 by a prosperous Bristol merchant.* It was elegant and palatial, situated in extensive grounds sloping steeply and adorned with flowers, shrubs, tulip trees, and elms. The view was magnificent, incorporating the towers and steeples of the many churches for which Bristol is famous, the truncated spire of St. Mary Redcliffe, and the tall masts of ocean-going ships in the harbour. Beyond were the hills of

---

*It is now a hall of residence for women undergraduates at the University of Bristol.

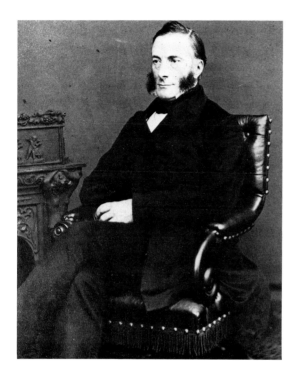

FIG. 1. John Addington Symonds, *primus*. (Courtesy of Wellcome Institute Library, London.)

Bath, with Dundry tower on the skyline and the Mendips sweeping southwesterly. Two fishponds were in the gardens, and there was stabling for eight horses.

Dr. Symonds travelled the Continent widely, visiting cathedrals, museums, art galleries, and places of archaeological interest. To utilize his vacations to the full, he journeyed by night, devoting the daylight hours to sight-seeing. He would return to his practice unrefreshed, however, and indeed in his late forties his health

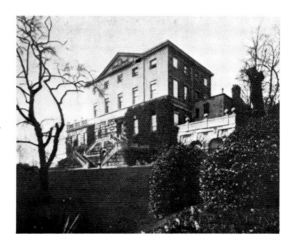

FIG. 2. Clifton Hill House.

deteriorated. Chronic diarrhoea led to loss in weight and exhaustion. Reluctantly he gave up clinical work but continued with his literary studies. In 1869 he presided over the annual meeting of the British Medical Association which was held in Bristol, giving the opening address. Death came in February 1871 at the age of 63.

The obituarist in the *Lancet* concluded with the words "probably no medical practitioner of our time ever conciliated more friendships, or inspired a wider respect for his character, his professional accomplishments and his refined tastes than Dr. Symonds, who so long represented in the provinces the science, the skill, and the liberal culture which are generally, but wrongly, supposed to be confined to the metropolis."

Sons are often unkindly critical in their evaluation of their parents. His son was, however, unequivocal in his appraisal of his father, for he realised how much he had learned from his fine and varied culture, his high ideal of purity in language, and his liberal philosophy of life.

The Good Physician

Dr. John Addington Symonds exemplifies that best type of physician who, inspired by Sir Thomas Browne, adorns the profession of medicine. Such a man had indeed been visualized by Hippocrates when he spoke of the association of the love of humanity with the love of his craft—*philanthropia* and *philotechnia*. With the advent of a scientific age, it has become increasingly more difficult to combine technology with the culture afforded by the humanities. "Without inspiration most expertise is sterile" is all too true. The possibility is there, however, as exemplified by such figures in our discipline—not too remote—as Sherrington, Osler, Cushing, Cajal, Geoffrey Keynes, and Fulton. These are household names, but, to quote Osler, "some there be that have no memorial, who are perished as though they had never been, and as though they had never been born." Such, I fear, has been the fate of that most erudite of physicians, Dr. John Addington Symonds.

John Addington Symonds, Fils

In 1840 was born the youngest member of the family who, like his father, bore the name of John Addington Symonds. At his birth he was privileged to receive the gift of gold, the frankincense of intellect, and the myrrh of artistic discrimination, but a wicked fairy darkened the scene. Her contributions were lifelong bodily and mental ill health, and sexual inversion.

His mother died when he was 4 years of age, and he grew up amidst three sisters for whom he cared little, an amusing but irritable aunt, a busy and rather reserved father, and a succession of nursemaid–governesses. Most of the last-named were ignorant, coarse, and superstitious; but finally came a refined German lady who taught him to speak her language fluently. His great-uncle Dr. Addington moved from Ashley Court to nearby Victoria Square and proceeded to teach him Latin when he was 4 years of age.

For schooling he attended a small establishment a mile away, run by the Rev. William Knight, who found him an eager and receptive pupil, except in elementary arithmetic. The daily journey from Berkeley Square took him through the squalor of Gallows Lane, where sinister figures stood at the doorways of wretched hovels, a daily walk that never failed to prove terrifying. Things were better for him when the family moved from their dark and cheerless residence to the majesty of Clifton Hill House.

The small boy, however, was underweight and weakly, afflicted by chronic diarrhoea and bed-wetting. Vivid and bewildering dreams tormented him remorselessly, and there were frightening tricks of light and shadow during the twilight hours. At night he would imagine he could hear weird noises; that a corpse in a coffin was underneath his bed; or that a devil lurked on the mat outside his father's bedroom. A phantom finger beckoned him as he lay asleep. His father often had to take his frightened son into his own bed, and he noticed how he would frequently talk to himself. Disturbing episodes of somnambulance also took place.

His father did what he could to assuage his son's fears. He would take him with him in his carriage on his many country calls, but none-the-less something was lacking. The young John Addington expressed the wish to learn the piano, but his father would not allow this, believing that music lessions might interrupt his schooling.

The youngster stoked the fires of his perfervid imagination by an almost compulsive reading of horror stories. He resented the routine attendance twice on Sundays at the evangelical chapel of the Blind Asylum and his being taken to hear the rantings of revivalist preachers.

A strange symptom began to recur, continuing well into adulthood. He referred to these attacks as "semitrances." They seem to have been ecstatic experiences with consistent prodromal sensations coming on while he was resting. Taking possession of his mind, they lasted what seemed to him an eternity. As they wore off he felt as if he were coming round from an anaesthetic. In later years Symonds said he could not describe them more explicitly; it was impossible for him to find the appropriate words. They entailed a swift and progressive obliteration of space, time, sensation, and the manifold factor of expression. At last nothing remained but a pure, absolute, abstract self. . . then, a feeling of approaching dissolution. Recovery began with the return of a sense of touch followed by an influx of familiar impressions. At last he would feel himself once again a human being, thankful for his return from the abyss. This description, based upon the patient's own observations, was made when he was in his thirties. He emphasized that he was straining the resources of the language at his disposal to portray the exact nature of these trance states. Description was not possible, for they were beyond the province of words. They reminded him of what Pindar called "a dream of a shadow of a man." Whether his behaviour altered at such times and whether these trance states were apparent to an onlooker he did not say.

What could have been the nature of these episodes? States of depersonalization of neurotic origin perhaps? Today a neurologist would certainly call for an electro-encephalogram.

At the early age of 11 John was sent away to Harrow where he remained for 6 unhappy years. Although younger than most of his peers, he was a year ahead of them scholastically. None of the masters at the school did he like or respect, save one. The vulgar behaviour of the boys distressed him, and he made few friends. He was too delicate to play games, but academically he did well, gaining the headmaster's scholarship and also the Botfield gold medal for modern languages. Because of his achievements he became head of his house. Years later he said that he had no high opinion of the academic level of Harrow, and that "all I owed the school was the corruption of my moral sense." Never did he revisit Harrow after he had left.

Proceeding directly to Oxford, he entered Balliol where the renowned Jowett was master and which at that time was one of the most scholarly colleges. He left Oxford with a double first class honours degree, having won the Newdigate prize for poetry (as Oscar Wilde was to do 18 years later). He was elected a Fellow of Magdalen but resigned after a year for personal reasons.

His academic success was followed by what was spoken of as a "nervous breakdown," for this was a pivotal period in young Symonds's development. During his last term at Harrow another boy confided in him that he had been having a love affair with the headmaster, the Rev. Dr. Vaughan, who had written him a number of indiscreet letters. These he handed over to the greatly shocked Symonds. At Balliol he showed them to one of the senior dons, who pleaded with him to let Dr. Symonds see them.

This John did, with devastating results. Dr. Symonds wrote to Dr. Vaughan, demanding that he resign his headmastership and return to the parochial life of a simple Anglican parson. Should offers of preferment come his way, he was to refuse them, under threat of exposure. Dr. Vaughan quietly resigned his appointment. Shortly afterwards he was offered the bishopric of Rochester. He was tempted to accept, but Dr. Symonds heard of the possibility and sent a warning telegram.

Meanwhile his son was going through a disturbing period of psychosexual maturation. He had immersed himself too deeply in the philosophies propounded by Plato, and he was being plagued by dreams of a Hellenic and homosexual nature. Unwittingly, too, he had developed a sentimental attachment to a choirboy at Bristol Cathedral, which lasted 2 or 3 years. This was followed by a similar attraction to a boy at Clifton College whom he was coaching in Greek.

Later Days

The vicissitudes of John Addington Symond's short but complex adulthood (Fig. 3) can be surveyed according to three headings: his emotional problem, his literary career, and his perpetual ill health.

1. *Emotional Problems.* He was steadily becoming aware that his *ethos* was likely to be dominated by his homosexuality. On medical advice and in a clinical

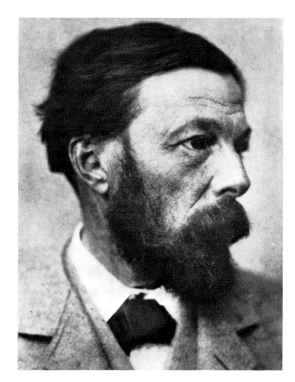

FIG. 3. John Addington Symonds, *secundus*, in 1886, at age 46.

fashion after discussion with his father, he began to ponder seriously if adjustment might come about within the framework of marriage. A passing flirtation with a Swiss tomboy of 15 years had come to nothing, but it had been a pleasurable interlude. With studied detachment, he selected and proposed to an acquaintance 3 years older than himself, Miss Catherine North. His overtures were accepted, not with obvious eagerness but after deliberation. How far Miss North was aware of what she was undertaking is not certain. In 1864 they married, and although the marriage endured for the rest of his days, and despite the blessings of four daughters, it became all too clear that this venture was not the answer to his problems.

His wife soon realised his proclivities, including his periodic descents into the seamiest regions of low society. As in the case of Oscar Wilde, the other half of the garden had its secrets which he was impelled to explore, for he shared Wilde's thrill at being among the evil things of life, finding their poison to be part of their perfection. Catherine soon learned of his attraction for the lowest class of partners. He kept an intimate diary, the contents of which did not come to light until 1964, for he had given instruction that the contents should be securely sealed for 50 years after his death.

Writing at a time when Freud was still a schoolboy, Symonds explained that his primary object as a diarist was to describe as accurately as he could a personality type which he believed to be not exceptional and yet not properly studied. He

wanted to supply material for an "ethical psychologist" by portraying a man of no
mean talents, of no abnormal depravity, whose life had been perplexed by passion—
natural, instinctive, healthy, in his own opinion—but in the view of society morbid
and abnormal, namely a persistent passion for the male sex. "As a secondary
object," he wrote, "I had in view the possibility of madness supervening on the
long continued strain, the lifelong struggle of this tyrannous desire, should the
worst come to the worst. I wanted to leave behind an *apologia pro mea vita*—no
excuses, no palliation, but an explanation of them."

No doubt this type of catharsis gave the writer no little mental relief, perhaps
even actual enjoyment.

2. *Literary Career.* It was thought fitting that Symonds should study law and
practise as a barrister. This was not a success, for he devoted more time to reading
and writing poetry than to his law books. He soon gave up his chambers in the
Temple and returned to Clifton in order to concentrate on literary pursuits, lecturing
perhaps, and a little teaching. He refused the Barlow Chair of Dante Studies at
London University. The vacant Chair of Poetry at Oxford attracted him, and for a
time it seemed likely that he would be successful, but it was not to be. A long
correspondence with Walt Whitman and Swinburne gave him much pleasure. Among
his close friends at that time were F. W. H. Myers, the author of *Phantasms of the
Living*; Alfred and Henry Sidgwick, the latter being one of the founders of the
Society for Psychical Research; Edmund Gosse, essayist and librarian to the House
of Lords; the notorious Frank Harris; and Horatio Brown, who was destined to be
the first of Symonds's biographers.

There is no evidence that Symonds and Oscar Wilde ever met, but they were
well aware of each other's writings. Wilde criticized quite warmly Symonds's study
of Ben Jonson and of Sir Philip Sidney, rating his essay on the latter superior to
that of Edmund Gosse. Indeed when Wilde was in gaol, he formally requested that
he be allowed access to some of Symonds's works. His petition was rejected.
Symonds, on the other hand, disapproved of Wilde, and when he received from
the author a complimentary copy of *Dorian Gray* he commented that it was a very
odd and very audacious production, unwholesome in tone but artistically and
psychologically interesting. He went on to say, "if the British public will stand this,
they can stand anything." On the other hand, he was a close friend of Wilde's evil
genius Lord Alfred Douglas ("Bosie"), who was delighted when Symonds sent him
an essay on Beethoven for publication in *The Spirit Lamp*.

Symonds never showed a wish to follow family tradition and take up medicine.
He always hoped he might pursue a career in literature. On coming down from
Oxford, he was sidetracked for a while into law, but the attraction of letters was
too strong. Because of his perpetual but fluctuating ill health, he spent much time
abroad, chiefly Italy and Switzerland, staying in hotels or rented villas. Such a life
style was ideal for that of a freelance writer of *belles lettres*.

Early preoccupation with the sexual mores of classic times determined the topic
of his earliest works. A *Problem in Greek Ethics* and *A Problem in Modern Ethics*
were printed and circulated privately and appeared anonymously in editions limited
to 50 and 100 copies, respectively.

His more orthodox work consisted in scholarly and beautifully written essays, as well as translations of some of the medieval Italian classics. He was not long in achieving a *succès d'estime*. His most important work was a study of the Renaissance in Italy which was published in seven volumes between 1875 and 1886.

3. *Perpetual Ill Health.* Ill health was to be his companion throughout the 53 years of his life. On this account he eventually left England altogether, to spend his remaining years in Davos and later Italy. The underlying pathology came to light when his father detected phthisis. He was then 25 years of age. The tubercle was ill-controlled and relentlessly worsened, extending from one lung to the other. His medical history, however, was fraught with many complications, mental and physical.

A paper by Dr. George M. Gould of Philadelphia (*Maryland Medical Journal* 47:281–291, 1904) dealt with the "life tragedy" of John Addington Symonds. This medical evaluation was written before Symonds's sexual deviation had been made public and is therefore far from an adequate appraisal. Gould emphasized Symonds's recurring headaches, which he regarded as migrainous; indeed he seems to have blamed migraine for Symonds's lifelong debility, his hypochondriacal preoccupations, and even his tuberculosis. Other complaints included mental and physical fatigue, inability to concentrate, forgetfulness, insomnia, photophobia, and a feeling in the eyes "as though they were boiled." Frequent colds and coughs weakened him still further, and a rise in temperature was a common occurrence. Symonds often remarked that the weakness of his eyes rendered systematic reading impossible, and he depended upon his wife's unfailing kindness to read aloud to him for hours.

Among the multitude of psychosomatic symptoms, Symonds mentioned an odd disorder of hearing which suggests the auditory perseveration encountered in some patients with a lesion in the temporal lobe. In his own words "in bed, but awake, thinking of death, desiring death, the bedroom suddenly seemed filled with music— the *Lontan Lontano* from Boito's *Mefistofele*. [The music] has not left my auditory sense—stays behind all other sensations."

During his life Symonds came under the care of many doctors. His family doctor in Clifton was Dr. John Beddoe, but while he was reading law in London Symonds consulted the eminent ophthalmologist Sir William Bowman, who every day instilled caustic drops into his eyes, charging a guinea each time. Because of "a terrible disturbance of the reproductive organs" he also went to see Dr. William Acton, a urologist who cauterized his urethra. He then sought advice from Sir Spencer Wells, surgeon to the royal household. Wells's advice was that he should either marry or have resort to a hired mistress. In 1877 he consulted the President of the Royal College of Physicians, Sir William Jenner, who darkly recommended him to put his affairs in order. At Davos, he was under the care of Dr. Ruedi and submitted to the fresh air cure.

In 1893 Symonds and his daughter Margaret were in Rome where he contracted influenza and a septic throat. Margaret called in Dr. Axel Munthe, the author of *The Story of San Michele*. Symonds was obviously desperately ill, and an English nursing sister was called upon to assist his faithful valet, an ex-gondolier with whom he had been associated for 12 years. A day later Symonds died and was buried in the Protestant cemetery close to the grave of Shelley.

Epilogue

John Addington Symonds *secundus* has had unconventional treatment at the hands of his biographers. In 1895 Horatio Brown, his close friend and literary executor, wrote a two-volume appreciation compiled from Symonds's diaries, notebooks, miscellaneous papers, an autobiography written towards the end of his life, and an extensive correspondence with Brown. Before it reached the printer, the manuscript was studied and revised by Symonds's family and two of his older friends.

A study of these volumes makes it obvious that a great deal of material is deliberately omitted. This is very evident whenever Brown quotes from the autobiography. Brown leaves the reader with the picture of a "highly analytical and sceptical intellect connected with...a profound sense of...a rich, sensuous, artistic temperament...[united] with a natural vein of sweetness and affection, an uncompromising addiction to truth, a passion for the absolute...."

In 1925 Symonds's daughter Margaret (Mrs. W. W. Vaughan), who had been at her father's side when he died, published under the title *Out of the Past* an account of her distinguished family and in particular the two John Addington Symonds. No allusion was made to her father's homosexuality.

Not until 1964 was the veil of secrecy discarded when Phyllis Grosskurth, having secured access to the material under embargo for 50 years, produced her biography. Thus was revealed to the world all that had been unknown save to relatively few. The subject matter released was also used by writers who were studying the *fin de siècle*, in particular Wilde and Alfred Douglas, as well as referring to Symonds as "an elderly, consumptive, homosexual scholar." Actually Symonds was only 53 when he contacted Douglas shortly before he died, and the commentators were in their seventh decade when they made their emotive remarks.

We are witnessing, therefore, one of those instances where knowledge of an unaccepted way of life has detracted unfairly from the appreciation which was due the individual. Wilde has now more or less been forgiven. After 20 years, is it not time for the rehabilitation of John Addington Symonds Junior?

Why Do We Laugh?

Man stands apart from the animal kingdom on several counts. He alone is endowed with language. His thumb can carry out the movement of opposition; he is more erect that most mammals; and he is relatively hairless. His brain, though smaller than that of an elephant, is unique by reason of its expansion in the regions of the frontal pole and the temporo-parieto-occipital carrefour. On a loftier plane we realise that man alone is capable of altruism, though not necessarily often displaying this quality. Perhaps Jules Renard hit the target when he declared that only man is plagued by financial worries.

To this catalogue let us tentatively add the phenomenon of laughter. Despite the claims for the hyena, the kookaburra, the New Zealand owl, the jaythrush, the Senegalese dove, and certain geese and gulls, laughter is the perogative of *Homo sapiens*. This equivocal privilege was expressly stated by Rabelais and more or less admitted by Aristotle too. Greville was more explicit by asserting that man is the sole creature endowed with laughter, being the only one who deserves to be laughed at. Such a conclusion is preferable to that put forward by Bulwer, who assigned laughter to man because animals do not possess the range of muscles of facial expression, though indeed he was correct in this statement.

What is this thing called laughter? To Samuel Johnson laughter was a "convulsive merriment; an inarticulate expression of sudden merriment." The *O.E.D.* informs us that laughter is "the action of laughing," which prompts us to turn to the word "laugh." Here we find "to manifest the spasmodic utterance, facial distortion, shaking of the sides, etc., which forms the instinctive expression of mirth, amusement, sense of the ludicrous, scorn, etc." The presence of these two *etceteras* in such close approximation hints darkly that there is much more to the topic that remains unsaid.

Common usage equates the act of laughing with the feeling of amusement. When abrupt it is believed to be precipitated by a sudden appreciation of things ridiculous or comic. Here again an explanation is required. When does a situation become ludicrous? One naturally looks for a triggering off by something unexpected and incongruous. This detonator may be situational or pictorial, but more often it is verbal, such as the unexpected bringing together of two ideas that are ordinarily quite disparate. The result is something of a shock leading perhaps to an audible gasp followed by Johnson's "convulsive movement." Herbert Spencer spoke of a "descending incongruity" as conducive to laughter, where consciousness is transferred from great things to small, an idea embodied within Thomas Hobbes's conception of a "sudden glory."

As we shall see later, laughter is a many-sided phenomenon and is by no means a manifestation of simple delight in the absurd. It has been asserted that laughter always contains an element of falsity or malice. To proclaim, for example, that an idea is laughable is to imply that it is not true. But for the time let us focus on the conventional and widely accepted equation of laughing with comedy, and in particular with its physical manifestations.

In the first place, laughter rarely takes place in solitude. Others must share the incongruity, if only one other person. A larger company is even better. In making this statement, I lay myself open to contradiction because of the idiosyncratic nature of the opinion: One can only speak for one's self. Certainly laughter in solitude is foreign to me personally, and I suspect to most others too. Does the editor of *Punch* or *Le Rire*, let us ask oneself, ever emit an audible spasmodic utterance, facial distortion, shaking of the sides when he solemnly scrutinizes the illustrations or wisecracks submitted for approval? It would be interesting to inquire of the respective editors. Did Mrs. Dorothy Parker, alone in her apartment, ever permit herself to smile, let alone laugh? I doubt it. She reserved it for her special corner at the Algonquin Hotel.

There is, I believe, an analogy with the laughter provoked by tickling. Aristotle asked, like everyone else who has thought about it since his day: "Why is it no one can tickle himself?"

On the other hand, laughter is typically associated with conviviality (Fig. 1). In such circumstances alcohol greatly facilitates its appearance—but not eating be it noted. Who has not been a solitary onlooker dining in a quiet corner of a restaurant? Outside in the bar foregathers a party of eight or ten enjoying preprandial cocktails. The noise level of voices punctuated by laughter rises and rises. Eventually the company take their places at a table reserved for them, and the comparative calm of the environment is shattered. Decibels continue to rise until the appearance of

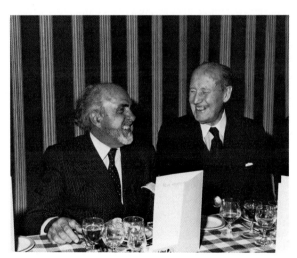

FIG. 1. Convivial laughter.

the first course. A lull in noise follows, and although wine no doubt circulates its effect is markedly buffered by the ingestion of food.

The social situation conducive to laughter may also be reduced to a matter of two persons. Here again the brake of good taste is released by the potent influence of alcohol. Upon the scene now comes the interchange of the inevitable "Have you heard this one?" How often does the detached onlooker observe that the narrator begins to laugh or titter long before he has reached his punch line, anticipating the reaction of the auditor, and continuing long after. Is it not also a fact that the listener, while awaiting the point of the joke, has on his own part recalled a *bon mot* and is only too eager for the speaker to finish so that he can score his own personal point?

The philosopher Mélinaud (1895) stressed that numerous factors, either singly or in combination, produce a situation in which laughter is readily detonated. Such include a state of well-being, youthfulness (for children are said to laugh more often than adults), recent success, achievement, or conversely a recent escape from peril. Mélinaud did not mention the most potent factor of all, namely alcohol.

Laughter is highly contagious. A thousand foregather in a music hall and await with pleasurable anticipation the entry of the comic. Long before he has opened his mouth the audience may laugh, their reaction being precipitated by the grotesque costume or physical appearance of the artiste. If the actor is well known and popular, laughter follows his simplest utterance, which, incidentally, may not be funny at all. Or it may be a stock phrase awaited by the expectant audience and hence devoid of any element of surprise. It requires only one isolated guffaw somewhere in the auditorium to precipitate a gale of appreciative hilarity. The experienced trouper knows this full well and by skilful timing he can provoke the audience to a crescendo of mirth. If less successful, the shrewd positioning of a claque or "shill" in key positions may serve to spark off the laggard house. At the same time, it is well known to touring comics that a geographical factor is all too significant, and certain cities in Great Britain are notorious as being the "comedian's grave."

In contrast to "live shows," the work of a comedian on radio is more difficult: He is invisible and is only a voice with its repertoire of wisecracks. A response is often artificially evoked by the employment of what is called the "laugh track," or the periodic interruption of the speaker with canned cachinnation. This is a dangerous technique, however, for to a more sophisticated and less naive auditor the laugh track is more likely to be an annoyance than an incitement.

That laughter is "catching" there surely can be no doubt. At the same time we do not adhere to the theory advanced by the irrepressible Ambrose Bierce. He quoted the alleged opinion of a hypothetical "Dr. Meir Witchell" to the effect that the infectious character of laughter is due to instantaneous fermentation of *sputa* diffused in a spray. From this peculiarity he named the disorder *convulsio spargens*.

Why is it that, on the whole, children laugh oftener than grownups? The disillusionment of age may play a role, but that is not the whole explanation. In our early years, everything around us is something novel, something unexplored, for

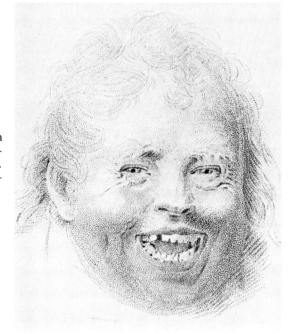

FIG. 2. Laughing child. (From Bell, C.: *The Anatomy and Philosophy of Expression*, 6th ed. Bohr, London, 1872, with permission.)

strong mental associations have yet to be forged. The *tabula rasa* is still to be filled, and things have not shed their cloak of wonder (Fig. 2). The child's mind is quick and more supple, and perceives the bizarre more readily. Some say that for like reasons women laugh more than men—as indeed they do, for they possess the agility and quick wit of a child to a greater extent.

Is laughter purposeful? Most philosophers have commented upon the fundamental ambivalence of its motor components, like the crackling of thorns beneath a pot. Its only possible rationale is to grease the wheels of communication in a climate of careless conviviality and so facilitate mutual harmony. Valéry had another idea. He regarded laughter as a way to avoid thinking. Philosophers as a class are said to be notorious for their avoidance of laughter. Democritus has been quoted as an exception derived from his cheery, outgoing personality, rare among the academics of the time.

The anatomy of the action of laughing deserves examination. There are of course numerous varieties, types, degrees, and manners of laughter, but certain fundamentals are common to all. In the first place there are the repeated, audible expiratory noises of the consonant–verb (cv) type. Typically, the c-component is an aspirate. This seems to be a *sine qua non*, for it is detectable even in those semiliterates who habitually omit the initial aspirate in their spoken speech. The vocalic component is usually, though not always, a short "a." Many years ago the anatomist Gratiolet said that men when laughing emit a *ha, ha, ha* or a *ho, ho, ho*, whereas women and children are characterized by a *hé, hé, hé* or a *hi, hi, hi*. His remarks are perhaps not too convincing.

Simultaneously there takes place a contraction of the facial muscles (Fig. 3). The *orbiculares oculorum* go into action. The mouth opens, widely so in the vulgar; flushing of the face and lacrimation occur when the laughter is extreme.

The musculature of the trunk and upper limbs undergoes changes in tonus. At first there is a spasm so that the neck and head are thrown back (Fig. 4). The truncal muscles, including the diaphragm and perhaps the elevators of the shoulders, contract and relax. Semipurposeful movements, unattractive to observe, may supervene whereby the laugher may slap his thighs, clap his hands, or violently nudge his neighbour. When laughter becomes excessive, a tonelessness develops that is not altogether pleasant to experience or to behold. In women the urinary sphincters may relax. The arms and trunk may flop forward helplessly, and it is not unknown for the lower limbs to become flaccid, causing a fall. Hence the expressions "to die with laughter," "to roll in the aisles."

Psychoanalysts have their own views about laughter, its origins and physical expression. They associate laughter with remnants of the magical pleasure of soiling, an intestinal catharsis, an orgastic ejection. As Meerloo put it: "Behind all laughter we find the defensive torsion movements of body. Such laughter may represent an anal or libidinal discharge effigy, without guilt or shame."

The foregoing represent the bare bones of the act of laughter. Some of the older descriptions have been more picturesque. Listen to Bulwer (1649):

> In this Dance of the Muscles performed by excessive Laughter upon the
> Theater of mirth, the Countenance, the Mouth seems to lead the Chorus;

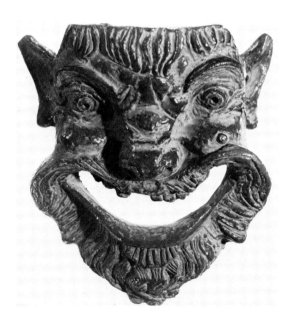

FIG. 3. Greek mask from Sicily representing comedy.

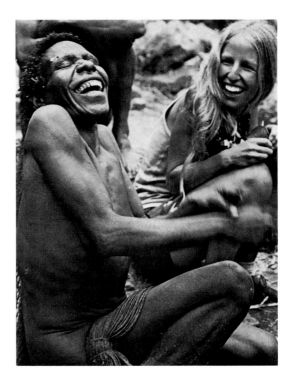

FIG. 4. Boisterous hilarity.
(From Morris, D.: *Manwatching*.
Jonathan Cape, London, 1977.
Courtesy of Bill Leimbach.)

for Laughter is a motion arising chiefly out of the Contraction of the Muscles of the lips, in which Motion of the Mouth, called Laughter, the parts about the mouth seem bounded out with certain lines called Rictus, whence Risus.

Bulwer went on to say:

In Laughter there is made, by reason of the Contranision, a certain corrugation or wrinkle about the angle of the eye, especially the outward angle, which in those that laugh often are supposed to grow habituall, which some Ladies fearing, will not laugh, lest they should contract wrinkles and looke old by breaking in that part which is near the Temples.

Armstrong (1709–1779) was more colourful than correct.

That palpitating of the stomach produced by hearty laughter, which thrills the whole body into a subtle and invigorating dance and sends the blood pulsing through the veins and arteries with a livelier and more sparkling flow, transmits a similar commotion to the mind. The mind flings open its doors and windows, its dim and dusty corners are filled with air and sunshine, its foul and secret places are ventilated and sweetened: it ceases to be a dark and complex thing and becomes airy and bright and simple.

Most writers on the subject of laughter have failed to dissociate the objective phenomena from the basic question of humour and wit. For example, Bergson in his monograph *Le Rire* rarely considered laughter per se but focused upon the physiological aspects underlying the ridiculous. He recognised three factors: repetition, inversion, and reciprocal interference of series. The third of these he explained by stating that a situation is invariably comic when it belongs at one and the same time to two altogether independent series of events and thus is capable of being interpreted in two entirely different meanings at the same time. The distinction between wit and humour was only touched upon. The comic thing is often evidence of exaggeration. To Alexander Bain comedy was, generally speaking, a species of degradation; to Gautier it was "the logic of the absurd." The preacher in *Ecclesiastes* was scathing: "I said of laughter, it is mad"; "Sorrow's better than laughter"; "the heart of fools is in the house of mirth."

Almost alone among philosophers who have pondered over the mechanism of laughter, Monro devoted thought to the mode of action of that purely material agency, so-called "laughing gas." He naturally found it difficult to coordinate a reaction to nitrous oxide anaesthesia within the medley of purely emotional or cognitive factors. To him it suggested a chemical phenomenon which might possibly conduce to a pleasant state of light-heartedness with a sense of relief from physical trauma. A euphoric attitude of mind makes it easy for some quite trivial stimulus to produce laughter.

Incidentally one wonders how often in fact laughter does follow nitrous oxide anaesthesia. It is probably far rarer than is popularly believed.

Among recent studies of laughter those of Pollio and his associates at the University of Tennessee are of interest. Here again they concentrated upon laughter as the paradigm of the funny man to the exclusion of other causes and circumstances. By studying the audience response to a comedian at work in the natural setting of a theatre as well as in a psychological laboratory, Pollio sought to record and then analyse the frequency, latency, volume, and duration of the laughing behaviour of the audience. He considered such variables as the size of the turnout, whether the auditors were strangers to each other or associates, and their sex. Incidentally, he did not examine the factor of age. He was also able to observe the considerable differences between the response to canned laughter and to that arising naturally. Pollio made no sharp distinction between smiling and laughing, regarding the former as both the setting and the aftermath of audible hilarity. This last point is discussed in the essay on smiling.

Pollio quoted from the literature two field studies among student volunteers. The circumstances conducive to laughter were explored. In 1937 Young recorded the frequency and causes of laughter among 184 college students. They were instructed to make notes of how often they laughed during a 24-hour period and to record the provocative incidents. On an average the female students laughed 13 times a day, and the males did so 19 times. The greatest single cause of laughter comprised jokes or wisecracks made by peers (62%). Humourous situations and incidents accounted for 15%, and unintentional antics amounted to 4%. The remaining 18% of the factors arose out of comic material in books, movies, plays, lectures, and radio programmes.

Young's results may be contrasted with the earlier findings of Kamboroupolou (1926) in a group of students at Vassar College. The participants were asked to keep a "humour diary" for a week in which each young lady recorded all the things she laughed at throughout the day. The number of laughs per day varied from 2 to 18, with an average of 4 to 5. Of the laughs, 25% were caused by clowning of others, whereas 33% were due to humourous remarks made by peers. The largest single category, amounting to 33%, was inspired by the mental inferiority, stupidity, or ignorance of another. In not one of the categories was there mention of droll situations in books, plays, or magazines. As Pollio et al. remarked: "It seems as if Vassar girls of 1926 never went to plays or read books or magazines for fun; or if they did, they never told anyone about it, least of all Kamboroupolou."

In neither of these field studies were we informed how many of the wisecracks or mirth-producing situations were of a bawdy or risqué type. We can but hazard a guess.

Pollio's own studies relied upon sound tracks. In that way any possible confusion between the auditory and visual precipitants of laughter was eliminated. A Bruel-Kjaer sound-level recorder was used so that it was possible to estimate (1) the latency, (2) the duration, and (3) the amplitude of each laugh. A sample record of this type is shown in Fig. 5.

The authors went on to compare the oscillographic tracings of dubbed as opposed to natural laughter. The tracings were seen to differ in many specifiable ways, such as in quality, latency, and waveform (Fig. 6).

A rather disturbing social study of laughter set off by witticisms was reported by Coser (1960) among the staff of a psychiatric hospital in Boston. The circumstances were the case presentations carried out by junior members of the staff. The group was made up of five senior staff members, six junior members, and six paramedical staff. Most of the badinage (90 of 103 incidents) was found to be directed at some target or other. Of these 90, 53 were perpetrated by the senior staff, 33 by juniors, and 4 by paramedical staff, even though junior staff members spoke more often than their seniors. As to the butts of these directed jokes, of the 53 senior staff witticisms 21 were at the expense of the junior staff, 9 were directed at patients, 4 at themselves, and 14 at no obvious target. Of the 33 junior staff wisecracks, 13 were aimed at patients, 12 at themselves, 2 at senior staff (but only in their absence), and 2 at no discernible quarry. Paramedical members told jokes only about patients (2) or about themselves (2).

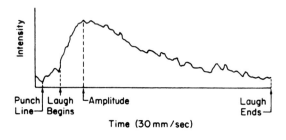

FIG. 5. Oscillogram of audience laughter during a movie performance. (From Pollio, H. R.: *The Psychology of Humor*. Academic Press, New York, 1972, with permission.)

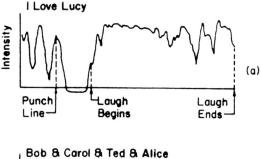

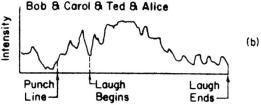

FIG. 6. Comparison of oscillographic tracings for **(a)** canned and **(b)** live laughter. (From Pollio, H. R.: *The Psychology of Humor*. Academic Press, New York, 1972, with permission.)

There seems to be a moral somewhere in these rather surprising findings. In any case, however, the phenomenon of joking and of wit lies somewhere outside our principal theme, which is the act of laughter.

The Physical Manifestations of Laughter

Let us admit that whether laughter fulfils a purpose, the performance is scarcely an attractive one. By him who laughs and his associates, this may pass unnoticed, the feelings engendered being those of hilarity and glee. The full measure of the situation, however, is all too obvious to the bystander who is just outside the circle of ribaldry. Those verbal comments which set off and maintained the boisterousness were unheard. When not shrill, the sound of laughter is raucous, unpleasing, and often annoying. The motor concomitants are inelegant, to say the least. Reviewers have taken me to task for my "emotionally charged" disapproval of the laughter of others. I am, however, unrepentant. A detached evaluation would support me. Meanwhile one reverts to the classics. "Nothing," said Catullus, "is sillier than a silly laugh." According to Congreve "nothing is more unbecoming a man of quality than to laugh." As one might guess, the Earl of Chesterfield was also unfavourably impressed. "Since I have had the full use of my reason, nobody has ever heard me laugh." And in a letter to his son he stated unequivocally that "nothing is so *illiberal* and so ill-bred as audible laughter." To Goldsmith loud laughter bespoke the vacant mind.

Such criticisms align laughter not only with silliness but also with noise, a concept which is reasonable. As an intrusion it therefore merits all the distaste which Schopenhauer expressed. "Noise is the most impertinent of all forms of interruption. It is not only interruption, but also *disruption* of thought. Of course, where there is nothing to interrupt, noise will not be so particularly objectionable."

It would not be difficult to offset such comments by quotations to the contrary. However, these are usually the expressions of those convivial hearties who are themselves addicted—laughaholics in fact. Nor are we impressed by sentimentalists such as De Quincy, who considered that the laughter of girls is, and ever was, among the most delightful sound on earth. Had he said the earthy sounds of delight he would have been nearer the mark. De Quincy obviously was never inveigled into a cocktail party, nor was ever the frustrated auditor of one going on next door. The philosopher W. S. Lilly (1896) was equally dewy-eyed. He referred to that ringing laughter of pure human happiness emanating sometimes from the lips of young girls. Was there any music like it? he asked, saying that they laughed as the birds sing.

So far we have dealt with laughter as the outward expression of sentiments of the comic and absurd. But there is much more to be said about the problem. For example, there is the alliance between laughter and tears. At first glance these two emotions might appear antithetical, but that is not so. Purely on the material side, laughter may proceed and end in the shedding of tears. Especially is this the case with pathological laughter, as we shall see later. Laughter may be a device for concealing tears, a comic mask behind which hides a tragic player. It may be a primitive and improbable means of expressing sympathy in circumstances where a display of grief would seem more appropriate to most of us. Anthropologists tell us that savages are apt to receive grievous news with laughter, this being their peculiar way of showing sympathy. In one of their fireside chats, the two learned Professors Whitehead and Lawrence referred to a party of Africans who returned from an expedition roaring with laughter. The explanation was that a crocodile had unexpectedly seized and devoured one of their company.

It has been alleged that in the Nazi concentration camps a nervous and contagious laughter often affected victims on their way to the extermination chamber. A veritable gallows humour in fact.

Many authorities have drawn attention to the relationship between *le rire* and *les larmes*. Goethe regarded laughter, weeping, joy, and grief as first cousins. Beaumarchais said he hastened to laugh at everything for fear of having to weep. Charles Lamb confessed he once misbehaved at a funeral, for anything awful made him laugh. Byron said "if I laugh at any mortal thing 'tis that I may not weep."

This relation between laughing and weeping applies even more when it is a matter of such attenuated forms of laughter as giggling or tittering. These types of mini-merriment represent not so much amusement as a cover-up for an uncomfortable state of embarrassment. This especially applies to giggling. The giggler is well aware of the inappropriateness of his behaviour. It distresses him, for he cannot control it. The more he tries to inhibit his unfitting conduct the more compelling it becomes, and the situation may eventually end in tears.

There is a third set of conditions which may conduce to laughter. This is the act of wilful ridicule. It is an ugly and deliberate thing which bears little if any relationship with enjoyment. What more unseemly sound is there in a supposedly solemn situation, as for example the U.S. congress or a parliamentary sitting, than the howling down of a speaker by a hostile pack. One of the few Old Testament references to laughter is of this type. It is to the effect that "All they that see me laugh me to scorn: they shoot out the lip, they shake the head." In his monograph *Le Rire* Henry Bergson emphasized the corrective function of laughter. "Being intended to humiliate, it must make a painful impression on the person against whom it is directed. By laughter, society avenges itself for the liberties taken with it."

"Not by wrath does one kill," wrote Nietzsche, "but by laughter."

Closely allied to the expression of ridicule is the cruel Homeric laughter engendered by the plight or discomfiture of another. Thus the *Iliad* narrates that the laughter of the Gods on high Olympus was unquenchable when they beheld the predicament of Ares and Aphrodite in bed, entangled inextricably in the net forged by Vulcan, the deceived husband. Only Neptune was not amused and intervened to liberate the guilty couple.

Sadistic laughter may betray gross indifference towards others, or even exultation over their suffering. It is the hallmark of one who wears all too often the smile of cruelty. The carnage suffered by Germans and French alike during the protracted battle of Verdun is said to have excited rather than horrified the Crown Prince Friedrich Wilhelm, who was indicted as the "laughing murderer of Verdun."

Personality Types

Individuals vary in their propensity to laughter. This is independent of any qualities of wit, humour, or drollery which they may evince. It is merely a matter of how inflammable is the individual, how easily he is set alight by the spark which evokes a conflagration of laughter. At one extreme is the one who giggles much— the hallmark of a fool, as the Latin proverb tells us. Certainly high-grade mental defectives laugh a lot, for it is their sole mode of responding to all sensations, so long as they are not painful.

Outgoing, extroverted, endowed with a warm but simple nature, friendly, and gregarious. These descriptions are usually applied to folk who smile a lot and are easily provoked to laughter. For some reason there is a correlation at times with obesity.

Conversely, there are others who seldom laugh and are often unapproachable and not gregarious. This judgement is not necessarily fair. Some nonlaughers are actually social, affable, and neighbourly. A witty conversationalist who was poker-faced provoked Max Beerbohm to speak of him as an "incomparable laugh-giver, he is not much of a laugher. He is vintner, not toper."

There is a personality factor as well. Thus the presentation of a witticism whether in print or by word of mouth (or in the form of a situational picture without words) may provoke one of a series of reactions. Thus Oscar Wilde's dictum that "work is the downfall of the drinking classes" may fail to hit the target in the case of the dull-witted. Others may recognise the paradox intellectually but fail to be amused. This type of response is, I submit, commoner in women than in men. The natural, and most usual, reaction is an appreciative sentiment of amusement. In some this evokes a smile; in a few an actual laugh.

Comic or unorthodox pictures are often employed as a clinical test in neurological practice. There is a drawing of a solitary skier descending a snow-covered slope. Behind him are the parallel tracks made by his skis. Half way down is an isolated tree. One ski track passes this obstacle on the left and the other on the right before approximating once more. When such a sketch is shown to a patient with some form of higher nervous disorder, the sheer ridiculousness of the situation is un-realised, the patient identifying the drawing as merely representing an Alpine skier.

Someone has pointed out that, as a class, philosophers belong to the nonlaughing category. Herbert Spencer, for example, was solemn and unsmiling and at times frankly depressive, and yet he wrote an essay on The Physiology of Laughter. Indeed the topic of laughter has been studied in cold blood by a number of other philosophers, particularly Hobbes, Hecker, Courdaveaux, Philbert, Penjon, Meli-nand, Bergson, Stanley Hall and Allen, Schopenhauer, Kant, French, Bain, East-man, Greig, Feibelman, Gregory, Kimmins, Kline, Leacock, Ludovici, McDougall, Krishna Menon, Sully, Monro, Koestler.

Tot homines, *tot sententiae*, for it is rare to meet wholehearted agreement among philosophers. Monro, perhaps the most readable, concluded his monograph with the words: "There are still many questions to be answered. If humour is the inappropriate, why should it cause the peculiar physical manifestations we call laughter? Why should the same manifestations be called for by tickling, by laughing gas and by nervousness? Any complete theory should answer these questions. I do not know the answer."

It was the opinion of Helvetius that were philosophers ever to laugh out loud no one would believe their dogmas. One at least went so far as to say that a perfect being—a Christ, for example—would be incapable of laughter for two reasons: He would be endowed with utter goodness which would exclude all malice, and being also omniscient he would perceive the absurdity of all our ways so clearly that they would become a commonplace and not amusing.

Whitehead, however, has drawn attention to an interesting point, namely the comparative rarity of any reference to laughter among the ancients. It seems to have been unknown among the earliest Hebrews and Greeks. Scarcely any allusion to laughter can be found in the Old Testament or in the works of Homer, except in that heartless attribute set off by ridicule. Aristophanes might have been a rare and striking exception, and the topical allusions in his comedies possibly proved up-roarious to his audience. Democritus might well have been merely benevolent and easy-going. Socrates was jocular towards his pupils, but he ended his own life. The Romans appear not to have been familiar with laughter until the second century AD, and indeed it was not until the Middle Ages that anything of a really hilarious nature can be traced in literature. Perhaps priority should be awarded to the publication of Rabelais' *Pantagruel & Gargantua* in the sixteenth century. Here, perhaps for the first time, we encounter wit, humour, and satire in abundance. Rabelais' extreme bawdiness may have been the idiom of his day, though one can but wonder about the reaction of his Benedictine brethren to his extreme salaciousness.

Clearly, too, factors of sex and age are important. If we concentrate for the moment on laughter engendered by a humourous situation, one can express the belief that although women tend to laugh more readily than men they lag far behind as perpetrators of wit. As Pollio and Edgerly put it: "Men talk and joke: women smile and laugh." Susceptibility to laughter was once gravely spoken of as the logic of the absurd.

Why Does Tickling Produce Laughter?

That tickling produces laughter is a commonplace phenomenon, no doubt familiar enough for thousands of years though rarely discussed. Children rather than adults are the usual recipients, though domestic animals obviously also find it pleasurable. But whereas humans respond by squirming and widespread movements of withdrawal accompanied by uncontrolled laughter, the reaction of a dog, cat, or horse is restrained and silent. Monkeys, it is said, may grimace and emit a chuckling sound when tickled in the armpits (Darwin). Cats purr, but it would be unsafe to equate that comfort sound with a human laugh.

Gratiolet (1867) believed some peripheral nerves to be more sensitive than others. The two areas in man recognised as ticklish are the armpits and the soles of the feet. To a lesser extent the depths of the outer ear and the threshold of the nares are sensitive and, to the right kind of stimulation, ticklish.

It has been alleged that these zones are areas ordinarily protected from tactile contacts. But that idea scarcely applies to the soles of the feet, which are in habitual juxtaposition with the ground. The stimulus, to be appropriate, must be light. This applies to the soles which are accustomed to pressure, but it scarcely holds true for the axillae.

Much that has been written about the connection between laughter and tickling is sheer nonsense. A lack of unanimity among writers is obvious. The ticklish areas of the body have been regarded as erogenous zones (Havelock Ellis, Greig); areas especially vulnerable in warfare, as well as to attacks by parasites (Louis Robinson); zones exposed to a special sort of teasing (Sully); and a conspicuous instance of a minor personal discomfort, falling short of pain (McDougall). Koestler spoke of tickling as "mock aggression."

It is said that babies begin to exhibit ticklishness at the age of 2 months. Researchers at Yale have found that laughter provoked by tickling takes place 15 times more often if the one who tickles is the mother rather than a stranger.

Neurologists with a considerable experience of tickling the soles of the feet in the search for a possible Babinski response would probably assert that laughter is a far less common reaction than an exaggerated withdrawal of the limb coupled with generalised squirming and verbal protests. The impression is that tickling of the soles is not, as a rule, a pleasurable activity. Often it provokes no reaction at all.

It is well known that one has difficulty tickling oneself. Darwin believed that the laughter of tickling arises from a background of pleasurable anticipation. If a child is taken unawares and his sole is stimulated by a stranger, the result is more likely to be one of fear and dislike. Darwin also believed that the precise point of stimulation must be known. For this reason, he believed, autostimulation is not effective.

Obviously, little is known about the physiology of tickling, and the purpose of the response by laughter is obscure. One cannot, therefore, submit a plausible reply to the question: Why does one laugh when tickled?

Pathological Laughter

When it appears without reason or at least insufficient cause, and when excessive in violence and infantile in character, laughter is a well-known symptom of a number of unrelated neurological diseases. Commonest among these cases of *Zwangslachen* is the pseudobulbar syndrome, the product of diffuse minor vascular insults. In addition to disordered motility, dysarthria, and difficulty in swallowing, there is a conspicuous degree of ready laughter and tears without any corresponding affect of amusement or grief. Hence the term "sham mirth." The patient who is an arteriopath and usually elderly displays a proclivity to titter, giggle, and then to laugh or cry uncontrollably. Sometimes the episode is set off by conversation, particularly if the term "laugh" is introduced. As a matter of experience, pathological weeping is commoner than pathological laughter. Often laughter continues until it turns to tears, and there is a period when it is difficult to determine whether one is witnessing laughter or crying. The pervading emotion is one of intense embarrassment.

Elsewhere I have referred to a patient of mine. He was an ageing arteriosclerotic who shuffled his way into a public park to seat himself on a bench. Suddenly he emitted a peal of loud, unprovoked, and ungovernable laughter. Onlookers summoned a policeman who escorted him to my hospital close by.

Something similar, though on a much attenuated scale, may be seen in patients with multiple sclerosis, where euphoria and ready though restrained laughter are characteristic. For that matter, such patients are also easily moved to tears.

Laughter is also known to be sometimes associated with epilepsy. It may appear as a component of an aura. When it has occurred often, it may act as a signal and lead to comment on the part of the victim. Thus in the case of "ictal laughter" recorded by Ames and Enderstein (1975), the patient periodically cleared his throat, laughed, and after saying "here we go again" lapsed into a minor seizure. Afterwards he would have no memory either of the turn or what led up to it. Sometimes the term "gelastic epilepsy" is used for outbursts of loud laughter culminating in a convulsion. Whether it bears any relationship to that neurological curiosity *Lachschlag* we have no idea.

Perhaps the most familiar association in the setting of epilepsy is for a patient with petit mal to giggle briefly at the end of an absence. Such a phenomenon is by no means uncommon.

Pathological laughter has from time to time been described as a symptom of cerebral tumour. The site of the growth seems to be so inconsistent that it would be foolish to endow this symptom with localizing import.

Another condition, fortunately rare, where uproarious laughter occurs is in the kuru of Papua New Guinea, especially in the terminal stages. It has also been described as a symptom of latah.

Tropical neurology holds yet another instance of uninhibited laughter. In Uganda and Tanga there have been outbreaks of epidemic unrestrained laughing particularly in schoolgirl communities. The most recent occasion was in Ghana as described by Addae and Kotei (1975). The "laughing disease," as it was called, was surprisingly regarded by the authors not as hysterical but as organic in nature, being associated with headache and fever.

Hysterical laughter is no great rarity. Its cardinal features comprise inappropriateness, extravagance, frenzy, an affect of distress, and its culmination in sobbing. Such episodes are triggered by sudden despair arising upon a background of protracted stress. An excellent example was depicted by Hugh Walpole in his novel *The Cathedral*.

Yet another well-known tie-up between laughter and neurological disease is met with in cataplexy. In narcoleptics some attacks of muscular tonelessness are evoked by sudden emotion, such as anger, surprise, fright. Most potent of all is laughter. When this takes place the patient's head falls forward and he slumps in his chair. Were he standing erect at the time he would buckle at the knees and probably fall. Although the patient is fully conscious, voluntary movement would be impossible for a minute or so. Neurologists who have witnessed these cataplectic attacks have observed a temporary loss of the tendon reflexes and extensor plantar responses.

The laughter which precipitates the cataplexy must be genuine. That is to say, the mock laughter of a play-actor would not produce an attack. Neither would a sudden feeling of great amusement unless it were accompanied by typical gelastic manifestations.

Substitute Laughter

By the term "substitute laughter" we refer to a form of invisible laughter that occurs during communication between two persons, neither being able to see the other or hear him speak. This happens in the case of two blind deaf-mutes where the notion of merriment is expressed by way of movement and touch. There is an even better example, all the more striking because the two participants are remote from each other and touch cannot be part of the communicative network. Wireless telegraphy offers such an example, especially when the Morse keyboard was used for transmitting messages by way of a code of dots and dashes. It used to happen—perhaps it still does—that during a slack period the sender and the recipient would engage in small talk or gossip over the air. This often led to the exchange of wisecracks or witticisms. At such times, the receiver would signal his amusement by tapping out MIM, MIM, MIM (- - · · · -).

Smiling

So much for laughter. The related topic of smiling merits an independent inquiry. In this essay one has concentrated upon the objective features of the phenomenon rather than those subtle gossamer things such as feelings of merriment and the sinister weapon of wit. Like shadows they tend to vanish when one submits them to the searchlight of science.

In his monograph *Le Rire*, Henri Bergson's approach was the opposite. His thesis covered the motives behind the physical expression. The philosophy of mirth and of the ridiculous he found elusive, but the reader is rewarded with his final paragraph which expresses in an engaging fashion the sheer mystery of his theme:

> Such is also the truceless warfare of the waves on the surface of the sea, whilst profound peace reigns in the depths below. The billows clash and collide with each other as they strive to find their level. A fringe of snow-white foam, feathery and frolicsome, follows their changing outlines. From time to time, the receding wave leaves behind a remnant of foam on the sandy beach. The child, who plays hard by, picks up a handful, and, the next moment, is astonished to find that nothing remains in his grasp but a few drops of water, water that is far more brackish, far more bitter than that of the wave which brought it. Laughter comes into being in the selfsame fashion. It indicates a slight revolt on the surface of social life. It instantly adopts the changing forms of the disturbance. It, also, is a froth with a saline base. Like froth, it sparkles. It is gaiety itself. But the philosopher who gathers a handful to taste may find that the substance is scanty, and the after-taste bitter.

The Land of Smiles

Having more or less disposed of the matter of laughter, let us turn to that cognate phenomenon the smile. Essentially it represents a mimic movement of the face consisting basically in retraction of the corners of the mouth and deepening of the nasolabial folds. In addition, an elevation of the upper lip may be observed which exposes the teeth. The palpebral fissures narrow, the automatic act of blinking may be momentarily halted, and the creases deepen at the outer corners of the orbits.

Smiling is not necessarily a deliberately conscious act, and it may not be purposeful. Ordinarily it is regarded as a "look of pleasure as opposed to a frown; a gay and joyous appearance" to quote Samuel Johnson's definition. This suggests that smiling represents an unpremeditated expressive facial contraction mirroring a particular affect or sentiment (Fig. 1).

In fact the matter is far more complicated, for smiling may connote many contingencies—or nothing at all. In other words, it may be little more than what Paul Valéry called *un pli de visage*, a crack in the face. When instructing artists in the elements of human anatomy, Charles Bell (1806) emphasized that a smile might convey a thousand different meanings. There was the placid smile of benignity; the arching of the lower lip to indicate contempt; the smile of sadness; the simper of conceit; the distorted grin of the toper; the leer of the bawd; and so on.

Anatomical Remarks

At this point it is appropriate to examine more closely the anatomy of the facial muscles that are concerned in smiling.

Many small muscles underlie the integument of the face and are usually referred to as the "muscles of expression." Their exact number is debatable, and it may be that there is some inconstancy in their morphology. Some regard certain fibre groupings as anatomical entities, whereas others regard them as but a part of a larger muscle unit. Hence discrepancies arose between Todd, who recognised 19 pairs of muscles plus one azygos muscle, and Moreau, on the other hand, who identified 55 distinct facial muscles.

The earliest contributions to this subject include those of Le Brun, Camper, Gratiolet, Charles Bell, Henle, Duchenne (who also made use of galvanic stimulation), Moreau, Lavater, Todd, and Charles Darwin. These facial muscles are obviously under the control of the nervous system but to a variable extent. Thus when the frontalis muscle is willed to contract, ordinarily both eyebrows rise, the forehead becoming corrugated. A few persons are able to raise one eyebrow only. In such cases the act is highly deliberate, and in the course of animated talk both eyebrows may rise from time to time, but never one alone. In the same way the ability to wink is a volitional act acquired in early childhood. Most persons can wink on either side, but a few on one side only. Many more can wink either eye but more easily on one side than the other. There appears to be no association with handedness, but there is a mild correlation with eye dominance. Thus out of a series of 153 dyslectic children, all above the age of 6 years, who could either close one eyelid only or else could close one more easily than the other, the preferred eye was the opposite one to the "preferred" eyelid in 98, whereas in 55 cases the master eye was on the same side as the "master" eyelid (Critchley and Critchley, 1978).

A few are also endowed with the ability to move voluntarily an ear, through a small range, either to and fro or in an up and down direction. Both ears or only one may be empowered in this way. Such a capacity is a highly voluntary one, for the movement does not take place automatically.

Can such exceptional unilateral movements be acquired by practice? In all probability they can, for we have the analogy of the learned skill of contracting one pectoralis major without moving the arm, or one quadrant only of the rectus abdominis, as in the case of tassel or belly dancers.

Similarly it is likely that one can cultivate the ability to contract all the facial muscles through an exceptional range. Such an accomplishment may attain the status of an "india rubber face," which may add no little to the art of the comedian (Dan Leno, Max Wall).

In addition to the variable degrees of awareness in the contraction of the muscles of expression, there is another phenomenon that we may refer to as "facial associated movements." This was a subject studied in 1924 by E. A. Carmichael and myself.

We examined more than 400 subjects and discovered at least six types of associated phenomena. Commonest was the oculoaural movement, which comprised a slow adduction of the helix of the ear on extreme lateral ocular deviation. This was found in 50 of 400 subjects. Usually the phenomenon was bilateral. If only one helix moved, it was the one on the side to which the gaze was directed. None of the subjects was able to move the ear voluntarily. Four in the series were patients with multiple sclerosis. Each one displayed aural "nystagmus" of the ipsilateral ear, even in the absence of ocular nystagmus.

In many subjects it became obvious that when their mouths were opened widely movement of the eyes to one side or the other would produce an oculolingual-associated movement, of which the individual was usually unaware. In other words, the tip of the tongue would deviate to the side to which the eyes were directed.

In one person an oculonasal-associated movement was observed, the gaze to one side or the other being accompanied by a flaring of the nostrils, equal on the two sides. One individual displayed an oculomandibular-associated movement. When the mouth was open and the eyes turned fully to one side, the point of the chin would move slightly to the opposite side. This phenomenon was particularly evident on rapid side-to-side deviation of the eyes.

One young woman was afflicted with an uncontrollable unilateral flickering blepharoclonus. This was associated with a synchronous, intermittent tinnitus within the ear at the same time, indicating (it was thought) an orbiculostapedial-associated movement.

The authors investigated the eye–ear movements of many animals in the London Zoo. In the higher primates (orangutang, chimpanzee) well marked oculoaural-associated movements were observed. There was no opportunity to test a gorilla. In the lower primates (mandrills, drills, baboons, spider monkeys, capuchins, woolly monkeys, geladas, and Japanese monkeys) oculoaural-associated movements were always witnessed though not to the same degree in the higher apes. Oculo-frontalis-associated movements were also present in many mammals, especially those with long, shaggy coats, as if to assist vision on lateral gaze.

It was considered that in *Homo sapiens* these associated facial movements were relics of a specialized alerting movement in animals with prominent mobile ears and forward-placed orbits.

The Smile of Amusement

The smile of amusement is the traditional type of smile, though not necessarily the commonest (Figs. 1 and 2). It betrays a quiet and restrained appreciation of drollery and, more especially, wit. In the latter context it can be looked upon as an intelligent response to an intelligent stimulus, for the creation of a witticism, in

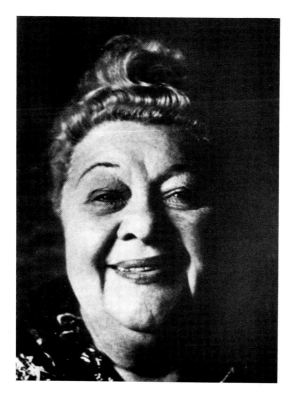

FIG. 1. A warm and genuine smile of amusement. (From Beaton, C., and Tynan, K.: *Persona Grata*. Wingate, London, 1953, with permission.)

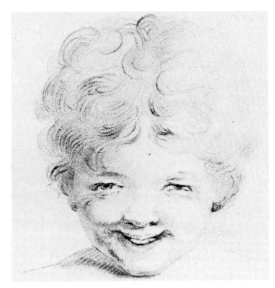

FIG. 2. Smiling child. (From Bell, C.: *The Anatomy and Philosophy of Expression*. Bohr, London, 1872.)

print or by word of mouth, is beyond the capacity of the dullard. Smiling is the thin and refined end of a wedge whose base is made up of boisterous laughter. It may take place in solitude. One may well picture oneself as smiling while quietly reading one of Oscar Wilde's comedies, whereas loud laughter would be expected only in a theatre (Fig. 6).

As we mentioned in the essay on laughter, Pollio et al. followed the precept of Darwin and emphasized the link between smiling and laughter, indicating that the former may precede the latter, or it may become inseparably combined with it. For that matter, it may linger after the latter has subsided so as to constitute a veritable Cheshire cat phenomenon. Perhaps Pollio and his colleagues went too far and somewhat overstated the role of smiling as a poor relation of laughter. In my opinion, they did.

The fundamental anatomy of the smile has been mentioned, but, as with the laugh, there are faint, restrained, fleeting smiles. Indeed in some persons an impending smile is heralded by a facial dimpling without any retraction of the mouth. At the other extreme, something broad and blatant, often spoken of as a grin, may become all too obvious. "When Farmer Oak smiled, the corners of his mouth spread till they were within an unimportant distance of his ears, his eyes were reduced to chinks, and diverging wrinkles appeared round them, extending upon his countenance like the rays in a rudimentary sketch of the rising sun" (Thomas Hardy, *Far from the Madding Crowd*).

The Social Smile

The social smile is the one that is assumed like a mask when two or more assemble. It is on a par with small talk, the purpose of which is to create a congenial atmosphere. The social smile contributes to that ambiguous attribute often summed up in the word "charm." Though a mask, it does not necessarily conceal a countenance of tragedy. Behind that smile, there may be the deadpan face of vacuity or even of evil.

Not surprisingly, the social smile is linked with personality, and some persons adopt it like a garment. Listen to what Stephen Birmingham had to say about the subject of his biography.

> Part of the insulation, the only part that showed, was the smile. The smile had changed enormously over the years. Early photographs show Jackie with a shy, tentative, uncertain smile. She seemed afraid to part her lips over her teeth. By her debutante days, however, she had developed a flirty, head-tilted-to-one-side coquettish smile. Later, posing campily with a hugely long cigarette holder, she had found a wicked smile, a smile that seemed to say she was a party to some splendidly naughty and delicious secret. But now the smile—and it had taken work—had perfected itself into something that was both radiant and ingratiating, enthusiastic and brave—a theatrical smile that was at the same time human. It was a smile of such quality that, when faced with it, there was almost nothing one could say or do. The smile of Jacqueline Kennedy Onassis was more than insulation. It was armor. Her smile had grown from a little-girl nothing to a big-girl something. The Jacqueline Onassis smile would become her trademark and her most effective weapon.*

Just as there are those who laugh more readily than others, so some persons smile easily and often. Up to a point it is an index of character, but one must not push the idea too far. Some warm-hearted and even witty persons habitually adopt a poker face, and in the case of the vaudeville comedian this is often a professional advantage.

In his study of gesture and kinesics, Birdwhistell is said to have identified a "smile belt" traversing the United States in close proximity to the Mason-Dixon line. (Some Americans have called it the "magnolia wall ".) Above this line the Yankees are regarded as tight-lipped and angry-looking, whereas below it the vivacity and warmth of the Southerners are said to be reflected in their tendency to smile a lot.

In contrast to the "smiler" is the mean-faced individual so well depicted by Dickens in the person of Uriah Heep. Heep never smiled; he could only widen his mouth and make two hard creases down his cheeks, one on each side, to stand for a smile. His thin and pointed nostrils, with dints in them, had a singular and most uncomfortable way of expanding and contracting themselves, that they seemed to twinkle, instead of his eyes, which hardly ever twinkled at all. Perhaps, too, Robert Peel belongs here, of whom Disraeli said: "The Right Honourable gentleman's smile

---

*Excerpt from *Jacqueline Bouvier Kennedy Onassis* by Stephen Birmingham reprinted by permission of Grosset & Dunlap from *Jacqueline Bouvier Kennedy Onassis,* © 1978 by Stephen Birmingham.

reminds me of the silver fittings on a coffin." Life-long ill-humour becomes moulded into a cast of sour insensitivity. As Louis Nizer remarked: "After 50, one gets the face one deserves."

The Spastic Pseudo-Smile

Sometimes one is deceived by the facial delineaments of an individual who appears to be continually smiling, even in sleep. All too often the impression engendered is one of sympathetic understanding towards all and sundry. No such attitude of warmth underlies this unwitting disguise. It is a *faux sourire figé*. Shakespeare's dictum "I saw his heart in his face" does not apply. The error in interpretation is produced by a perpetual and meaningless spastic contraction of the muscles of expression, so that there is a deepening of the nasolabial folds. The effect seems to be one of a warm and genial smile. The eyes, however, do not participate (Fig. 3), but this fact is rarely noticed, and so misunderstanding results.

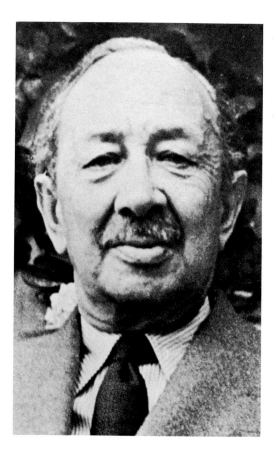

FIG. 3.   A spastic pseudo-smile.

Volume VI of *Munk's Roll* contains photographs of 284 recently deceased Fellows of the Royal College of Physicians. At least 10 display a definite and quite unposed, spastic pseudo-smile. The spastic pseudo-smile must not be confused with the *risus sardonicus*, which is a highly pathological facies provoked by the convulsive spasms of tetanus.

The Incongruous Smile of Politeness

A discrepant social smile is exemplified in the one with which some individuals impart or receive news of a potentially distressing character. It is reminiscent of the giggling or the laughter that may occur in similar circumstances, particularly in cultures not our own. This particular facial gesture is well seen in what is known as the Japanese smile, or *mikoniko*. For a deep and understanding account one should consult the writings of Lafcadio Hearn, that eccentric Greek-Irish-American author who after much travelling finally settled in Japan where he became naturalized. He pointed out that a Japanese can smile in the teeth of death, and usually does. His smile does not denote defiance, or hypocrisy, or resignation. It is part of an elaborate and long-cultivated etiquette, part of a silent language in fact. Laughter is not encouraged, but the smile is there always, whether the occasion be gay or grave. To a Japanese it is a rule of life that one should always display to the outer world a mien of happiness, conveying to others, as far as it is possible, a pleasant impression. To look serious or unhappy is rude, for it may cause distress to others. Whenever painful or shocking news *must* be imparted to or by the sufferer, he must do so with a smile or even a low, soft laugh. The key to the mystery of such behaviour is politeness.

I have drawn at some length upon what Lafcadio Hearn has written, but with some qualified thinking. Perhaps he oversentimentalized the phenomenon, believing, as he explicitly stated, the Japanese to be the happiest people in the world. But Hearn died in 1904, and so many cataclysmic happenings have taken place since then that he probably would not recognise or understand the Japanese of today. Nevertheless, despite the changes they have shown to others and have experienced themselves, they still display their incongruous smile though to an extent that is now less puzzling to Occidentals.

The Enigmatic Smile

The enigmatic smile is something quizzical or mysterious. The impression it imparts is one of knowledge not shared by the onlooker. In the *Colossus of Maroussi*, Henry Miller described this type of enigmatic smile as the culminating expression of the spirited achievement of the human race. Frankly such a remark means little, and one is left wondering what he was trying to say.

Something like an enigmatic smile can be seen in *La Gioconda* as depicted by da Vinci. Gautier was perhaps exaggerating when he referred to *"un sourire vague, énigmatique et délicieux: le regard qui promet des voluptés inconnues et l'expres-*

sion devinément ironique" (the vague, enigmatic and charming smile, that look which promises untold things, that divinely ironical expression). One reason for the reams of speculation that have been written upon the *Mona Lisa* is the sheer rarity with which the human face was ever represented as smiling by the classic masters of medieval art.

The enigmatic smile has also been associated with the weather-worn features of the sphinx of Ghiza, which probably represents King Chephren of the Fourth Dynasty. It seems likely that confusion exists between the not too convincing smile of this Egyptian sphinx and its alleged riddle. The latter, of course, undoubtedly applies to the female winged sphinx of Thebes who set a conundrum to her visitors. When they failed to solve the puzzle she devoured them. Oedipus, however, was successful, whereupon the sphinx destroyed herself.

Important differences exist between the Egyptian and the Greek conceptions of a sphinx. The former was always a male figure symbolizing the god Horus or Hor-en-Khu. The latter comprised the winged body of a lion, and the foremost part was that of a woman. This variant probably took origin in Assyria and was emblematic of the esoteric forces of death. Both the Egyptian and the Greek versions of the sphinx were allegedly endowed with a smile, faint and serene and none too obvious in the former but broader in the latter. One is a smirk, the other a grin. The mysterious smiles of some of the great statues of ancient Egypt (e.g., the calf-bearer 570 BC and the Rampin head 560 BC) have been written off as "artistic clichés," rarely seen in later works. Recently in Corinth a white marble sphinx has been unearthed with an unusually expansive smile.

The Smile of Portraiture

Not until the beginning of this present century were portraits commonly represented as smiling. Throughout the Middle Ages the themes were largely religious in nature, and neither laughter nor a smile was appropriate. With the introduction of secular motifs, the same tradition continued. Exceptions such as the *Mona Lisa* were rare and hence conspicuous. Other such exceptional instances include the painting *Venus, Cupid, Folly, and Time* by Angelo Bronzino (1503–1572), where Folly is wearing a faint smile. The same artist also painted a child with quite a merry smile. This is the Don Garcia dei Medici, now in the Uffizi Gallery. Drunken leers were sometimes seen in the Dutch–Flemish school of art, and there is also an excellent example in *Topers* by Velasquez (1599–1660).

The tradition of facial repose in serious portraiture persists to the present as far as painting is concerned. Striking exceptions came about, however, with the introduction of photography. Here again there was a delay before broad meaningless smiles became conventional. One has only to turn the pages of a family album or a work of biography to observe that grandparents and those before them maintained a serious pose when being photographed. Not so in the camera portraits of more recent years. The same phenomenon can be observed in group photographs. At the turn of this century, sporting teams, classroom photographs, family reunions, even weddings were the occasion for a dignified seriousness. This does not suit modern photographers, who insist that their victims adopt a spectacle of mass grinning. So far this convention has spared the funeral scene, but one wonders for how long this will be so. At present, too, amateur photographers are worse offenders than the professionals, whose portraiture consists in a tasteful play of form, light, and shade. The result is a dignified work of art.

Another innovation which leads to the ubiquity of broad but vacuous grins is the advertising business. No product, however mundane—beverages, detergents, cigarettes, even the motor show—can exist without the interpolation of a young and attractive girl wreathed in smiles. In the case of cosmetics the smile is dispensed with in favour of a sultry, seductive look. We who are old enough can trace the beginnings of this phenomenon in Great Britain to the once-famous "five-boys" advertisement for Fry's chocolate. A series of five likenesses of the same youngster were labelled "desperation," "pacification," "expectation," "acclamation," and "realization," respectively. The last three of these displayed the dawn of a gentle and restrained smile.

No doubt the motive behind this advertising technique is not only to capture the gaze of the hurried reader or television viewer but, more especially, to suggest a state of utter satisfaction on the part of the customer. Then again, smiling is infectious. A smile, even when displayed pictorially, is more likely to engender empathy than indifference in the mind of the beholder. Perhaps this practice is being abused, and the public may well be on the edge of boredom. The concept may have been taken too far when there is little relation between a picture and its caption.

Not only is smiling uncommon in official paintings as opposed to camera studies, it is rarely seen in sculpture. One exception, so extreme as to be unforgettable, is the statue of Voltaire in the foyer of the Comédie Française.

In the full flowering of Greek civilisation it was, of course, a common practice linked with the theatre to carve out of wood or stone twin masks depicting tragedy and comedy, respectively. The latter was in the guise of a satyr-like face with a broad toothless grin, the mouth being curved upwards in an extravagant fashion. These became popular and were reproduced consistently over the centuries. At times the expression in the Greek mask was so improbable as to be equivocal, and tragedy and comedy were not easily distinguished (Fig. 4).

Masks are always worn in the Japanese Nōh plays. Usually they are almost expressionless, whether used to represent males or females. An exception occurs in the Kyogen masks, which are assumed by comic actors during the intervals in the course of a lengthy Nōh play. Or they may be reserved for the Okina, which is the ceremonial introduction. The Kyogen masks are characterized by three facts: They have a separate and movable lower jaw; stiff hairs are embedded within the woodwork of the mask to represent eyebrows and beard; and the expression is one of broad smiling or even laughter with open mouth and narrow eye-slits.

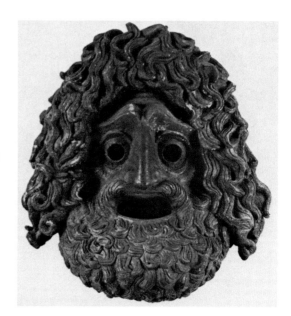

FIG. 4. Greek tragic actor's mask from Piraeus 350 B.C.

The Cruel Smile

Just as laughter can be a weapon used to connote scorn or ridicule, so also a certain movement of the face may be recognised as a smile of contempt, of malicious enjoyment, or *Schadenfreude*. The smiler is demonstrating his sadistic pleasure at the predicament or discomfiture of someone else. It may represent the response of something that has been said to him. It is a sneer that scoffs, taunts, and holds up to scorn an idea, more often another person. Pope had this type of smile in mind:

> Damn with faint praises, assert with civil leer
> And, without sneering, teach the next to sneer;
> Willing to wound, and yet afraid to strike,
> Just hint a fault and hesitate dislike.

Anatomically speaking, this unpleasing variety of smile is different. The mouth is more likely to turn down than to curve upwards. The lips do not part. Usually the eyelids droop as if in disdain. Most important of all is a flaring of the nostrils. This is generally accompanied not by a sniff—which is an inhalation of air through the nostrils—but a faint expulsion of air, for which I know no term. Persius expressed it, however, when he wrote *Rides et nimis naribus indulges*, which literally translated means "You laugh and indulge too much in curling of your nostril (i.e., sneering)."

Pathlogical Smiles

Just as laughter can manifest itself as a symptom of neurological disease, the same experience applies in the case of smiling.

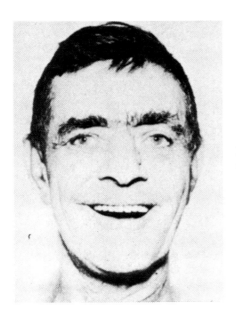

FIG. 5. Smile of euphoria in a patient with a frontal lobe tumour.

Perhaps the most blatant example is met with in patients with hepatolenticular degeneration (Wilson's disease). In this condition a state of extrapyramidal rigidity involves the facial muscles, causing a perpetual widely gaping mouth. Such a "smile" is pathognomonic of this disorder and immediately betrays the diagnosis.

Patients with tumours of the frontal lobe, especially in the nondominant hemisphere, often display a surprising lack of insight into the gravity of their condition. They are even euphoric and may utter facetious and inappropriate witticisms. The Germans speak of this as *Witzelsucht*, or the joking malady. While not engaged in futile chatter the patient may sit with a fatuous grin on his face (Fig. 5).

Abnormally smiling patients are sometimes encountered in psychiatric practice. One circumstance is schizophrenia, especially of the hebephrenic type. Here the patient may indulge in odd posturing and attitudinizing accompanied by broad grins (Fig.6). Often this type of behaviour takes place in front of a mirror.

Autistic children also display at times a smile which in many ways is specific in appearance. The smile is faint, that is, small-ranged; often the eyelids are closed. One gets the impression that the patient is listening to phantom voices or indulging in thoughts, either of which is pleasing in nature and not shared by others. The term "secret smile" is appropriate to such a phenomenon.

A secret smile is also not uncommonly witnessed in mental defectives, particularly those with an overlay of a primitive psychosis. It has been observed in some patients with tuberous sclerosis (Critchley and Earl).

Can We Ever Visualize Vulgarity in a Smile?

Alas yes. Laughter that is coarse and in bad taste is common enough, but ordinarily a smile is something different. As a rule it is inviting and signals a

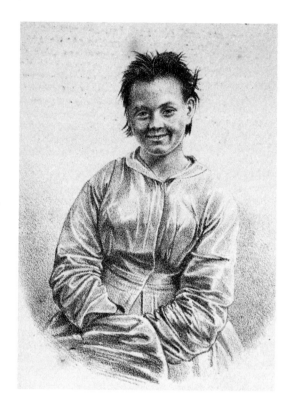

FIG. 6. Smile of a patient with puerperal mania.

feeling of sympathy and warmth. But there is also that other type we have dwelt upon at some length—the artificial, mirthless smirk utilized so often by advertisers in their work. Here one begins to encroach upon the province of the pin-up.

Within this latter category is a small but unselect group where the smile is in distinctly dubious taste. The circumstances are readily defined. One need not be a male chauvinist to assert that the vulgar smile is confined to the opposite sex, and to the young and dollybird representatives at that. We do not meet it in males or in the elderly, the plain, or even the handsome, serious members of the female sex.

Hallmarks of a vulgar smile are a gaping, wide-opened mouth displaying too many teeth. The eyes and the upper part of the face do not betray mirth, fun, or amusement. The bodily posture as a whole may be unnatural, unusual, suggestive, and the facial appearance is that of one who is screaming or perhaps merely about to devour an apple.

Smiles Unseen

Not everything in the land of smiles is necessarily obvious. As in the country of the blind, smiling may be transmitted unseen, detectable nonetheless by a momentary change in the voice. Broadcasters know this, for they are taught the art of speaking in such a manner as to project the image of one who is smiling.

In psychiatric practice, aberrations in sense perception occasionally involve the act of smiling. To some patients, for instance, the world around may seem to be peopled by persons wearing a sinister, menacing grin. The notion is not a pleasant one, for the grimaces appear to be personally directed, hostile, and evil. This is the phenomenon of *le faux sourire* of paranoia.

There are also states of delirium wherein the victim feels disembodied, "surrounded by beckoning shadows and airy tongues." One example will suffice. Laurie Lee, that magical word-spinner, using prose more like poetry, has recalled the high fevers that beset his boyhood, and what they entailed.

> Out of the ceiling, advanced a row of intangible smiles; easy, relaxed, in no way threatening at first, but going on far too long. Even a maniac's smile will finally waver, but these just continued in silence, growing brighter, colder, and even more humourless till the sick blood roared in my veins. They were Cheshire-cat smiles, with no face or outlines, and I could see the room clearly through them. But they hung above me like a stain on the air, a register of smiles in space, smiles without pity, smiles without love, smiling smiles of unsmiling smileness; not even smiles of strangers but smiles of no one, expanding in brilliant silence, persistent, knowing, going on and on...till I was screaming and beating the bed-rails.

Defective Pictorial Interpretation: A Pervading Deficit in Patients With Higher Nervous Dysfunction

My distinguished friend Professor E. Herman and I are both of an age to confirm Hughlings Jackson's dictum that it takes 50 years to establish a new idea within neurological teaching. Neither of us is quite old enough to corroborate his rider—that it takes twice as long to eradicate a fallacy.

My plan therefore is to restate some observations with which I have familiarized my students, though rarely are they mentioned in the literature. First, I will reemphasize the hidden fundamentals of the clinical profile of patients with a cerebral lesion irrespective of its site, extensity, or sidedness. Secondly, I wish to draw attention to the habitual inability of such a patient to identify the overall meaning of pictorial subject matter. Thirdly, I will mention some rare and extreme defects of visual perception.

For almost a century it has been suspected that the symptoms of highest level brain disorder are twofold in type. In addition to the focal manifestations that depend upon the location of the disease process, other important though subtle features exist which are not related to the location of the pathology. The latter constitute the *Grundstörung*, or common denominator, that pervades the clinical picture. Hughlings Jackson had this idea in mind when he described "the four factors of the insanities." (By "insanity" he was referring to what would nowadays be spoken of as a higher nervous disorder.)

Configurational psychologists identify the *Grundstörung* in the patients's characteristic inability to make a clear distinction between figure and background. Gestaltism is perhaps more a matter of faith than of science and for that reason is as difficult to disprove as to substantiate. There is, however, one relatively simple clinical test which baffles many subjects with brain disease. I refer to Tongonquay's camouflaged photographs. Pictures are taken *en pointillisme* of various common objects: a teapot, cup and saucer, an apple. The background is made up of "visual noise" of increasing magnitude, so that eventually a normal person can scarcely distinguish the picture from the background. In pathological cases there is extreme

---

Originally written in commemoration of the 90th birthday of Professor E. Herman of Lødz.

difficulty in identifying the object even when the visual noise is low, and the foreground should ordinarily be conspicuous.

It is not necessary to describe or even enumerate the various other clinical tests, some of them quite simple in character, which highlight this figure background confusion.

Other attempts have been put forward to recognise a *Grundstörung* in patients with cerebral lesions. Perhaps the best known is the subordination of an abstract mode of thought to one which is wholly concrete in nature, so eloquently propounded by Kurt Goldstein.

In this essay I particularly wish to draw attention to another clinical manifestation which is rarely absent in patients with cerebral pathology. This symptom comprises an inability to interpret the total meaning of a figurative or representational picture, such as Georges Marlier described as "textual." It matters not whether the illustration is coloured or in black and white. Ordinarily the patient seems unaware of his shortcoming. Occasionally, however, he will confess that watching television brings him no pleasure, the panorama moving too fast for him to comprehend.

The task of apprehension particularly applies to those pictures which "tell a tale," so popular during the last century. Portraits, a still-life, an abstract, or surrealistic art are unsuitable for testing purposes. Pictures that are appropriate for demonstrating this symptom have been the work of many of the postimpressionists, as evidenced by Manet's *Dejeuner sur l'Herbe*. The title must of course not be shown to the patient. A comparable decoding defect was described by Wolpert as *Simultanagnosie*, though the term is not altogether a happy one.

It is a revealing experience to watch how the patient operates when asked to explain the meaning of an illustration presented to him. Although he may slowly name a minute detail here and another one there, the motif as a whole is either unintelligible or misunderstood. Just why particular components should be recognised is obscure, for they are rarely the most significant ones, nor optically the most conspicuous. Some patients eventually achieve a measure of interpretative success, not by resort to the "critical detail" of Birkmayer but by proceeding slowly in a piecemeal or bit-by-bit fashion. More often the interpretation continues to elude the patient, even though this item and that may be understood.

The visionary poet William Blake proclaimed that a fool sees not the same tree that a wise man sees. The latter might be expected to recognise here a forest, there a copse, a grove, an arboretum, thicket, orchard, or spinney, while the one who is brain-damaged detects little more than leaves and twigs.

Various suggestions have been put forward to explain this phenomenon. It has been attributed to a defect of *Ueberschauen*, or the art of surveying the scene as a whole, but this is merely to describe and not to elucidate what is taking place. Hillebrand spoke of a disorder in the "flow of attention," but Pötzl preferred to visualize a "change" of attention. Neither conjecture is convincing.

A more subtle and more consistent variety of this "defective pictorial interpretation" comes to light when the patient is shown an "equivocal" illustration such as a cartoon, a caricature, or a humorous drawing. Some attempt at explication

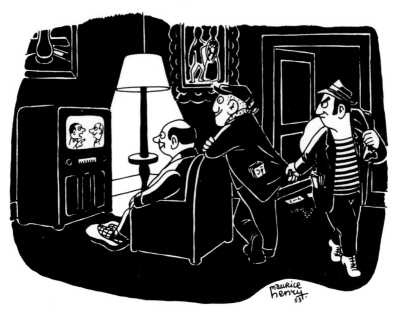

FIG. 1. Cartoon that requires the individual's interpretation. (From *Liberté Chérie*. Fernand Hazan, Paris, 1955, with permission.)

may be forthcoming, but an unsatisfactory one, for the patient will probably have missed the "point" of the picture, that is, its inner or ultimate meaning—what has been called "the last refinements." A comic drawing without a caption that depends for its wit upon some situational incongruity (Figs. 1–3) fails to evoke a smile. Indeed the patient may not realise that the sketch even purports to be humorous or a caricature.

The normal ability to recognise a two-dimensional likeness of a person or a solid object may be a faculty that is acquired late. The cave art of the upper palaeolithic stage, approximately 20,000 years ago, was symbolic rather than representational. True realism came much later. Pictorial recognition is virtually confined to *Homo sapiens*, for only a few domesticated animals ever appear to identify a picture of a familiar object, though life size and in natural colour. If motionless, recognition is still less likely. Occasionally a dog betrays some fleeting notice if confronted by its reflection in a mirror or if it sees a horse, a cat, or another dog on a television screen. The interest is short-lived, however, for it is not really deceived. A baby does not smile at its reflection in a looking glass until 2 months of age, and a child betrays no curiosity in picture books until at least a year old. When illustrations begin to attract interest, they do not delude. Thus the normally developing infant goes through the perceptual stages of recognising its mother; then itself in a mirror; and later still large photographs of itself as well as its mother. At no time does the facsimile appear real.

Ontogenetically, therefore, visual interpretation is an acquired endowment and one that is relatively vulnerable. It is often lost in patients with brain damage

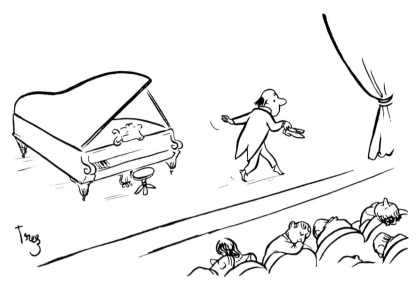

FIG. 2. Cartoon that requires the individual's interpretation. (From *Liberté Chérie*. Fernand Hazan, Paris, 1955, with permission.)

wherever the lesion. For example, it may happen that the patient fails to identify a picture of a common object, especially if it is drawn or photographed from an unusual angle, at a time when he can recognise the object itself. Incidentally, his performance improves when objects stand in isolation. Thus he may recognise an apple but be confused when confronted with a basket of fruit, being unable readily

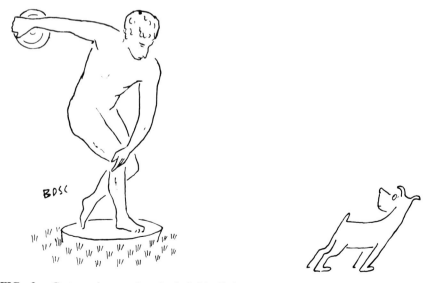

FIG. 3. Cartoon that requires the individual's interpretation. (From *Liberté Chérie*. Fernand Hazan, Paris, 1955, with permission.)

to select the apple. Something similar is met with in a developmental dyslexic of young age: He may be able to name each cut-out letter he sees, but when a dozen or more of these letters are placed at random before him he finds it difficult to pick out a particular letter to command. The defect seems to lie not in visual recognition but in the act of search, whereby he has to find a particular item among many others.

The piecemeal technique which occurs in a patient who is unable to detect the theme of a picture may also be demonstrable in those who are slow in identifying an actual object or who fail to do so altogether. This can be made evident by studying the exploratory movements of the eyes. Yarbus of Moscow, working with Luria, devised a technique for recording the ocular movements carried out in identifying the picture of a single object, e.g., a house. Whereas in normal circumstances recognition is achieved at a glance, and tachistoscopically speaking a fleeting glance, a brain-injured subject can be shown to carry out numerous exploratory movements of the eyes, proceeding, be it noted, in no orderly system of search but in a haphazard fashion. If identification is ultimately achieved, the process has been measurably slow.

Finally, one may mention those extreme cases of visual imperception. These include the so-called visual object agnosia. Then there are cases where the patient cannot recognise an object either by looking at it *or by handling it*. Lastly, we recall those patients who fail to recognise their own mirror-image, an extreme example of prosopagnosia. The foregoing probably possess a focal rather than a general connotation. But what of the patient who, gazing into a looking glass, sees nothing at all? This is the *signe de miroir*, met with in psychotics more often than in patients with brain damage.

Mythical Maladies of the Nervous System

What an ebbing and what a flowing in the tide of clinical neurology has one witnessed over the years! Hypotheses have been mooted, only later to be demolished or, more often, to wither from inanition and neglect. Take, for example, that slippery and tragic disorder multiple sclerosis. For 60 years one has been confronted with a considerable number of so-called cures. Where are these remedies now? The relief of migraine is little better than it was 70 years ago, though more elaborate. And yet, although new correctives are being extolled almost daily with much pride and publicity, a stalemate is the outcome.

How often is a disappointed practitioner frank enough to publish his subsequent disenchantment? Perhaps editorial waiting lists are too long for disconcerting disclaimers. Surely there is room for a *Journal of Fatuous Findings*, a *Revue de Neurologie Manqué*. The late Professor Henry Miller, the gadfly of the North, was full of horse sense on this idea.

Such periodicals would be a worthy vehicle for those would-be Marco Polos of neurology who imagine they have stumbled upon some novel syndrome or a physical sign fit to be mentioned in the same breath as the Babinski phenomenon.

These preliminary and cynical reflections encourage one to ventilate a long-projected idea of expressing certain doubts about the status of a number of neurological fancies which smack more of romance than of reason. Here are a few:

Orbital periostitis. This rare but familiar combination of circumocular pain with paralysis of a group of cranial nerves suggested to James Collier of London an inflammatory lesion narrowing the fissure through which emerge the third, fourth, and sixth cranial nerves. Collier was a brilliant clinician, but unreliable. His penchant for deliberate exaggeration earned him the soubriquet "Truthful James." In 1922 Frederick Price had published his *Text Book of Medicine*, a volume which attained enormous popularity throughout Great Britain. The section on diseases of the nervous system was entrusted to James Collier, with the help of his disciple, W. J. Adie, who was fated to die prematurely. The Collier–Adie contribution was outstanding, a pinnacle in the textbook. Here was Collier's opportunity to ventilate his idea of an orbital periostitis, claiming that he had seen 40 cases, all patients recovering completely. The trouble, he thought, might result from exposure to the cold, from septic conditions in the nose and accessory sinuses, and sometimes from no obvious cause.

Collier's syndrome was never confirmed by autopsy. Since arteriography has become a commonplace, we have preferred to invoke some local pressure proximal to the sphenoidal fissure by an aneurysm of the anterior communicating artery.

Pyknolepsy. We owe this term to Jean Baptiste Edouard Gélineau of Paris. In 1880 he applied it to a syndrome comprising extremely frequent minor epileptic absences. Although these patients did not respond to the current treatment (sux-imide-troxidone coming much later), the outlook was believed to be unexpectedly favourable. The attacks were said to cease spontaneously, never to return, and the episodes disappeared without detriment to personality or to intelligence. Gélineau's work long antedated electroencephalography, and in retrospect we can reasonably doubt whether or not there was any essential difference between pyknolepsy and petit mal. Most modern textbooks ignore the topic.

The conception of pyknolepsy would probably have died from natural causes and vanished from memory had it not been for Adie, whose nose for the outlandish caused it to be exhumed in 1925.

Phakomatosis. In 1913 Van der Hoeve the Dutch ophthalmologist, noticed a similarity between the white patches in the retina in some cases of von Recklig-hausen's disease and those in patients with tuberous sclerosis. He went on to assume a histological identity but without any supporting evidence. Furthermore, he be-lieved that the *phakos* (plate, birthmark) was the hallmark of an aetiological bond between these two widely disparate entities, namely generalized neurofibromatosis and Bourneville's disease (or epiloia), as tuberous sclerosis was often termed. Nor was that all, by any means. A whole volume in our classic *Handbook of Clinical Neurology*, edited by Vinken and Bruyn, was dedicated to the topic of "the Phakomatoses." Under this umbrella were relegated Lindau–von Hippel's disease as well as the facial angiomatosis of Sturge and Weber. Here too were later squeezed—like students packing a telephone kiosk for fun—odds and ends such as ataxia telangiectasis and such eponyms as the syndromes attached to the names Krabbe, Cobb, Ullmann, Bregeat, Riley, and Smith. No wonder Dr. Jules François was apologetic when introducing the volume as *Phakomatosis*.

Vasovagal attacks. Not for a moment would one have dared question the bona fide of this syndrome during the lifetime of Sir William Gowers, whose wrath would have been devastating. It was in 1907 that this giant of neurology published in the *Lancet* the text of a lecture that he had delivered on Vagal or Vaso-vagal Attacks. Within this term he included a number of unusual episodes. Other authors had briefly referred to these attacks under various terms, e.g., the "angina vaso-motorica" of Northnagel, the "vasomotor angina" of Douglas Powell, the "*pseu-doangine neurosique*" of Herchard, and the "*syndrome médullaire*" of Bonnier. Gowers traced an analogy between these attacks and what he called "extended epilepsy." For their relief he advocated nitroglycerine.

Gowers was not dogmatic as to the pathogenesis of these attacks, and he looked upon them as belonging to the "borderland of epilepsy." Electroencephalography came much later, and vasovagal attacks are being increasingly looked upon as syncopal. Monographs on epilepsy have more or less ignored these turns.

This must be the one and only instance when Gowers—that masterly clinician—seemed to put a foot wrong. *Quandoque bonus Dormitat Homerus.*

The theme of neuromythology could be extended considerably to include some other syndromes that have been described but where growing doubts lead to an attitude of scepticism short, however, of frank disavowal. In such a batch belong Devic's disease; neurasthenia; railway spine; infective myelitis; Costen's syndrome; facioplegic migraine; otitic hydrocephalus; ataxic paraplegia; acroparaesthesia; senile paraplegia; pseudosclerosis; olivorubro-cerebellar atrophy, and many others.

May I also submit that there is a growing tendency to overemploy certain diagnostic labels for some clinical disorders where no pathological evidence is forthcoming? Two such examples are Alzheimer's disease and the Jakob–Creutzfeldt syndrome. These mellifluous labels have rather belatedly become fashionable tags to attach to puzzling cases in the clinic. These are not mythological entities, but they are somewhat in the way of rarities. Many commoner types of presenile dementia exist than the one associated with the name Alzheimer.

Visual object agnosia. This is something I have been accused of disclaiming, as by my good friend the late Denny-Brown. I plead not guilty: What I dispute is the allegation that the imperception (a better term, one coined by Jackson and Gowers) occurs against a background of normal vision and a clear sensorium. On the contrary, there is always some qualitative or quantitative disorder of sight or some mental confusion, and frequently both. The idea of such an entity as visual gnosis must surely be a fantasy.

Some mythical maladies are not so much old wives' tales as neurological fossils. The idea may be sound but of such remote ancestry as to be cloaked in archaic terminology. Today the result is noncomprehension, perhaps rejection. Thumbing through the pages of Romberg's *Nervous Disease of Man* (1840–1846), one chances upon many unusual terms. Some of them are obsolete versions of accepted concepts; in other cases the concept itself is outdated. Today, how many would be able to pass a neurological quiz containing such items as: Compare and contrast "chasmus" and "oscedo." Write short accounts of (1) "neuralgia coelica" and (2) "hebetude visus." What are the indications for "accubitus"? Such a catechism would probably floor most who aspire to a career in the neurosciences.

More than enough has been said upon this topic. *L'art d'ennuyer c'est de tout dire.*

. . . .

May I change the subject and finish with one or two guides to would-be pioneering writers?

1. When publishing a case report, a cure, or an unusual sign or symptom, never assume that the relevant literature began only 10 years ago. Almost certainly it did nothing of the sort, and facts that are significant may stem from at least the nineteenth century.

2. Search the literature scrupulously, as well as personally. Do not depute this job to your secretary or even to the librarian. Cicero said: "Not to know what has been written before is to remain always a child."

3. Avoid petty theft. Do not lift great chunks from someone else's writing without (1) using quotation marks and (2) giving the name of the author you are citing.

4. When quoting someone's opinion, avoid using the present tense. How ridiculous it is to say "Oppenheim believes....." He died 65 years ago.

5. Do not confine your library research to the literature of your own country or even to the English language. Almost certainly you will find something relevant among the medical writers of France and especially in the work of the German giants prior to 1933.

6. Check your references. If you have made a mistake in the date or the number of the volume, or if the pagination is inaccurate, everything else in your text becomes suspect. If you have misspelt an author's name, you have read the reference with insufficient care. Readers will discredit you, believing, perhaps correctly, that you have not read the paper at all. And you will earn the scorn of the author if he is still alive.

7. Before rushing into print with news of a novel idea in clinical neurology, consult carefully the *Manual of Nervous Diseases* by William Gowers. The chances of your "discovery" being at least briefly anticipated, perhaps in a footnote, are 50–50. This two-volume masterpiece is still the "bible of neurology."

The Present Status of Our Understanding of Aphasia

Let us first recall the four principal attributes of articulate language. They are: antiquity, specificity, individuality, and imperfection. How language originated cannot be understood, and I will obey the edict of the Linguistic Society of France formulated in 1866 and not even mention the problem further.

Phylogenetically speaking, language was a latecomer, though we do not know and are unlikely to discover the precise point at which it began in the transition from ape to man. The Magdalenian who adorned the walls of his cave in Lascaux certainly used language: That takes us back 10,000 years. Can we go further? Were Pithecanthropus and Neanderthal man endowed with a true symbol system, or were they limited to a few crude grunts and gestures; communicative perhaps, but scarcely language?

The specificity of language means that it is confined to *Homo sapiens*. Just as there is no animal invested with speech, so also there is no race of man, however savage, that does not possess the ability to talk. The *Homo alalus* of the philosopher is a myth.

In man, language ripens to become a firmly built-in aspect of Self, constituting a personal identity. Not only is language man's prerogative, it is something specific for each and every individual. Hence the term "idiolect," which implies that no two persons share the same word bank.

As units of meaning, however, words are unfortunately imperfect and imprecise. They are loaded with mental and emotional associations, complex undertexts and overtones. Words are said to be as moody as prima donnas, for they cannot be relied upon to mean the same thing at different times, or at the same time to different listeners. Often they cannot be satisfactorily translated from one tongue to another. And how fickle, mischievous, potentially dangerous they may be. Words constitute the deadly weapons of propaganda, and they are the stock in trade of the lawyer, the theologian, and the sales promoter.

At the same time, one cannot go all the way with Du Maurier who wrote, doubtless with tongue in cheek: "Language is a poor thing. You fill your lungs with wind, and shake a little slit in your throat, and make mouths; and that shakes the air; and the air shakes a pair of little drums in my head—a very complicated arrangement with lots of bones behind—and my brain seizes your meaning in the rough. What a roundabout way! And what a waste of time!"

How futile, I submit, to try and allocate such a fundamental, all-pervading endowment as language—as opposed to speech—to a limited and sharply demar-

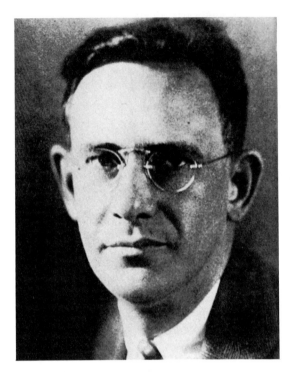

FIG. 1. E. Sapir, linguist; of New Haven, Connecticut.

cated cluster of nerve cells in the brain. As the linguist Sapir (Fig. 1) wrote: "Language as such is not, and cannot be, definitely located, except in that general and rather useless sense in which all aspects of consciousness, all human interest and activity may be said to be 'in the brain.'" All the same, we know that one-half of the brain takes precedence over the other insofar as articulate speech is concerned. Why? We cannot confidently reply: It seems to be somehow related to manual preference. Here then, it might be argued, is already localization of a sort. Forty years ago, however, I was suggesting that the minor hemisphere also played some part in language function. At the time, neurologists were sceptical or else not interested, but since then this idea has attained respectability and acceptance.

Let us realise that language (including speech)—a latecomer in comparative neurophysiology—is a vulnerable function, as clinical experience shows. All four of those attributes of language I mentioned influence the pattern and prognosis of speech impairment as seen in neurological practice, and the factor of individuality implies that no two cases of aphasia are identical.

In patients with brain atrophy the faculty of speech, not surprisingly, shares in the general intellectual decline. More relevant to our present discussion are the syndromes of aphasia, or partial speech loss, which accompany certain limited cerebral lesions.

In 1800 the suspicion arose that the most anterior lobes of the brain were in some way associated with speech. There was, however, no unanimity in this belief,

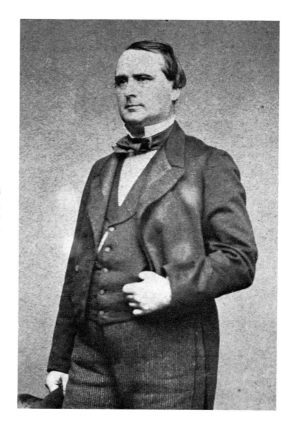

FIG. 2. Dr. Ernest Auburtin (1825–1895), Physician of Paris, Son-in-Law of Professor Bouillaud, Dean of the Medical Faculty.

although strongly supported by the formidable dean of the Faculty of Medicine in Paris, Professor Bouillaud. In 1861 the problem seemed almost to be solved, for, at the newly established Société d'Anthropologie, Bouillaud's son-in-law, Dr. Auburtin (Fig. 2), delivered on 4 April an address entitled *Sur le Siège de la Faculté de Langage* arguing in favour of this association. The secretary of the Société was the surgeon Paul Broca, who was stimulated to invite the speaker to visit the Bicêtre and see along with him a patient named Laborgne, a feeble-minded man for many years hemiplegic and bereft of speech. He had been referred to Broca because of a cellulitis which proved fatal a day or two later.

At the next meeting of the Société a month later, Broca produced the brain where, sure enough, there was an obvious scar in the frontal lobe. The controversy now seemed to be at an end, especially when, a month later, Broca was able to exhibit another brain with a frontal lesion from another patient called Lelong, who during life had had a speech defect. His colleagues were now convinced, even though their attention was focused exclusively upon the frontal lesion, ignoring the fact that the scar (in the first case in particular) obviously extended way back through the temporal lobe. Not until the present century was a horizontal section made through that brain, showing even more clearly that the scar was one of considerable size. But it was the frontal lesion which attracted attention, so that when other pathological specimens accumulated it was suggested that the region at the foot of F3 be designated "Broca's area."

When colleagues continued to refer to him patients with disordered speech or relevant pathological specimens, Broca complained that unwittingly he had come to be looked upon as the discoverer of the centre for speech.

Thus, in retrospect, this way of thinking took origin in at least one misconception.

For a hundred years our textbooks have identified certain patterns of impaired vocalization as "Broca's aphasia," and yet this alleged syndrome as described today is quite different from the clinical model in Broca's original case where the speech defect was one of unusual severity.

Later, neurologists described other aphasic syndromes representing isolated derangements of language; mild perhaps, or maybe severe, as in the so-called Wernicke's aphasia, but rarely was the patient utterly mute. The practice then arose of correlating the character of the disorder with the precise situation of the lesion, which, incidentally, was almost always confined to the major cerebral hemisphere. The localisers, however, did not always agree. At one time there was a conflict between those who thought in terms of cortical lesions and those who placed greater emphasis upon involvement of the fibres connecting one gray area with another. Although these rigid localizers were often in dispute about exact clinicopathological correlation, they rarely lacked dogmatism. Such thinking was didactically tidy and easy for students to follow, so it led to ready acceptance.

But, as Hazlitt said, all great men know how little they know, in comparison with what they do not know. Over the past century, quiet voices were being raised in protest, pointing out that the brain does not function like the keyboard of a piano, each ivory note corresponding with a particular word. Hughlings Jackson never referred to any definite site of lesions associated with "disorders of expression," to quote his term. Henry Head, too, was a reluctant localizer. In Philadelphia Allen Starr pointed out that the same type of aphasia could follow lesions differing widely in position.

Thus neurology became involved in a hundred-year war between the advocates of structuralism and those of holism. May I make a challenge and submit that the wisest and deepest thinkers inclined to the latter group? Professor Aaron Smith of New York recently complained "Broca is alive and well, and living in Boston; Jackson still lives, too, but all over the world."

But, you may say, why become embroiled within this battle of words for, today, where is the problem? In 15 minutes a technician can pinpoint the aphasia-producing lesion by means of a computerized scintiscan.

Let us pause for a moment. How much wiser are we because of this precision tool? True, we can direct the surgeon where to plan his incision; tell him what to expect and how much time he should assign for the task. But let us admit our shortcomings. In some respects, the brain scan has been a disservice to our discipline. It may tempt us to dispense with the deeply probing history-taking and the searching, detailed clinical examination. It may tempt us to play down the clinical skills derived from experience, intuition, and judgement. It may tempt us to refrain from thinking. Even though we have discovered *where* the fault is located, do we really understand any more the *modus operandi* of the patient's faltering speech? After all, the scan has merely displayed the whereabouts of a clump of dead cells within the complex structure of the brain. Dead cells, however, have no function. As Jackson said, they are no more than "dirt in the brain." How then do we explain the nature of our patient's halting and fragmentary speech? Why are some aphasiacs relatively voluble but barely understandable? Why are others laconic, perhaps even limited to a solitary word or phrase? In such a case, why does that particular word or phrase survive to the exclusion of all others? Why can so many patients utter nothing except a vulgar interjection? Why, on the other hand, does a particular patient say nothing but "yes" and another nothing but "no"? Do not tell me that the brain is a mosaic and that the lesion has spared one tiny component or tessera representing "yes" or "no" as the case may be. The brain does not operate in that way. Why does yet another patient keep uttering some such unlikely remark as "ace of spades"? Or, as in Professor Alajouanine's patient, *"bonsoir les choses d'ici bas,"* something which the author called "an insignificant spar from the shipwreck of speech". Not always are these recurring utterances meaningful; sometimes they are a repetitious scrap of jargon. To Jackson these recurring words were the ones the patient was about to emit when struck down by his apoplexy. Hence his term "a stillborn proposition." Gowers thought somewhat differently; to him they were the *last* words the patient had spoken just before losing consciousness.

Is the locality of the aphasia-producing lesion of the brain identical with the region wherein speech is believed to be organised? (Or as we often carelessly say, "represented"?) Do we not really mean the "site of speech vulnerability"? Should we not logically drop the term "speech centres" in favour of "centres of destruction"? We must not forget the distinction between speech and language, realising that the latter is a function of the brain as a whole.

Neurologists are sometimes confronted with a patient without an obvious aphasia whose brain scan is negative. But he is a sick man, and deeply probing tests of language function may bring to light something not quite as it should be. Such a patient may have what we may call an "impending aphasia" or "protoaphasia." If the lesion is a progressive one, a marked speech defect will in time become obvious.

Let us consider another variety of aphasia, where the flow of speech is suddenly interrupted by a word block, especially if the patient is shown an object and asked to name it. The aphasia presents an extreme example of the commonplace "tip-of-tongue" phenomenon which assails all of us at times. As Marcel Proust wrote: *"Nous sentons dans un monde, nous pensons, nous nommons dans un autre, pouvons entre les deux établir une concordance mais non combler l'intervalle".* ("We feel in one world, we think, we give names to things in another; between the two we can establish a certain correspondence, but not bridge the interval.") What is it that hampers the patient, and why is his problem immediately solved should his eye happen to catch the missing word in a printed list placed before him? Sometimes in mild cases of naming difficulty, the aphasiac eventually finds the word and then, as if in an effort to overcompensate, proceeds to elaborate with some barely relevant comment. Thus, shown a coin he may eventually say "a quarter" and then go on to proclaim: "Not that you can buy very much with it nowadays." This is the phenomenon of "gratuitous redundancy." Or he may perseverate and for a time persist in calling every other object shown him, "a quarter."

Often, an aphasiac glibly attaches a wrong name to an object or a concept and fails to notice his mistake. Thus shown a spoon he may confidently call it "a fork." But the next day he may get it right or perhaps call it "a table knife." This inconsistency is typical and difficult to explain. The patient may talk far less well with the professor than he did earlier the same day with the first assistant. And better still with his wife than with his business partner. And best of all when alone with his pet dog.

Under the term "preverbitum" we refer to all the complex cognitive operations that take place between the impulse to speak and the act of exteriorisation. In different types of aphasia the defect probably occurs at different levels within this preverbitum.

Surely it behoves us neurologists not to rest content once we have demonstrated the situation of the lesion. We must continue with eagerness and enthusiasm to explain how our patient manages to utilize the *intact* areas of the brain so as to deal as best he can with the highly artificial task facing him at that particular moment.

When determining the pattern of a given case of aphasia, three factors must obviously be taken into consideration: the site of the lesion, its size, and its rate of expansion or shrinkage, as the case may be. These are not the only variables, however, and perhaps not even the most important. For instance, the age of the patient is surely significant. Perhaps also the sex, for the use of language is not the same in men as it is in women. *The most intriguing aspect of all is the literary status of the patient before he was taken ill. This factor, intangible though it be, may well be crucial. Prior to the illness, was the patient uneducated and barely literate? Or was he a highly cultured academic, familiar with several languages? Was he an avid reader? Did his vocabulary match the size of his library and be measurable in ten of thousands of items?

Premorbid literacy must surely affect the type and severity of the resulting aphasia. Yet we do not know whether the influence of literacy is auspicious or inauspicious. When struck down by a stroke, is a man of letters at an advantage prognostically—or at a disadvantage? What little evidence we have is both anecdotal

---

*In this connection we recall the words of Dean Swift: "The common fluency of speech in many men and most women is owing to a scarcity of matter and scarcity of words; for whoever is a master of language and hath a mind full of ideas will be apt in speaking to hesitate upon the choice of both; whereas common speakers have only one set of ideas and one set of words to clothe them in; and they are always ready at the mouth. So people come faster out of a church when it is almost empty than when a crowd is at the door."

and contradictory. Perhaps the size of the lesion is the key factor here. A small defect may perhaps prove devastating to one who is of mediocre literacy, whereas someone with an unusually rich vocabulary may manage to conceal his handicap by resorting to his bountiful word bank of synonyms, alternatives, circumlocutions, and periphrases. A bigger lesion, on the other hand, may prove more catastrophic to a writer or orator than to one who has never been a scholar. Perhaps erudition also implies vulnerability. We simply do not know, but as neurologists we should set about exploring this matter.

Yet another aspect of language must, I submit, affect its susceptibility. I refer to the purely aesthetic properties, what is referred to in the Bible as "apples of gold in pictures of silver." This is something which attracts the ear rather more than the eye. Some fortunate souls are under the spell of the sheer magic of words. Their euphony, their allurement, their marvel hold them captive, so that they take pleasure in selecting, matching, and linking them as if they were gems lovingly assembled to form an exquisite piece of jewelry. Such a sensitive obsession with words must surely influence the clinical picture of an aphasia and its prognosis. Whether favourably or not I am uncertain. Mindful of Jackson's distinction between superior and inferior levels of language and the susceptibility of the former, I cannot conceal my concern about the outlook in a poet or literary stylist who becomes aphasic.

So far everything we have been discussing has been pure neurology, the product of the thinking and the labours of generations of great figures within our discipline. Let us, I beg of you, keep it that way. Do not relax because the brain scan has done so much for you. Much still needs to be done, and there is a promise of exciting projects for us to explore.

More than 40 years ago I was deploring the lack of interest on the part of professional academic linguists in our topic of language pathology. I knew that we could help them, and I also believed that they could assist us. Today the scene has changed, and we have witnessed the rapid growth of that young branch of soft science, psycholinguistics. The cooperation of its practitioners and of neuropsychologists has been valuable, without any question, but we neurologists must not capitulate before their enthusiastic inroads into our province. Circumspection on our part is necessary. Sometimes I feel that I have opened a Pandora's box. Unlike the pioneer philologists of last century, many modern linguists seem to concentrate on the mathematics of language at the expense of clarity and style. In neurolinguistics, neologisms multiply so that a professional jargon threatens to sully the serene, unambiguous prose of neurology. As F. L. Lucas wrote: "A research student may turn his life into a concentration camp, he may amass in his own field a staggering erudition; but he cannot write. And where the words are so muddled I suspect that the mind is muddled too." The same author reminded us that obscurity comes from fumbling with thoughts or fumbling with words, and generally the two go together.

Nor have we followed Head in shattering the image-makers of the last century to make room within our domain, aphasia, for complicated geometrical psycholinguistic models.

I have almost finished, but there is so much to be said about aphasia and so much for us neurologists to unravel. May I just mention three outstanding examples of continuing obscurity: classification; intelligence; and "contrastive linguistics" in relation to aphasia.

As yet no satisfactory classification of the aphasias exists. Long ago Jackson was deploring that the issue was obscured by classifications that were partly anatomical, partly physiological, and partly psychological. Such confused sorting, said he, is as scientifically wrong as to group plants into endogens, Graminaceae, kitchen herbs, ornamental shrubs, and potatoes. Classifications based upon eponyms such as Broca and Wernicke are not adequate. Ambiguous terms such as "central aphasia," "deep dyslexia," and "category specific access dysphasia" should be discarded, along with many others. The erudite Roman Jakobson devised his own linguistic taxonomy, which fortunately did not survive, for I suspect that he himself had encountered very few aphasic patients. We refuse to accept the invitation to comply with at least a dozen varieties of dyslexia, as well as terms such as coding, encoding, decoding, and transcoding.

How soon we have forgotten what Gowers said—that Nature is prone to ignore our divisions and to blend that which we distinguish. No wonder that some of our wisest neurologists postpone all attempts and simply refer to "the aphasias" in expectation of some eventual scheme of classification that will be scientifically appropriate.

The second problem I had in mind for neurologists to tackle concerns the question of the extent to which aphasia entails a disorder of intelligence. We cannot accept too seriously the retrospective descriptions of aphasiacs who have recovered their speech. They often minimize any change in their intellectual powers during their period of ill health. Clinicians know well the common unawareness, forgetfulness, or repression of past handicaps of cerebral origin.

So far the comments of neurologists and psychologists on the intellectual status of aphasiacs have been cautious, evasive, even quibbling. What we forget is that the hair-splitting of the schoolmen might any moment be challenged by the stark and straightforward problem of an aphasic patient who wants to make a will, or to alter an existing will, or to continue to attend to his financial affairs. What sound advice can we, as philosophers of language, put before the highest courts of law in such cases—advice that would stand up to the cold logic of the legal profession, as opposed to our less demanding colleagues? How much weight would a judge of the Appeal Court be seriously expected to place upon the jargon and indecisiveness, or perhaps the overconfidence, of the so-called expert witness? Very little I can assure you, and rightly so.

Lastly, let us realise that 95% of the work on aphasia has been in French, German, English, Italian, or Spanish. These belong to the S.A.E. or standard average European group of tongues, all of which are built upon a fundamental subject–predicate system. But what of aphasia affecting the millions who speak one of the many tongues of Africa, Asia, and Amerindia, where the basic construction is vastly different? For example, the Hopi, Navaho, and Nootka dialects of the

Amerindians differ radically from the languages of Europe in the way in which they are designed. Thus there may be no clear expression of notions of time, or of space, or even of number. Some authorities speak of "the principle of linguistic relativity" and believe that the structure of a language mirrors the intrinsic mode of thinking. What an opportunity for a young and venturesome neurologist to undertake fascinating field work into the pattern of aphasia among the local population. If discouraged by considerations of distance, close by are millions of potential aphasiacs whose mother tongue is Arabic, Farsi, or Hebrew. What is known of how they respond to a language disorder? Nothing.

A final plea to my neurological colleagues: Do not, I implore you, forsake the perplexing and intriguing problems that aphasiology presents. It is *you* who will have to care for those "uncommunicating communicators" who are your patients. It will be *your* task to release their walled-in intelligence, and I believe it will ultimately be *your* privilege to solve the riddle of language disorder.

I believe the rewards will be great if we neurologists keep a firm grip upon the tiller of aphasia.

If not, not.

1884–1984, A Century of Endeavour

A dramatic event took place 100 years ago, constituting a landmark in neuro-science. The occasion was momentous, for it confirmed what Ferrier had long been proclaiming—that the coverings of the brain are not sacrosanct. Hitherto the attitude towards cerebral tissues had been one of *noli me tangere*: keep off.

Let us also recall that before 1884 the diagnosis of brain tumour was made only rarely; localization was not feasible; and its therapy was nonexistent. Despite all attempts at palliation the patient would sooner or later perish on this account. The infrequency with which a new growth was even detected, whether during life or at autopsy, is strange, especially when we remember that tuberculomas, gummas, and parasitic cysts were commoner than they are now. It is difficult to escape the suspicion that the incidence of glioma, meningioma, and metastatic carcinoma has increased. Of course some of these may have masqueraded under terms no longer in use, such as local cerebritis, red softening or white, focal engorgement, or sarcoma. The only cerebral space-occupying lesions which could be both diagnosed and treated were the abscesses, which had been yielding to the bold technique of William Macewen in Glasgow.

The year 1984 marks the centenary of a spectacular occurrence in the annals of neurology—the first removal of a glioma, one that had been both shrewdly diag-nosed and accurately pinpointed. The venue was the Hospital for Epilepsy & Paralysis then located near Regent's Park where it stood for 30 years, that is, until 1903 when it moved to Maida Vale where we know it today.

Who were the players in this great spectacle? Of the two stars, the first was Dr. Alexander Hughes Bennett, a distinguished but modest physician who was not only on the staff at Regent's Park but also, since 1877, at the Westminster Hospital, then a conspicuous edifice in Broad Sanctuary. It was to Bennett that the patient had been sent from as far away as Dumfries. The case was subsequently recorded in a paper read before the Royal Medico-Chirurgical Society and published in its *Proceedings*. It is outstanding because of its detail in which we observe the clinical acumen and skill prevalent in those days. The contemporary shortcuts such as x-rays, arteriography, EEG, and brain scan were in the future.

Hughes Bennett was the son of a professor of medicine in Edinburgh. After qualifying at that medical school, he came to London. His contributions to our discipline were few but able, and he gave promise of an important future in his profession. Unfortunately, he had to resign his hospital appointments at the early age of 45, having developed an obscure neurological disorder from which he died in 1901 at the age of 53.

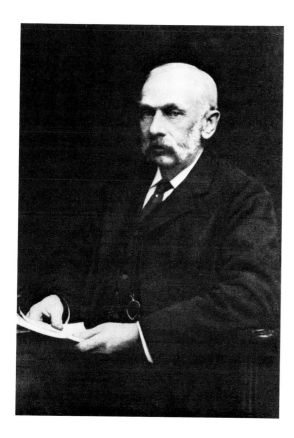

FIG. 1. Sir Rickman Godlee. (Courtesy of Wellcome Institute Library, London.)

His surgical co-star and another pioneer was, as we are all aware, Rickman Godlee (Fig. 1), for several years on the staff of University College Hospital as well as Regent's Park. It is ironic that he had already retired from the latter hospital and had been succeeded by Alfred Pearce Gould. However, it was not convenient for Gould to take up his appointment at that vital moment in November 1884, and Rickman Godlee was continuing to stand in for him.

Godlee was of Quaker stock, a nephew and ardent disciple of Lord Lister and hence a cousin of Marcus Beck. He had the privilege of being born at No. 5 Queen Square, a house which Hughlings Jackson was to occupy 20 years later. Though on the staff of Regent's Park, it was as a general surgeon, and after the drama we are discussing he did not continue with cranial surgery but devoted himself to his considerable practice. At U.C.H. he was admired for his simple, didactic teaching and his routine handling of patients. Though somewhat reserved, critical, and outspoken at times, he was highly respected; and in 1912 and 1913 he was president of the Royal College of Surgeons (Fig. 2). After serving as surgeon to Queen Victoria's household, he was appointed surgeon to King Edward VII and to George V. He was not interested in research, like his junior colleague Victor Horsley, and was in no way an academic.

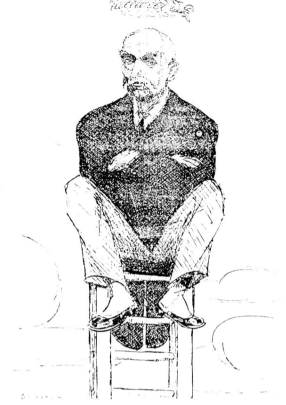

FIG. 2. Caricature of Sir Rickman Godlee.

He had followed his uncle to London and acted as his personal assistant. Having served on various hospitals, such as Charing Cross, the Victoria Hospital for Children, and the Brompton, he joined his cousin at University College Hospital. If, indeed, he nursed any specialized surgical interest, it was in diseases of the lung. Like his uncle, he was a brilliant medical artist and, in the same way as his colleague Gowers, a keen botanist. Little is known about the relationship between himself and his dynamic junior colleague Victor Horsley.

He retired to Whitchurch, near Reading, where he died in 1925 at the age of 76. His widow, who had been a daughter of Seebohm the banker, died in 1950, aged 91. There were no children.

The third and most important participant in this drama was, of course, the patient concerned—that individual who is so often an anonymous but indispensable stagehand. He was an otherwise healthy young farmer of 25 years, bold and cooperative. His advisers had made known to him the hazards of this hitherto untried procedure and with his eyes wide open he unhesitatingly took the risk. His name was Henderson, and his home was in Dumfries.

What induced this young Scot to make the long and costly journey to London when close by in Glasgow was Sir William Macewen working miracles with brain

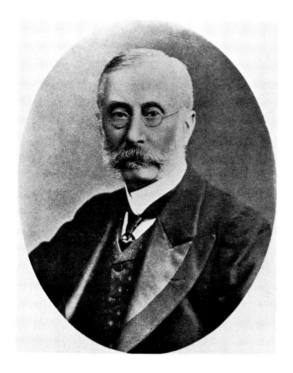

FIG. 3. Sir David Ferrier.

surgery, or in Edinburgh redolent with the results of Lister's research? I believe it was the instigation of Sir James Crichton Browne, also from Dumfries, that brilliant and silver-tongued alienist, who, from the Wakefield Asylum in Yorkshire, was supplying anatomical material as well as considerable support to David Ferrier (Fig. 3). Indeed, if Hughes Bennett and Rickman Godlee were stars in this performance, the director was Ferrier, inspired by Hughlings Jackson. Crichton Browne will return to our story a little later.

It was the clinical genius Hughlings Jackson who indicated that some measure of localization lay within certain cortical areas. His beliefs were confirmed by the animal experimentation of his younger colleague David Ferrier. It is thought that Hughes Bennett sought Ferrier's advice before calling on Rickman Godlee's skill, though he does not specifically say so. Certainly both Jackson and Ferrier were present at the operation, and possibly Victor Horsley too, then aged 27 years.

What was the clinical problem which confronted Hughes Bennett when Henderson arrived at the Regent's Park Hospital on 3 November 1884?

For some 2½ years the patient had been noticing every day peculiar twitches at the corner of the mouth on the left side. In addition, he had developed frequent lapses of consciousness, the nature and duration of which we are not told. Both of these occurrences grew worse. Six months before leaving home, he found involuntary twitchings also appearing in the left hand and forearm. Episodes were now daily, affecting alternately either the face or the upper limb. The next development was an epileptiform seizure ushered in by a peculiar feeling in the left half of the face and tongue, then the hand, spreading up the arm and down the leg on that side. During the next few days Henderson began to complain of headache.

Soon after, he noticed that the left hand was weak, a symptom which increased day by day until, in August 1884, he could no longer work. By now his headaches had become intense in severity and lancinating in character. He began to drag the toes of the left foot when he walked.

During the early days of his admission to the Regent's Park Hospital his focal attacks continued. The headaches increased in violence in a manner quite unusual in patients with a brain tumour.

Hughes Bennett's clinical examination was a model in thoroughness. His detailed case notes are rarely bettered even today. Without any adventitious aids except an ophthalmoscope, he diagnosed a cerebral tumour which he localized to the middle third of the precentral convolution on the right side. An interesting sign, often neglected nowadays, was an area of tenderness in the scalp or skull bone overlying that region of the brain under suspicion.

Matters were becoming desperate, and the patient was demanding that surgical intervention, however hazardous, should be carried out without more delay. Operation was set for 25 November 1884.

After the head had been shaved and the scalp thoroughly prepared according to Listerian dictates, carefully measured markings were made to indicate the position of the underlying fissure of Rolando (Fig. 4). Three trephine holes were drilled and a piece of skull bone removed to reveal a bulging dura. When incised, a convolution was exposed with a large blood vessel running posteriorly. A ¾ in. cut was made into the cortex; this disclosed ⅛ in. below the surface, a solid tumour the size of a walnut, lobulated, transparent, and encapsulated. With the aid of a

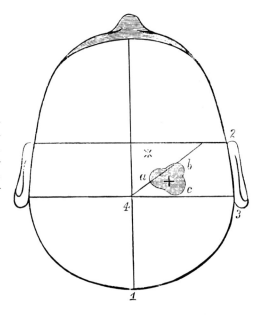

FIG. 4. External surface of the scalp. *(1,2,3,4)* Lines to determine the position of the fissure of Rolando. *(+)* Theoretical and actual position of the tumour. *(*)* Tender spot on scalp. *(a,b,c)* Position and order to trephine openings. (Courtesy of Wellcome Institute Library, London.)

spatula and a Volkmann's spoon, Rickman Godlee removed a growth, conical in shape with base upwards. When all haemorrhage had been controlled, the dura was sutured. Dr. Hebb examined the growth microscopically and proclaimed it to be a glioma.

The operation had lasted 2 hours. Thirty minutes later the patient was able to answer questions. The left upper limb was paralysed. Next day the patient was complaining of headache and occasionally he vomited. Some facial twitchings were still evident.

Considerable interest was aroused by this surgical event. On 17 December a brief report was sent to the *Lancet* and appeared in the 20 December 1884 issue. A lengthy, elegantly written letter was published in *The Times* on 11 December 1884, signed "F.R.S." It opened thus:

> While the Bishop of Oxford and Professor Ruskin were, on somewhat intangible grounds, denouncing vivisection at Oxford last Tuesday afternoon, there sat at one of the windows of the Hospital for Epilepsy & Paralysis in Regent's Park, in an invalid chair, propped up with pillows, pale and careworn but with a hopeful smile on his face, a man who could have spoken a really pertinent word upon the subject, and told the Right Reverend Prelate and a great art critic that he owed his life and his wife and children from bereavement and penury, to some of these experiments on living animals which they so roundly condemn.

The letter was long-winded by today's standards and ended:

> The medical profession will declare with one voice that he [i.e., the patient Henderson] owes his life to Ferrier's experiments without which it would have been impossible to localize his malady or to attempt its removal, and that men and women will henceforth, there is reason to anticipate, be saved from prolonged torture and death by a kind of treatment that has been made practicable by the sacrifice, under anaesthetics, of a few rabbits and monkeys.

Two anonymous leading articles in *The Times* followed over the course of the next few weeks, and no fewer than 64 letters were published supporting or denouncing the operation and the broader subject of animal experimentation in December 1884 and January 1885. Excitement had spread to medical circles. Dr. Hughes Bennett read an account of the case at the Royal Medico-Chirurgical Society of London on 18 May 1885, and the discussion which followed was printed in the *Proceedings* a little later (Fig. 5).

Meanwhile, what of the patient himself? All was not going too well. He was hemiplegic and was developing a hernia cerebri which had to be resected at least twice. Headaches were still present, and at times he vomited. He became listless, dysarthric, and feverish.

Two days after the roseate picture drawn in *The Times* by "F.R.S." the patient's temperature was 103.6°F, and he was delirious and incontinent. As Wilfred Trotter was to remark some years later, "he was young, intelligent, courageous, and he was to die." The end came on 23 December, that is, 4 weeks after operation.

CASE

OF

CEREBRAL TUMOUR.

BY

A. HUGHES BENNETT, M.D., F.R.C.P.,

PHYSICIAN TO THE HOSPITAL FOR EPILEPSY AND PARALYSIS, AND ASSISTANT
PHYSICIAN TO THE WESTMINSTER HOSPITAL.

THE SURGICAL TREATMENT

BY

RICKMAN J. GODLEE, M.S., F.R.C.S.,

SURGEON TO UNIVERSITY COLLEGE HOSPITAL.

Read May 12th, 1885.

[*From Vol. LXVIII of the 'Medico-Chirurgical Transactions,' published by the Royal Medical and Chirurgical Society of London.*]

LONDON:

PRINTED BY

J. E. ADLARD, BARTHOLOMEW CLOSE.

1885.

FIG. 5. Title page of published paper concerning the patient Henderson.

Autopsy revealed a septic basal meningitis which, to Lister's nephew and devotee, must have been a source of discomfiture. There is no record of Rickman Godlee ever again embarking upon cranial surgery, although he continued on the staff of University College Hospital for another 30 years.

Despite the outcome, the impossible had been achieved and the Rubicon crossed. The coverings of the brain were no longer impregnable, and Ferrier appears to have been the principal one vindicated. Godlee seemed perhaps disillusioned, but neurologists were encouraged by the thought that a diagnosis of brain tumour might no longer represent a sentence of death. True, Henderson had not survived, but his demise was due not to neoplasia but to sepsis. Perhaps Lister's carbolic spray was not the complete answer to bacterial invasion. Surely there must be other techniques to keep microorganisms at bay.

So confident were neurological physicians that they invited Victor Horsley, that young man of promise, on 9 February 1886 to join the staff of the National Hospital,

Queen Square. His first operation there took place 3 months later. The patient was, again, a young Scot who had traumatic Jacksonian epilepsy and a mild hemiparesis. Horsley exposed and removed a mass of scarred brain tissue from the ascending frontal convolutions. With his paper in the *British Medical Journal* for 9 October 1886, on Brain Surgery, he established himself as the world's pioneer of neurosurgery. Indeed, during his first year on the staff of the National Hospital, he operated upon 10 patients with only one fatal outcome.

Fifty years ago, on 28 November 1934, the staff of the Maida Vale Hospital organized a jubilee dinner at the Dorchester Hotel to commemorate the 50th anniversary of Sir Rickman Godlee's operation. Lord Horder presided. Dr. Wilfred Harris proposed a toast in memory of the surgeon, who had died in 1925, and Sir Charles Ballance responded.

The most outstanding speech, however, was delivered by Sir James Crichton Browne (Fig. 6), then 94 years of age, the only survivor of the medical drama of 50 years previously. Though he had not been able to attend the operation he had obviously been the *deus ex machina*. He had known the patient personally, a fellow townsman, and he had probably engineered the consultation in London. Crichton

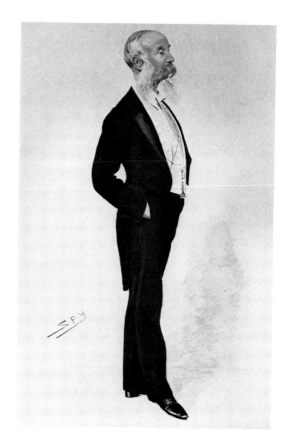

FIG. 6. Spy cartoon of Sir James Crichton Browne. (Courtesy of Wellcome Institute Library, London.)

Browne admitted to having written the anonymous letter to *The Times* signed "F.R.S." One of the most polished after-dinner speakers in the country, he talked of the great strides in neurology over the previous half-century. He quoted the case of an army officer from whom Sir Frederick Treves had resected a large amount of damaged brain tissue. Several years later they met at a party, but Treves avoided the officer. "You don't seem to remember me," the officer said to Treves, who replied that he did but in view of the operation had been rather diffident about greeting him. "That's all right," replied the officer, "I am now head of the Intelligence Department." In 1934 *The Times* again rose to the occasion and gave a full account of the dinner at the Dorchester as well as of the various speeches.

Two other papers must be mentioned. One was from the pen of Sir D'Arcy Power (1932), that well-known historian of surgery, giving an account of the operation. The second was Wilfred Trotter's masterly article couched in the prose one associates with that supreme philosopher-surgeon. In the *Lancet* for 1 December 1934 under the title "A Landmark in Modern Neurology," Trotter described this event of 50 years earlier as a "nodal occurrence that marked the convergence of two distinct processes, the evolution of operative surgery on the one hand, and of neurology on the other." He concluded with two important remarks. "[The operation] was fought in the strength of three great principles—the antiseptic system . . . the precise projection of the cerebral markings on the surface of the skull; and the doctrine of the exact localization of cerebral function. The first two," he went on, "have long been abandoned by the surgeon, and I should be sorry to have to define the present position of the third."

That last remark I personally welcome, being in many respects somewhat of a holist in my thinking, for as Ramon y Cajal said: "The human brain is a world consisting of a number of explored continents and great stretches of unknown territory." It strikes me that had Henderson's glioma been sited anywhere in the brain other than the ascending frontal gyrus, we would not today be commemorating the centenary of its removal.

. . . .

This drama of 1884 has been spoken of as the "dawn of neurosurgery." We must not, however, forget the false dawn which had been glowing for some time 400 miles away in Glasgow. In 1879 William Macewen had operated upon a 14-year-old girl with a dural tumour which he successfully removed (Fig. 7). The presenting symptom had been twitching of the right arm, and there was a conspicuous signpost in a limited area of cranial hyperostosis. In retrospect, this must surely have been a meningioma. The patient died 8 years later from Bright's disease.

Of even greater significance was Macewen's earlier case of a boy with a fissured fracture of the skull, an infected wound causing an intracranial abscess. Macewen localized the lesion within Broca's lobe and advised surgery. The parents refused permission, and the patient died. At autopsy, an abscess was, sure enough, found in the base of the third frontal convolution on the left side; it would certainly have yielded to simple aspiration. This was in 1876.

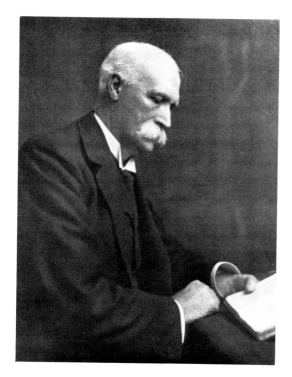

FIG. 7. Sir William Macewen.

Over the following 7 years Macewen operated upon seven patients in whom he had diagnosed circumscribed cerebral lesions, septic or haemorrhagic; not one, however, neoplastic.

The Present Situation

What is the present status of tumours of the brain? Dramatic advances in hygiene and in pharmacology have made extreme rarities of tuberculoma, syphiloma, and parasitic cysts. The incidence of the gliomas, meningiomas, and metastatic growths may have increased; certainly that is one's impression. At the same time there have been outstanding advances in anaesthesia, the prevention of infection, and the control of haemorrhage and surgical shock, coupled with an increased sophistication in operative technique. Immediate mortality, which was 50% at the beginning of this century, fell to 7.6% when Cushing retired. Mellan of Chicago has asserted that it should now be virtually nil.

Meanwhile the development of ancillary diagnostic aids afford us not only confidence in localization but also a shrewd guess as to the pathology of the space-occupying lesion. This is all-important, for it allows the surgeon to select or reject, which while improving his operative statistics has, however, bypassed the majority of patients with malignant brain tumours.

Godlee's operation therefore did two things. It opened the door to a surgical approach, and at the same time it served as a challenge to the neurologists and neurosurgeons of today to extend the duration of postoperative survival; to improve the quality of that existence; and, above all, to tackle seriously the problem of the malignant and inoperable growths. Perhaps the scalpel and the trephine are not the ultimate answer, and surgeons may cooperate with physicists to perfect laser techniques for this unhappy minority. As Peter Schurr recently declared in his presidential address to the neurological section of the R.S.M: "A future is envisaged in which immunotherapy of glial and other tumours will replace radiotherapy, and surgical treatment will be confined to biopsy and cyst aspiration."

Medical progress is a relay race where the torch is passed from one hand to another. The Ferrier–Bennett–Godlee team is unforgettable in that therapeutic Olympiad.

Posthumous Papers of the Hexagon Club

Private, intimate, and self-selected dining clubs abound within the older universities at all academic levels. Whether they exist in the bazaars of neurology I cannot judge. I have personal knowledge of only one, the Hexagon. It was certainly intimate—there were only six of us; and it was private in that the outside world knew nothing of our existence. Friendly and informal, it was made up of five neurologists and one neurosurgeon. The idea was to dine in private somewhere neutral and where the cuisine was above criticism. Rules? We had none. In practice we took turns in alphabetical order to ventilate some neurological topic of the speaker's choice for 20 to 30 minutes, after which a frank, fierce, but friendly discussion went on well into the night. Before and during the carefully selected dinner, the conversation was general and ranged over anything but medicine.

Many a paper which eventually found its way into *Brain* had been tried out as an immature, unpolished, and tentative contribution to the Hexagon, where it was debated, censured, and modified; it was later to appear in print complete with the advantage of second thoughts. Sometimes the gestation period was so stormy that the foetal version never went to term.

The original idea of the Hexagon was, I believe, an inspiration of C. P. Symonds. Certainly it was at dinner in his house in Wimpole Street that we first met to discuss the project.

As the name implies, there were six of us: Russell Brain, Hugh Cairns, myself, Derek Denny-Brown, George Riddoch and Charlie Symonds. We decided we would meet in a private room in that capacious station-hotel The Great Central, now no more, this building being today the headquarters of the British Railway.

At that time Russell Brain was the junior neurologist at the London Hospital and physician at the Hospital for Nervous Diseases, Maida Vale. Hugh Cairns, after a stint with Cushing, was neurosurgeon to the London Hospital. Although he had also been appointed to the National Hospital, he did not operate there as the facilities were at that time inadequate. I was then the junior neurologist at King's College Hospital and physician to outpatients at the National Hospital, Queen Square. Denny-Brown was an assistant physician at Queen Square but spent much time in the department of physiology in Oxford. George Riddoch and Charles Symonds were both senior to me at Queen Square. The former was also senior neurologist at the London Hospital, and the latter, neurologist at Guy's.

The date of the original dinner party in Wimpole Street was 30 April 1930, and in the Minute Book, now in my possession, is listed as the first meeting of the

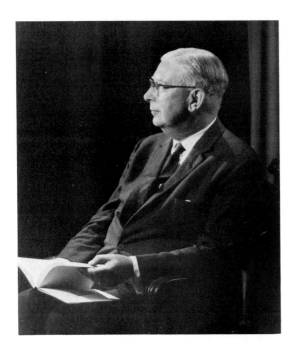

FIG. 1.   Russell Brain.

FIG. 2.   Hugh Cairns.

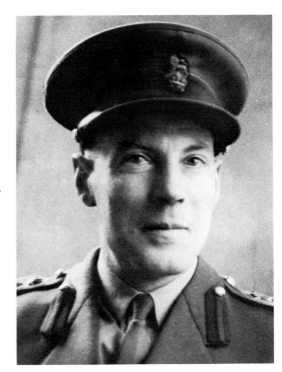

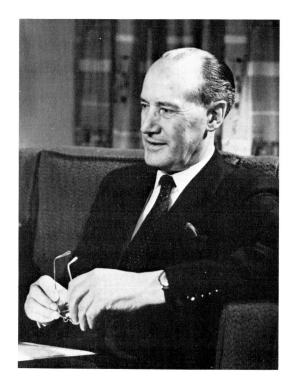

FIG. 3. Macdonald Critchley.

FIG. 4. Derek Denny-Brown.

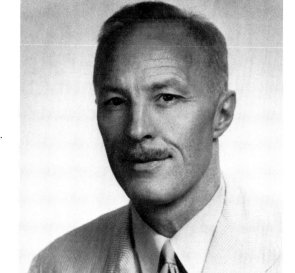

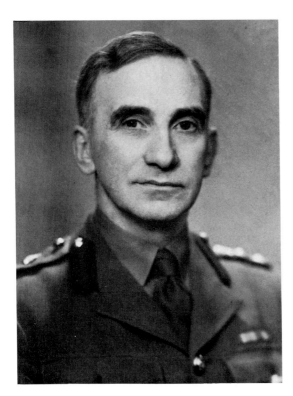

FIG. 5. George Riddoch.

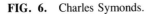

FIG. 6. Charles Symonds.

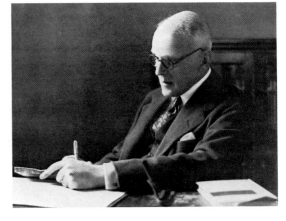

Hexagon. By lot, Denny-Brown obtained the privilege of opening the discussion at the next meeting. The rotating chairman was to be the one who had previously been the opener. Cairns was appointed secretary for the ensuing 12 months. Thereafter the secretaryship would change according to the alphabetical order of our names.

The second (or first true) meeting was held at the Great Central Hotel on 27 June 1930, when Denny-Brown gave a talk on the Relationship of Cerebellar Signs to Cerebellar Function. After this had been delivered and discussed frankly and at length by the rest of us, Hugh Cairns spoke quite briefly on Changes in the Symptomatology of Tumours of the Vermis after Cerebellar Decompression. The meeting finished at 11 p.m. Unfortunately, no record was kept of the menu of this or indeed any of the subsequent meetings; this is a pity, for he who does not mind his belly is apt not to mind anything else, as Doctor Johnson so wisely said.

On 31 October 1930, the third meeting was taken up with the discussion of two papers. The first was by Russell Brain on the Grasp Reflex of the Foot. This was followed by Symonds' talk on Disorders of Mood. Symonds had once worked with Adolf Meyer and regarded psychiatry as a poor relation of neurology.

Over dinner on this occasion, Henry Head's name was raised. At that time he had retired in the country, severely incapacitated by Parkinson's disease for which he stoutly refused to take any medication, fearing that drugs might blunt the keen edge of his intellect. It was agreed to send him, from all of us, a warm letter of Christmas greeting. As the secretary, Hugh Cairns drew up a letter which we all signed. On 28 December 1930, Henry Head dictated to his wife Ruth the following reply:

> My dear Cairns,
>
> Your letter with its kind expression of goodwill from all the members of the Hexagon have touched and pleased me more than I can tell you. In my days of enforced inactivity it [is] so good to have for my solace thoughts of you six friends in all your young vigour carrying on the work that lies nearest my heart, and I realise with thankfulness that you include some of a past generation in your plans for the present day in which I am convinced your club will bear a helpful and increasingly important part.
>
> With my grateful thanks and good wishes to every member of the Hexagon.
>
> Believe me,
>
> Ever your sincerely,
Henry Head (p.p. R.H.)

On 27th February 1931 Riddoch opened with a talk on Reflex Reactions in Paraplegia, a subject which had been dear to him since World War I. The address must have been lengthy, for the meeting did not break up until 11:38 p.m.

It was over dinner that evening that we realised that Professor Otfried Foerster of Breslau was due to visit London in April. It was therefore decided to hold a special meeting of the Hexagon and to invite him to attend. As the new secretary, I was deputed to write and invite him to the dinner and simply talk, rather than give a formal paper.

This took place on 1 May 1931. According to the minutes, "During the dinner and afterwards, a most delightful and informative talk of an informed character took place on a variety of subjects of neurological interest."

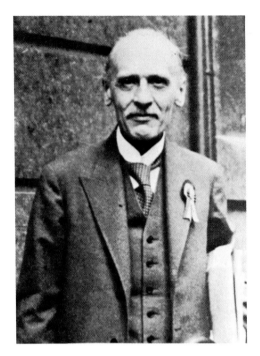

FIG. 7.   Professor Otfried Foerster.

The occasion was unforgettable. The professor, a delicate, frail figure (Fig. 7), delighted us with his quiet charm while astonishing us with his erudition. We touched upon this topic and that, and the talk ranged from cabbages to kings. However way-out or esoteric the subject that was raised, Foerster was able to bear refreshing and novel ideas. *Nullum quod tetigit non ornavit.* In this respect he reminded us of S. A. Kinnier Wilson.

Gradually the conversation turned to that famous patient of his, Lenin, who had died in 1922. For the last 2 years of his life Lenin had suffered from a severe and progressive cerebral arteriopathy. No longer trusting the neurologists in Moscow and Petrograd, he sent for Foerster. Here was someone who inspired in the patient both confidence and liking, and indeed the friendship became mutual, Foerster finding him highly intelligent and, strange to say, modest. Lenin begged Foerster to stay on in Moscow to take charge of his case. Because of his university commitments Foerster demurred, but at the highest diplomatic level he was directed by the German government to accede to Lenin's request. Foerster sent for his unfinished manuscripts and in the Kremlin over the ensuing months spent his free time in writing his monograph on the peripheral nerve injuries among the German troops during World War I.

Lenin's condition steadily worsened. One stroke followed another until he was left with a double hemiparesis and a severe aphasia in which a recurring expletive constituted his only utterance. As in the case of Mencken and Baudelaire, these lords of language were stricken devastatingly in their powers of speech. During his last days he was afflicted by a vast number of focal seizures.

We raised the question whether Lenin had had G.P.I., as had been suggested by some of the newspapers in the West. Foerster emphatically denied this idea, pointing out the arteriopathic nature of his last illness.

Foerster was particularly kind to me personally on this and later occasions. Hearing that I was shortly to make an extensive tour of Russia he gave me a warm letter of introduction to Lenin's widow Krupskaya. Needless to say, when I reached Moscow I was successfully prevented from meeting this lady.

The next (i.e., sixth) meeting of the Hexagon was on 26 June 1931, when I spoke on Some Aspects of Pain. On 13 November 1931, Russell Brain discussed Exophthalmos of Central Origin, after which C. P. Symonds briefly spoke about Absent Reflexes in Cerebral Contusion. At the next meeting on 8 April 1932, Hugh Cairns spoke on Pituitary Symptomatology, dwelling especially on the variations in the development of the diaphragma sellae and of the position of the optic chiasma. The effects of operation upon the physical signs of acromegaly and on the sex hormones were described. On 24 June 1932 when the Hexagon met again, it was announced that as Professor Foerster was revisiting London in order to deliver the Schorstein lecture, he should be once more a guest of the Hexagon. The business was taken up with Denny-Brown's paper on Infective Polyneuritis followed by an enthusiastic and sometimes critical discussion.

Professor Foerster wrote on 15 July 1932:

> Dear Dr. Critchley,
> I have your letter of June 27th and thank you most sincerely for your kind invitation. I myself have in *[sic]* the most delightful memory [of] the evening which I spent with you and the other members of the Hexagon Club during my last visit to London and I look forward with the greatest pleasure to a repetition of that more charming party. Friday, Oct. 19th will suit me very well.
>
> With my kindest regards
I am yours very sincerely,
Otfried Foerster

The date of this occasion was Friday, 19 October 1932. Once again Professor Foerster kept us all intrigued with his brilliance and originality of thought. Apparently this was the type of occasion he enjoyed, for we are told that in Breslau he would sit in a café with a group of his disciples drinking German champagne and talking until closing time.

The 11th meeting was held on 4 November 1932. It was decided that in future the time spent in dining should be shorter and the price reduced. Charlie Symonds gave an informative talk on The Disturbances of Cerebral Function in Head Injuries, which was discussed in depth. It was obvious that Charlie was making cerebral trauma a topic to which over the years he was to contribute much. The next meeting was on 10 March 1933 when Georgie Riddoch spoke on Chronic Subdural Haematoma. According to the minutes, his views received a mixed reception, but the discussion was lively and interesting.

I was ill and unable to attend the next meeting, which took place on 30 June 1933. The other members of the Hexagon were kind enough to send me "a cheery note." Three short communications were delivered on this occasion, Cutaneous Pigmentation in Nervous Diseases (Russell Brain); Visual Discrimination in Homonymous Half Fields (George Riddoch); and Lightning Pains in Syphilitic Nervous Disease Other than Tabes (Denny-Brown). It was at this meeting that it was agreed to invite Harvey Cushing to attend.

The following letter to Riddoch was received from him:

> Peter Bent Brigham Hospital
> July 22 1933
>
> Dear George,
>
> Nothing would give me greater pleasure than to turn your famous Club into a septagonal one some evening in November. But whether it will be before the 6th, when I must be in Paris, or afterwards I cannot now tell. I hope it won't inconvenience you if I delay coming to any decision in the matter until later on. My past recollections of this delightful dinner club are such that the prospect of meeting them again would justify my whole trip abroad.
>
> Do give my affectionate greetings to the Heads when you see them. I certainly must run down to pay them a visit.
>
> Always sincerely yours,
> Harvey Cushing

This letter suggests that Cushing had attended some earlier meeting of the Hexagon, but there is no record of such an event in the minute book, nor can I recall his attendance.

On 27 October 1933 I was back in harness and addressed the club on the topic of Reflex Epilepsy. Russell Brain was the speaker at the 15th meeting of the Hexagon on 2 March 1934 and he talked about Papilloedema and Consecutive Optic Atrophy in conditions other than brain tumour. The Club by now had tired of the Great Central Hotel and decided that the next meeting, to be held on 29 June 1934, should start with a short dinner in a private room at Pagani's restaurant in Great Portland Street. Afterwards the members would repair to 101 Harley Street, the rooms of Dr. H. M. Worth where he and Dr. Montagu Jupe (another neuroradiologist) would, in association with Hugh Cairns, display and discuss a series of interesting x-rays. In closing, a few cases illustrating the value of ventriculography were described.

Pagani's restaurant was again chosen as a venue for the next meeting on 2 November 1934. Denny-Brown gave a paper on Problems Concerning Micturition. It was agreed that a special meeting should be held on 16 November at the same place and that Professor Lhermitte should be invited as our guest. Pagani's restaurant, which was located between Soho and the medical enclave around Harley Street, was a famous Italian restaurant furnished with many private rooms, consequently in great demand by Masonic Lodges. It was, alas, totally destroyed by a bomb during the war and was never rebuilt.

George Riddoch, meanwhile, received the following letter from Dr. Jean Lhermitte (translated):

Paris
2 October 1934

Dear Dr. Riddoch,

You are very kind to write me so graciously on the occasion of my next trip to London and I most willingly accept and will participate in the intellectual revels *[agapes spirituelles]* of your Hexagonal club on 16th November.

As you have informed Dr. Macdonald Critchley I am due to lecture to the Listerian Society* on the 14th and another on the 15th at the Neurological Society. For the first I have suggested to Critchley "Charcot, His Life and His Time"; for the second, "Cortical Cerebellar Atrophy, Clinical and Pathological Anatomy".

My papers will be illustrated with slides.

For the Hexagon club, as you wrote, it would be a pleasure to participate in a talk about spinal concussion. This of the two [suggestions] would interest me.

I am very happy at the thought of seeing you again but I hesitate to accept your kind hospitality, fearing that if my wife comes with me we shall be in your way. We have not yet made any arrangements for we will be returning to the Basque coast where we have spent 2 months.

My wife joins me in telling you and Mme. Riddoch for we are touched by your thoughts and in renewing the expression of faithful and sincere friendship.

J. Lhermitte

The special meeting called to welcome Professor Lhermitte took place as arranged. According to the minutes, "a most enjoyable evening was spent diagnosing spinal concussion. Dr. Lhermitte had microphotographs of histological lesions in concussion and demonstrated their resemblance to those of the phrenic nerve after avulsion and twisting of the nerve. The same swelling and irregularity with occasional destruction of axons could be seen, along with the myelin sheaths."

This brief note hardly does justice to the occasion. Jean Lhermitte (Fig. 8), the admirable Crichton of neurology, was probably the most learned and versatile expert in Europe in diseases of the nervous system. Eloquent, excitable, vivacious, infectious with his perpetual enthusiasm, he was a man of tremendous learning who brought deep philosophical thinking to almost all aspects of neurology. I stress "almost all" because, as I once pointed out to him, he left untouched the tremendous problem of language and its disorders. As if to compensate for this hiatus, his brilliant son, Professor François Lhermitte, became one of the very greatest living aphasiologists. I number him among one of my most admired and stimulating friends.

On 1 March 1935 short papers were read, namely, A Peculiar Form of Headache (Symonds); A Case of "Aphasia" in a Deaf-Mute (Critchley); and Two Unusual Cases of Subacute Combined Degeneration (Riddoch). At the following meeting

---

*The Listerian Society was run by the students of King's College Hospital. Each year a member of the honorary staff served as president. In 1934 that was my privilege.

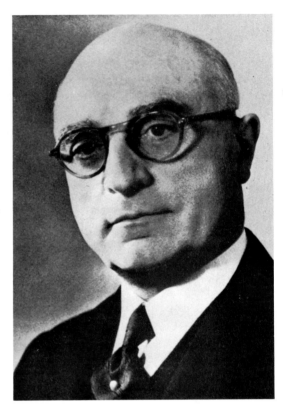

FIG. 8.   Dr. Jean Lhermitte.

on 5 July 1935, Symonds spoke about The Effects of Head Injury Remaining After One Year.

It must be borne in mind that during September the Second International Congress of Neurology was held in London with Gordon Holmes presiding; Sherrington, being the honorary president, did not take any active role. At the banquet Holmes had invited as his principal guest his old friend Foerster, who had originally been elected to head the German delegation. But since 1933 Germany was in the grip of Hitler, and Foerster was replaced by a neurological nonentity. Holmes insisted that Foerster should be at the top table, and he refused to sit next to the Nazi nominee. During the course of the Congress, Foerster delivered the Hughlings Jackson Lecture for which he received a gold medal.

Friday, 22 November 1935 was the date of the next meeting, where Riddoch discussed Radiculitis of the Cauda Equina. It was agreed to invite as guest Professor Brouwer of Amsterdam at a special meeting. Here is his reply:

6 January 1936

Dear Dr. Symonds,
    In receipt of your letter of January 3rd I have the pleasure to inform you that it will be a great honour for me to assist a dinner of the Hexagon

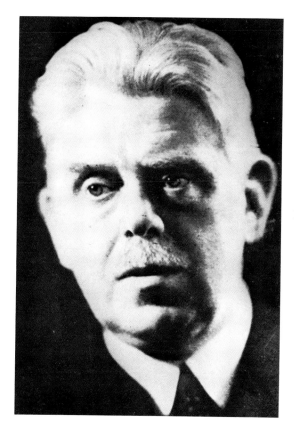

FIG. 9.   Professor B. Brouwer.

Club. I hope some of you will also be present at my lecture, because I like to know what the English neurologists think about amaurotic idiotie [*sic*] and on pseudosclerosis.

Yours sincerely,
B. Brouwer

Brouwer (Fig. 9), it can be recalled, was another of the neurological giants of that time and a close personal friend of Gordon Holmes. A giant in body as well as in mind, his status in neurology was outstanding. His interests embraced the normal and pathological anatomy of the nervous system as well as clinical neurology. Psychiatric and psychological aspects he left to others. There was something attractively boyish about him, and he spent his Saturday afternoons as a referee at football matches.

At the Hexagon he ate heartily, and sat and talked entertainingly upon a diversity of topics—angiomas of the nervous system, hypotonia in cerebellar disease, the definition of the motor cortex, and much else.

The 23rd meeting of the Hexagon took place on 23 February 1936 when I raised the question of Endogenous Factors in the Aetiology of Disseminated Sclerosis.

On 2 June 1936 Russell Brain spoke on Acute Optic and Retrobulbar Neuritis. At this meeting a guest was present, Dr. S. P. Bedson.

At the 25th meeting I was asked to invite Professor Kroll of Moscow to attend as a guest for he had also been invited to address the neurological section of the Royal Society of Medicine. It was he who had headed the Russian contingent at the International Congress of Neurology where he had impressed all by his profundity of thought and his great personal charm. Unfortunately, Professor Kroll never replied to the invitation of either the Hexagon or the Royal Society of Medicine. Follow-up letters met with no response, and we could only assume that he was either incommunicado or else not alive. It was at this meeting that Cairns discussed Colloid Cysts of the Third Ventricle.

Symonds discussed The Symptomatology of High Cervical Tumours, and Russell Brain read a paper on Some Rare Varieties of Optic Atrophy. The occasion was 17 February 1937.

The minutes of the 27th meeting contained the note that Riddoch and Critchley should ascertain whether suitable accommodation for the club could be found elsewhere. Why we were becoming disillusioned by Pagani's I cannot recall. It was then, too, that Denny-Brown gave vent to two papers, viz. Sensory Incoordination of the Eye Muscles and Construction of the Retinal Arteries in Patients with Hypertension.

On 29 October 1937 Riddoch and Critchley reported their failure to find suitable accommodation elsewhere for the club. Symonds then spoke on Conditions Simulating Brain Abscess. Short papers were read at the next meeting; Denny-Brown on Olivopontocerebellar Atrophy and Symonds on Obscure Cases of Horner's Syndrome. On 24 June 1938 Riddoch spoke on Hypothalamic Autonomic Attacks. He received a mixed and guarded reception, the club remaining "open-minded" on the subject.

The minutes of the Hexagon end here, but apparently two more meetings were held. The war then came, and the Hexagon was a casualty. Half-hearted attempts to revive it were made in 1946, but Denny-Brown was then in Boston; Cairns had died; and George Riddoch was a very sick man.

"And All the Daughters of Musick Shall Be Brought Low"

I need not remind my readers that the words of the title are from Ecclesiastes or, as expressed in Judaism, the Koheleth. Using highly symbolic prose, the preacher is describing the physical attributes of senility. The "daughters of musick" represent speech, and being "brought low" signifies the disordered diction of the aged.

Were the man in the street questioned as to what he would regard as the distinctive features of spoken speech in old persons, I suppose the answer would be a high pitched, quavering, croaky voice production. Such qualities inspired Shakespeare to describe the lean and slippered pantaloon whose big manly voice reverted to a childish treble, piping and whistling in its sound. Earlier still, Aristotle asserted that old men's voices tremble and did so because they cannot control them, just as when invalids and children take hold of a long stick by one end, and the other end shakes. Cicero was less critical and said that the style of speech which graces the old man is subdued and gentle *(quietus et remissus)*, and very often the sedate and mild speech of an eloquent old man wins itself a hearing.

But speech is merely the wind instrument played upon by something more organismic, namely language, the co-partner of thought. Examination here will uncover phenomena which are far more subtle, and more significant. To begin with, let us take stock of the common belief that talkativeness is characteristic of the aged. *"Senectus est natura loquacior,"* as Cicero wrote. According to Sir Thomas Moore, "A fonde olde manne is often as full of woordes as a woman." Perhaps all of us have had the experience of serving on administrative bodies where the chairman, a very senior colleague, has hogged the proceedings by such loquacity as to allow junior members little opportunity to make comments or suggestions. Sometimes this has happened in the high courts of justice where the presiding judge has exasperated counsel by his interpolations and even by usurping the function of interrogating witnesses.

As Ambrose Bierce wrote when defining "dotage": "an imbecility from age, commonly manifested in loquacity. The word was originally 'anecdotage,' but those of whom it is the characteristic virtue, haven't time to speak the entire word, they are too busy talking."

Unkind, and not really true.

I submit that garrulity as a hallmark of senescence has been exaggerated, and that a commoner state of affairs is the reverse, namely a relative parsimony of speech. This is on a par with a similar paucity in the sphere of movement *(Motorik)*, a relative hypokinesis.

From Critchley, M. (1984): *Archives of Neurology,* 41:1135–1139, with permission.

My suggestion is that in senescence (which sooner or later we will have to distinguish from senility) a poverty of speech is more usual. In committees and assemblies it is the young who usually do the talking. The elderly members are apt to sit quietly and modestly until specifically invited to express an opinion. As Dante put it, *"parlaver rado, con voi soave"* (seldom they spoke, with voices calm and low). Dipping into the deep well of experience and wisdom, they then reply, and in few and considered words. Even in social circumstances, older men are on the whole laconic. They have shed their former verbal expansiveness, though anecdotage may be close on their heels. Another characteristic of the diction of the elderly is a slow rate of talking, pondered and deliberate. Precipitancy and rapidity of utterance suggest impetuous thinking, something which is foreign to the elderly. As we read in *De Senectute*, had the mental qualities of reflection, reason, and judgement not been characteristic of old men, our fathers would not have called their highest deliberative body the "senate," or assembly of elders.

Continuing this train of thinking, we can follow the linguistic habits of the aged into the realms of pathology, at the limit of which lie the language disorders of senile or presenile dementia. Interesting speech patterns may then be seen and striking analogies exist with what I have described as "ingravescent aphasia" or "proto-aphasia" as observable in one who has a slowly expanding lesion within the left frontal pole.

We are now touching upon a subject which has been neglected by those whose very business it is to study speech usage. I refer to what we might term the "unlearning of language." A longitudinal analysis of an individual's use of words from childhood to the grave would not be difficult if we were to concentrate upon the purely written work of that individual. I know of only one such investigation, namely that carried out by D. P. Boder, who studied the *Journals* of Ralph Waldo Emerson from 1820 until 1876 when he was 73 years of age. Work of this nature might reanimate the dullest of biographies by an alchemy which transmutes the lead of narrative into the silver of neurolinguistics.

But it is first necessary to consider what we might term the *norm*, that is, the qualities of speech in the mature, healthy, educated adult, and then turn to a comparison with the picture that tends to appear with advancing years. In all our discussions we must always bear in mind that speech shows itself in two principal ways, the spoken form and the written form, and that linguistics tends rather to ignore that which one commits to paper.

Let us deal with the purposes or objectives of speech, and then with the question of vocabulary.

Silence is broken in one, at least, of four circumstances, viz., to make a statement, to pose a question, to formulate a request, or to emit an interjection. Three of these apply to written speech, exclamatory phrases being rare. Another classification of speech is into "mands" versus "tacts," depending upon whether or not some action is expected of the listener. If it does, it is a tact; otherwise it is a mand. More easily understood is a dichotomy into transitive versus intransitive speech.

The term "speech vocabulary" needs amplifying. A scholar may amass a word bank of many tens of thousand terms. There are words he recognises when he meets them. But not all of them are words that he is likely to employ either in speech or in writing. In addition to the large available vocabulary, there is therefore a smaller one which is in constant use, one which we may term the "utilized" as opposed to the "utilizable" vocabulary.

With these considerations in mind, one may ponder on the taciturnity of the aged. Are his relatively infrequent remarks capable of statistical analysis? Provided we have adequate data in the way of tape recordings or written material, the answer is yes.

As to the circumstances in which the elderly speak, it is clear that transitive types of utterance outnumber the intransitive. Or, using the fourfold classification, requests and exclamations more and more outnumber the declarative and interrogative types of utterance. The change is a progressive one, reflecting the growing reliance upon others.

It is possible to measure yet another individual employment of the word bank, especially in writing, and that is a test of verbal diversification. This is the type/token ratio. Let me explain. A chunk of written or spoken speech comprises, say, 100 words. These are technically called "tokens." Of these 100 tokens, some are used more than once, e.g., the articles, the prepositions, and certain nouns and verbs according to the subject matter. Consequently there may be only, say, 60 *different* words appearing in the text of 100 tokens. These different words are referred to as "types." Let me give an example.

Take the lines:

> Here am I, homeward from my wandering,
> Here am I, homeward, and my heart is healed.
> If I was thirsty, I have heard a spring,
> If I was dusty, I have found a field.

Here there are 34 words, or tokens. But several words appear twice (*if, am, was, homeward*), and the personal pronoun *I* crops up six times. In fact there are only 21 different words within this piece of verse. Hence the type/token ratio (or TTR) is 21/34, or 0.617. Provided one is scrutinizing packages of data which are not excessively long, we can assert that the simpler the sample, the greater is the proportion of recurring words, and the TTR is low, approximating to, or even falling below, the 0.5 mark. If every word used were different, then the number of types and tokens would be the same, and the TTR would be unity. In experience, however, this is met with only in sentences which are brief (e.g., "No, it is not so. Over that wall the grass is greener"). Were a TTR of unity to apply to lengthy pieces of prose, the text would approximate to jargon or bafflegab.

In old age and in dementia the TTR is low. May I borrow a brief speech recording of the utterance of a presenile dement studied by Schwartz, Marin, and Saffron? Their patient was reported as saying:

> Oh yeah, she's real nice. She, you know . . . she tells me something and I say Oh Oh Oh and she says "Hon . . . why don't you say that?" and I say "Well ah!". . . . Then when she says it, I say "Oh yeah!" But Oh Lord my other-ah-girl, you know, my gal that I have, she says "Mom, now you tell me something!" and I say "Oh I can't tell you anything." She says "Ma!" cause she's so excited.

Out of the 79 words or tokens of this quotation there are 35 types. The TTR is therefore 0.44.

Let us compare this with an extract from the actual paper wherein this patient is described. Taking a passage of the same length, i.e., 79 words, we read:

> . . . underlying categories. On a nonverbal match-to-sample procedure, for example, dogs were treated as exemplars of the cat family. Evidence for the breakdown of semantic knowledge was not limited to picture labeling paradigms. Thus, we found that the subject was unable to utilize semantic context in the written disambiguation of spoken homophones but could, at the same time, use even minimal syntactic cues as the basis for proper lexical selection. This last result was consistent with other lines of evidence. . . .

On scrutinizing the prose we find that the number of types is as high as 63, and the TTR is therefore almost 0.89. This high ratio not only reflects the difference between written and spoken speech, it can also be taken as evidence of complexity. It carries no implication of clarity either of exposition or of thinking, stylistic elegance, or even readability; indeed on the contrary.

While still on the topic of the written language of the ageing individual, we may bring up the matter of the *adjective/verb ratio*. It has been suggested that adjectives are indices of a qualifying category of speech, whereas verbs refer to a more active style. It was this ratio that Boder studied in the writings of Emerson, finding that his use of verbs tended to increase with age, the adjective/verb ratio changing from 1:2 to 1:3, but in an irregular fashion.

According to G. A. Miller, dialogue in plays entails nine verbs to every adjective (1:9), whereas scientific writings showed only one verb to three adjectives (3:1). Legal statutes have five verbs per adjective (1:5). A master's thesis contains 15 verbs for every adjective (1:15), whereas with Ph.D. candidates the ratio is 1:1.

Although this change has been tentatively associated with the degree of emotional stability of the writer, the most important single factor must surely be the type of writing under scrutiny.

I have tested this AVR (adjective/verb ratio) in the writings of a few individuals all of whom were of high intelligence, early readers, endowed with exceptional memories, and much practised in the use of words. The results obtained are shown in Table 1.

It seems that the data are as yet insufficient to justify any conclusion about the effect of ageing upon the employment in writing of these two particular parts of speech. So far, the available information has been too imprecise, too diverse, and too lax in standardisation. One needs guidance as to exactly which words rightly

TABLE 1. *Adjective/verb ratio (AVR) according to age*

Subject	First evaluation		Second evaluation		Occupation	Remarks
	Age	AVR	Age	AVR		
Samuel Johnson	9	1.75	71	2	Writer	
Francis Galton	14	1	89	2.3	Scientist	Could read at 2½
Hughlings Jackson	28	0.5	74	0.9	Neurologist	
Arnold Bennett	29	3	62	1.4	Writer	
H. G. Wells	14	2.5	80	0.81	Writer	
Hilaire Belloc	8	1.6	72	0.6	Writer	
Compton Mackenzie	14	2.5	79	1.6	Writer	Mnemonist
Rudyard Kipling	18	0.73	71	2.2	Writer	
H. H. Asquith	12	1.6	74	1	Politician	
G. Bernard Shaw	52	1.4	93	1	Writer	
Charles Dickens	23	1.21	58	0.75	Writer	
Winston Churchill	8	0.54	79	0.34	Statesman, writer	
Lord Randolph Churchill	14	1.7	44	0.71	Politician	
			45	4.5	←————————{ Rapid dementia	
Wilkie Collins	15	2.3	65	1.75	Writer	
George Meredith	21	1	81	2.3	Writer	
Oscar Wilde	14	0.75	46	0.27	Writer	

fall into the categories spoken of as "adjectives" as opposed to "verbs." And yet this linguistic approach gives promise of being a project worth pursuing, given a bigger set of more reliable variables.

Still other tests of the personal use of language might yield interesting results if studied longitudinally, so as to extend into old age. For example, one might investigate the question of *sentence length* as measured in either syllables or words. Idiosyncratic factors of style are naturally involved here and must be taken into account.

Yet another influence of age on verbal diversification can be detected in the increasing employment of a favoured word or phrase, something which reveals to the percipient reader the identity of the author. When this reaches an unacceptable stage it amounts to *verbal contamination*, something which is also met with in the writings of some mild aphasiacs, and it is something which can be quantified. Occasionally when revising his text the writer becomes aware of this irritating verbal overusage and makes erasures. Rarely, however, does he detect and expunge all of the surplusages, for scotomas are not always visual.

As Shakespeare proclaimed, "old men forget"—a truism but underlying something for which we should be grateful. It is, however, an unusual kind of forgetfulness, one which spares remote events but hinders the retrieval of day-to-day trivia. In part this is due to lack of interest in the passing scene. The *tabula rasa* of the young child has become so overcrowded as to leave very little room for new material. The clinical picture differs from Korsakov's syndrome, for recent memory is less severely affected, and confabulation is rare.

Childhood memories are not necessarily accurate. Not only are some experiences repressed in the aged, but temporal and even spatial elements are apt to be distorted. Proust spoke of the "translucent alabaster" of our memories, which we cannot display for we alone perceive them.

This impairment of memory is reflected in the speech. I refer to the phenomenon of *verbal standstill*, whereby the easy flow of talk is arrested in midstream because a word suddenly and inexplicably eludes the speaker. Should the missing term be offered to him either by the interlocutor or by reference to appropriate reading matter, it is promptly identified and irrelevant alternatives are rejected at once. Proper nouns are more often the offenders than common substantives, and nouns rather than any other unit of grammar.

Anomia is not limited to the elderly. It may also afflict younger subjects, especially in circumstances of stress or fatigue. Occasionally it is a verbal mannerism or idiosyncrasy stamping an individual as an eccentric. Unlike the erudite aphasiac, paraphasic errors are uncommon, and the aged do not unwittingly employ verbal substitutions.

Forgetfulness for proper names is a social embarrassment which may demand the ingenuity of a Disraeli to conceal. Whenever he was buttonholed by someone whose identity escaped him, after a pause of 15 seconds he would inquire, "And how is the old complaint?" In this way the situation was saved.

The person whose name escapes one may be an old friend or a recent acquaintance, a well-known individual or a nonentity. There is no quality which one can isolate which causes the proper name to be elusive. Often one has a misty image of the name. It may be realised whether the missing name is a short one or a long one; a commonplace name or one that is out of the way; one that is monosyllabic such as Smith, or an articulated one such as Van den Bergh. One may even be aware which is the initial letter of the elusive word.

I know of no study of the linguistic effects of ageing upon those who throughout their long lives have been endowed with exceptional memory. Does the faculty of total recall, or photographic imagery, withstand the senescent processes better or worse than the average? Luria did not live long enough to inform us of his mnemonist's abilities in old age. I remember the writer Compton Mackenzie, whose gift of total recall induced him to publish the first of a 10-volume autobiography on his 80th birthday, a work he had embarked upon the previous year and which he completed when he was 88. His reminiscences are fantastic in their detail, and as an octogenarian he showed none of the obvious blemishes of senescent speech. He possessed two life-long qualities which may have helped preserve both his memory and his ability to communicate. In the first place he was a synaesthetic with vivid colour associations. Secondly, words fascinated him. As he explained, "Words had such a tremendous significance for me that the name of an object or of a person was in a way more real than the object or person it described."

Incidentally one would like to know something of the ageing processes of speech in such individuals as the chess masters, the musical prodigies, arithmetical freaks such as Bidder, and other members of that small *corps d'élite* who are endowed with exceptional memories. For my part I know of one well-known "memory man" of the vaudeville who died demented, but to what extent alcohol or syphilis played an aetiological role I can only guess.

Reverting to the *lapsus memoriae* of the aged, one can identify one or two side effects. One is *repetitiousness*, which derives from a loss of awareness that some vivid experience has already been recounted to a particular person. Perhaps it has, possibly more than once, and this becomes embarrassing.

The other side effect is the habit of leaving a sentence unfinished, the necessary verbal counters being temporarily unavailable. Grammarians refer to this conversational trait as "*aposiopesis.*"

In extreme cases this leads to *incoherency*, which may become embarrassing when speech-making is obligatory. Several samples can be cited by political historians of a dementing statesman becoming more and more rambling, uttering vague parenthetical clauses to the extent of bringing to an ignominious end a long and distinguished parliamentary career.

Yet another indication of linguistic breakdown is a modified form of aposiopesis, whereby a speaker relies increasingly upon the employment of *imprecise generic substitutions* such as "whatsisname," "thingummybob," "whatyoumaycallit," or *tout court*—"things." The last-named may occur as a mannerism in the prose of some affected, mannered writers still in their youth. Oscar Wilde is a case in point, with his references to "frightened forest things," "scarlet things," a "foul thing," and many others.

In pathological old age, namely, in cases of senile or presenile dementia, the truncated speech may reach its peak in the phenomenon of *echolalia*. Here the patient merely repeats the words put to him, with or without a change in pronoun. The frontiers of sanity have been crossed, for it is essentially a psychotic symptom. Echolalia implies a defective recall of verbal symbols, extreme suggestibility, identification with the interlocutor, lack of insight, an impulse to maintain social contact through speech, and loss of supralinguistic inhibition.

An allied phenomenon is that of *verbigeration* whereby the patient emits, in a compulsive fashion, an inappropriate recurrent utterance. So do some aphasiacs in their desperate effort to communicate. In the dement the words constitute a verbal tic. Thus in season and out, the demented person may give vent to such interjectional absurdities as "Oh my God, what shall I do"; or "And the Lord shall prepare a niche in the rock." These I quote at random.

Dickens, who had an uncanny knowledge of medical oddities, was aware of senile verbigeration, and he gave us two choice examples when he wrote *Bleak House*. The dementing Mrs. Smallwood at one time kept saying "Over the water! Charley over the water, Charley over the water, over the water to Charley!" Her other speech iteration was "Fifteen hundred pound. Fifteen hundred pound in a black box, fifteen hundred pound locked up, fifteen hundred pound put away and hid."

At this point one might mention the phenomenon of *defective exemplification*, something which is not apparent to the patient himself or to those with whom he converses. It comes to light only on appropriate exploration. Although the patient can readily name objects and pictures of objects in front of him, he cannot quickly reel off a satisfactory list of examples belonging to some particular category, e.g., vegetables, animals, makes of automobile, girls' first names, and so on. Only haltingly does he come up with an inventory which is all too brief, his words emerging at increasing intervals. He may unknowingly repeat himself. The test can be made still more searching by switching from a concrete to an abstract attitude by requesting the subject to specify those articles which share a common property, e.g., colour, size, texture. These manoeuvres comprise a delicate test of a waning accessibility to the innate vocabulary.

Let us pause for a moment to consider the subject of nonverbal communication in the aged. Gesture is a contrivance employed wittingly or unwittingly by a speaker to emphasise or embellish his words. Occasionally in the elderly this becomes exaggerated, so that automatic movements of the face or upper limbs take on a greater flamboyance. The contrary is commoner, however, and an increasing hypomimia strikes the observer. Gestural as well as volitional movements become increasingly infrequent and slow, leading to a bowed, statuesque posture reminiscent of something between pomposity and parkinsonism. The face loses its play of expression and, as we read in Isaiah, "becomes set like a flint."

At the same time one must not overlook the occurrence of involuntary movements in senility, such as tremor and the oral dyskinesias, but these are not communicative. Neither, for that matter, are the variegated psychomotor activities of the dements with their sucking, grasping, groping, picking, fumbling, and patting movements.

Terminology

What is the most suitable expression to use when referring to the mild or severe changes in language which characterise old age at one end of the spectrum and dementia at the other? It is tempting to speak of an "aphasia," and yet to most neurologists that term implies a focal as opposed to a diffuse lesion of the brain. "Generalised aphasic difficulty" and "nonaphasic speech impairment" have been suggested but are clumsy. Schwartz et al. described their patient as showing "dissociations of language function in dementia." "Pseudo-aphasia" might do or, alternatively, "alogia" or "dyslogia", though Kleist tried to commandeer these terms for quite another purpose.

The Contribution of Linguistics

Linguistic analysis of the language used by the aged and by senile dements may contribute something to the vexed question whether ageing is a natural, unavoidable process of involution or the result of a summation of multiple minor pathological insults. Or, could it derive from a combination of the two processes? More than

50 years ago I discussed this problem in some detail and quoted the contrasting viewpoints of two American experts, Warthin and Tilney. The former favoured a physiological conception of old age. "The senescent process is potent from the very beginning. . . . Involution is a biologic entity . . . an intrinsic, inherent, inherited quality of the germ plasm." Tilney, on the other hand, thought otherwise. Senescence was pathological and hence could be shelved, postponed, held back, even evaded. In his own words, "The brain in aged people may present certain morbid changes but these are in their turn incident to many pathological assaults upon the tissues sustained during life. . . . old age has a pathological background. It arises from definite conditions which may be combated or corrected."

My studies of long ago upon the neurology of old age preceded—I like to think— the beginnings of gerontology. The potential importance of that subject is overwhelming, and I believe linguistics can make an important contribution.

The Case for a Brain Institute

I started this discussion with a quotation from Ecclesiastes. May I conclude with another, to the effect that . . . "better is the ending of a thing than the beginning thereof"?

Nevertheless, it would be wrong if I did not also quote Tilney again: "Some day, people will awaken to the fact that they have been missing the greatest constructive opportunities. . . . One liberally supported and effective brain institute would prove an incomparably more profitable investment for civilisation than the most powerful battle-fleet that ever sailed the seas. The political party which will have the foresight and humanity to introduce into its platform an article advocating and supporting the longer and better use of the human brain will offer a worthy issue to its electorate."

Records of Some Famous Migraineurs

The "Grievous Head Pains" of Anne, Viscountess Conway

The case here presented is that of Anne Finch, born 16 December 1631 of noble origins, being descended from Henry Fitzherbert, Chancellor to Henry I (Fig. 1). She was born and brought up in Kensington House, which became Kensington Palace after its purchase by William III. Of an intellectual calibre that placed her within the category of a "gifted child," she profited from an appropriate standard of scholarship, excelling at mathematics, Latin, and Greek. When she was older her writings on philosophical themes brought her in touch with Henry More, Fellow of Christ's College, Cambridge, with whom, over a period of many years, she exchanged a copious and scholarly correspondence.

When barely 19 she married the Third Viscount Conway and Killultagh, a member of the famous Seymour family who in due course became the first, and last, Earl Conway.

At the age of 12, after a pyrexial episode of obscure nature, she developed headaches which continued intermittently throughout her life. As might be expected, her family attributed these, at first, to "overzealous reading."

The headaches were often precipitated by quite minor disturbances, but sometimes they arose spontaneously. They were usually unilateral, affecting either side of the head, though at times the pains were generalised. Each "fitt" or bout would last 1 to 4 days and was disabling in character. She would retire to her bed in the dark, disallowing visitors, shutting out all noise, and rejecting food and drink. Often she would vomit. Until the cessation of the attack she was wakeful, but afterwards she would fall into a deep and protracted sleep. Such episodes recurred every 3 weeks at first, but later they increased in frequency and eventually became almost continual.

Her symptoms were considerably aggravated in 1657 when she was pregnant but abated somewhat after the birth of her son, Heneage. Sadly, he died from smallpox before he was two, and Anne never again became pregnant.

Not surprisingly, Her Ladyship came under the care of many physicians and apothecaries. One of the first who attended her was Sir Francis Prujean, later to become President of the Royal College of Physicians. Indeed at his own expense he erected the college building at Amen Corner, later to be destroyed in the Great Fire of London. Prujean referred the viscountess to his close friend William Harvey,

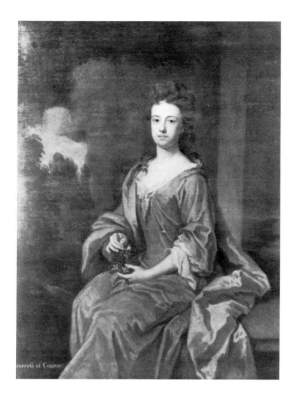

FIG. 1. Anne, Viscountess of Conway. Portrait attributed to Kneller. (From *Migraine Matters*.)

who happened to be a distant relative of hers by marriage. Her Ladyship willingly fell in with this suggested consultation, for she had "heard him much commended, and they say he knows very many secrets in physicke unknown to other physicians." Yet John Aubrey has told us that, after the publication of his classic *De motu cordis*, "he fell mightily in his practize, and that 'twas beleeved by the vulgar that he was crack-brained. . . . " Harvey could only suggest that she visit France and submit to trepanation, a procedure which her Ladyship, after much thought, wisely refused. Again we are reminded of Aubrey's comments about Harvey, that "all his Profession would allow him to be an excellent Anatomist, but I never heard of any that admired his Therapeutique way. I knew severall practicers in London that would not have given 3d. for one of his Bills; and that a man could tell by one of his Bills what he did aime at."

Sir Kenelm Digby was also consulted, even though he was better known as a naval commander and diplomat than as a doctor. According to Professor Hope Nicolson, the genial Sir Kenelm knew everybody, read everything, and was the centre of more gossip and rumour than any other Englishman of the early century. What Sir Kenelm prescribed we do not know, but we suspect that it might have been the volatile salt of vipers, which was one of his most favoured remedies. We can shrewdly surmise that he at least mightily charmed Her Ladyship. His epitaph proclaims what manner of man he was:

Under this Stone the Matchless Digby lies,
Digby the Great, the Valiant, and the Wise;
This Age's Wonder, for his Noble Parts;
Skill'd in six Tongues, and learn'd in all the Arts.
Born on the day he died, th' eleventh of June,
On which he bravely fought at Scanderoon,
'Tis rare that one and self-same day should be
His Day of Birth, of Death, of Victory.

Another unorthodox adviser was Mercurius, the son of the Belgian J. B. van Helmont and who was as much of a mystic and an alchemist as his father. He visited the viscountess at her country house, Ragley Hall, near Alcester in Warwickshire. How successful was Mercurius' treatment we are unaware, but the patient had a high personal regard for him and left him in her will the sum of £300. He in turn presented his patient with a portrait of himself painted by Sir Peter Lely. This hung in the library at Ragley until comparatively recently when it was sold by the seventh Marquess of Hertford, and is now to be found in the National Gallery.

Lady Anne also sought the advice of that "skeptical chymist" the Hon. Robert Boyle, 14th child of the Earl of Cork and hence an ancestor of the gallant admiral the Earl of Cork and Orrery, better known throughout the service in two world wars as "Ginger Boyle." Though his special interests lay in matters scientific or even theological rather than medical, his wise and caring personality doubtless brought temporary solace to her Ladyship to a greater extent than his *Ens Veneris.*

Of particular importance from the standpoint of diagnosis were her visits to the famous Thomas Willis, who graphically recorded her symptoms but without mentioning her by name. In his own words, "Although the Distemper most grievously afflicted this noble Lady, above twenty years, when I saw her, having pitched its tents near the confines of the Brain, had so long besieged its regal tower, yet it had not taken it: for the sick lady, being free from a Vertigo, swimming in the Head, Convulsive Distempers, and any Soporiferous symptoms, found the chief faculties of the soul sound enough."

Even today, patients plagued by chronic headache are easy victims to charlatans, quacks, qualified faddists, and practitioners of fringe medicine. Wealth, book-learning, and worldly wisdom do not protect them: Indeed such endowments seem to make them all the more gullible, as every doctor knows. It is not surprising, therefore, to hear that Lady Conway became prey to the ministrations of "the touch doctor Valentine Greatrakes," also known as "the Irish Stroker." Travelling from Waterford to Ragley Hall he practised his art upon her *coram publico* day after day for some weeks. The onlookers comprised an august company of members of the Royal Society, theologians, and philosophers. No relief followed.

Anne Conway and Henry More exchanged ideas as to management and treatment, and this doctor and that was recommended to her. Exercise in the open air was advocated, as well as avoidance of fruit and restriction of fluids. In 1658 she was advised to indulge in lamprey pies, for her health's sake. Many drugs were suggested until More began to protest about "overmuch medication." Among the medicaments that were tried were coffee, tobacco, and the *Ens Veneris* of Robert Boyle. When pregnant, she was advised to carry on her person an *aetites*, or eaglestone. Two well-known London chemists—Charles Hues and Frederick Clodius—ran into serious trouble, the former for allowing Her Ladyship to contract a dangerous degree of mercurial poisoning. Long-continued dripping of water onto the head was at one time advocated, but it is doubtful whether Her Ladyship was stupid enough to submit.

Meanwhile, the headaches worsened, and we find the patient writing in 1664 to her friend: "I cannot dissemble so much as not to professe myself very weary of this condition."

In 1669 both Anne Conway and Henry More began to evince an interest in Quakerism or some variety of that discipline. Typically, too, More was tempted to admit in his letters to numerous minor aches and personal disabilities, for nothing is so seductively contagious in correspondence or in conversation as the interchange of symptoms.

The disorder now rapidly augmented. Headaches became more frequent and more violent. More spoke of them as "agonies." Generalised physical weakness supervened until she became bedfast. Her pains seem to have spread beyond the confines of the cranium, and in written reports from the Steward at Ragley to Lord Conway there are references to alimentary complications. Other than sips of small beer, she could take no nourishment. Then came frequent nosebleeds, and later still it was noted that her arms had become weak. Consciousness was intact, however. A terminal oedema of the lower limbs ushered in her death on 23 February 1679, when she was 48 years of age. She was buried in the country church at Arrow, near Alcester.

Discussion

The nature of this lady's ill health is an interesting topic for conjecture. It is difficult to escape the conclusion that her periodic attacks of severe hemicrania were migrainous in nature, even though they worsened rather than abated when she was pregnant. Willis' description is too realistic and too detailed to allow any alternative. However, migraine in itself cannot account for her final illness, and it seems probable that Lady Conway was a chronic migraineuse whose symptoms steadily became overlaid by some intractable and lethal disorder. At her age the possibilities of either malignant disease or of hypertension cannot be dismissed.

Even before she died the nature of her ill health had been a matter of speculation. Her brother, John Finch, proclaimed: "I cannot guess at any other cause than what I formerly told unless it should come from the closenesse of the sutures in your head which may hinder the perspiring vapours." Translating this notion into terms of raised intracranial pressure, John Finch may well have been right. As an alternative hypothesis we can but admire the perspicacity of Henry More when he judged his friend's malady as being "mainly complexionall." This is as shrewd an explanation of migraine as any conception held today.

Epilogue

Anne's bereaved husband, now an Earl, soon married again, first to Elizabeth, daughter of Lord Delamare, who died in childbirth. Earl Conway then wedded Ursula Stawell, niece of Baron Stawell. She brought a dowry of £30,000 but produced no heir. Four years after the loss of the Lady Anne, the Earl died and his estates devolved upon Francis Seymour-Conway, the title becoming incorporated within the present Marquisate of Hertford.

Blaise Pascal: Was He a Victim of Ophthalmic Migraine?

The background of the brilliant seventeenth century scientist, theologian, and philosopher Blaise Pascal has intrigued his numerous biographers. Dr. Cabanis (1930) questioned whether he belonged to that category of *demi-fous* or *dégénérés supérieurs* where outstanding intellectual stature is coupled with emotional instability. In 1949 Dr. René Onfray raised the hypothesis that Pascal was a lifelong victim of recurring attacks of migraine associated with transient fortification figures and a hemianopia. His contention was supported by the evidence afforded from a study of the manuscripts of the *Pensées* preserved in the Bibliothêque Nationale of France.

Blaise Pascal was born in 1623 at Clérmont-Ferrand, where his father was a respected and prosperous lawyer. A sickly infant, he was afflicted when 12 months of age with an illness characterized, it is said, by marasmus, languor, and softening of the bones. Apparently this was a not uncommon syndrome in young children at that time and went under various names. Such patients seemed not to belong to the caring family circle and were regarded as being *tombés en châtre*, that is, "imprisoned." Another label in common use was "*carreau*," and the disorder was ascribed, on no convincing evidence, to a tuberculous affection of the mesenteric glands.

Symptoms continued for about a year and were followed by some unusual neurotic manifestations. Thus Pascal would be greatly upset by the sight of water, which caused him to fly into ungovernable rages. Another symptom worried the family. Although affectionate towards his mother and father individually, he could not tolerate seeing the two of them together.

These phobias—regarded by neighbours as the result of witchcraft—continued for about a year. As he grew older it became obvious that young Blaise was what we would now call "a gifted child." By the age of 12 he had, unaided, mastered the 32 propositions of the first book of *Euclid*. At 16 he wrote a thesis on conic sections. Following Torricelli's inventions, he determined the weight of air and also showed that barometric pressure readings were an indication of altitude. He invented a hydrostatic press and a calculating machine, as well as devising theories of probability and of differential calculus. It is not surprising to learn that he was introduced to Cardinal Richelieu as "the wonder boy."

At 18 his health deteriorated. A general lassitude was accompanied by continual pains, including headache. In 1654, when he was aged 31, he became immersed in

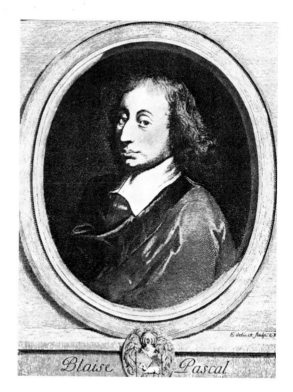

FIG. 2. Blaise Pascal. (From *Migraine Matters.*)

theology and he spent some time in the Jansenist Abbey of Port-Royal where his sister was a novitiate.

When he attained adulthood it was obvious that he had a mild facial asymmetry, the left side being a trifle smaller than the right (Fig. 2). This is well shown in his death mask.

Two important events are recorded. At the age of 24 he suddenly developed a weakness of the legs from the waist down, rendering him almost incapable of walking. Both legs were stone-cold and required friction with *eau de vie*. The nature of this temporary paraparesis is obscure, most authors favouring a psychogenesis. This symptom was followed by difficulty in swallowing cold liquids. Fluids had to be warmed and then sipped cautiously.

The other incident, given prominence by all biographers, was an alarming one, although Pascal escaped physical injury. He was enjoying a country ride in a coach drawn by four horses (some say six). They came to a narrow, unguarded bridge at Neuilly spanning the river Seine. The two leading horses swerved and fell into the water. The carriage itself remained on the bridge but tilted precariously. The date of this incident, which was much publicised, was 8 November 1654, when Pascal was 31 years of age.

Six years later the news got around that Pascal had become prey to a recurring phobia wherein he suddenly became aware of a yawning chasm on one or other side of him, usually the left, which threatened to engulf him. Thus arose the notorious legend of *l'abîme de Pascal*. The nature of this imaginary ravine or chasm was widely debated, and some regarded it as a hallucinatory symptom of a mental illness. At first it certainly terrorized Pascal, who would shift the surrounding furniture so that a chair would stand on one side of him as a mark of reassurance. At this time his health had worsened, and he was suffering intense headache, periodic fainting attacks, and colic.

Nonetheless, he continued to write his celebrated and masterly *Pensées* as a preliminary, it is believed, to a projected full-scale *Apologia*.

His health was never restored and at the early age of 39 he was critically ill. A sudden agonizing pain in the head was quickly followed by a violent convulsion. Other fits occurred in the ensuing days, and the end came on 10 August 1662.

An autopsy was performed. The liver and stomach were shrunken *(flétris)*, and a length of bowel was gangrenous. No evidence whatsoever of mesenteric tuberculosis could be found. The brain was characterized by a terminal intraventricular bleeding. Particular notice was taken of the skull bones where no trace of any sutures could be seen. At the point where the anterior fontanelle had existed in infancy was a localized bony overgrowth. (This finding may conceivably represent a limited degree of intracranial hyperostosis interna.)

Discussion

Such is the story of Blaise Pascal. That he had been a life-long migraineur had never been mooted prior to the monograph of Dr. R. Onfray (*L'Abîme de Pascal*. Imprimérie Alençonnaire, Alençon, 1949). The contention is an attractive one, for it explains the notorious "abyss" on the basis of a recurring hemianopia. That he was plagued by headaches there can be no doubt.

The diagnosis of migraine was confirmed in Onfray's opinion when he inspected the original manuscripts of *Les Pensées*. On 89 sheets of paper, the handwriting fills the page, leaving only a margin of the usual width on the left-hand side. There are, however, at least 30 sheets where the handwriting starts close to the left edge but the lines do not extend completely across to the right. In this way a compensatory broad and irregular margin is present on the right. It was Onfray's belief that such pages were written at a time when Pascal was in the throes of a right hemianopia.

Although Onfray did not comment, it might also be alleged that the handwriting on such sheets of paper was particularly untidy with a greater number of erasures. It could be argued that there were indications of a relative visual and intellectual malaise at such times, not severe enough, however, to incapacitate the writer completely.

The illustrations in Onfray's monograph unfortunately do not include any manuscript sheets that afford a plausible indication of a *left*-sided hemianopia, that is, pages with an excessively wide margin on the *left*. This is unfortunate because most of the accounts of Pascal's dreaded chasm refer to its being on his left-hand side. Pascal was also in the habit of writing brief observations either on small scraps of paper or on papers that were subsequently trimmed by scissors to a small size. These scraps would then be pasted onto the usual folio sheet. Here again the left-hand alignment was usually more accurate than the right.

Some of these scraps of paper would be covered with writing consisting of no more than three or perhaps four words to a line, and other lines would follow each other in a columnar fashion. This practice is difficult to explain.

As an additional piece of evidence favouring the diagnosis, Onfray drew attention to zigzag scribbles interrupting the text. There were two such phenomena on Fol. 251 of the manuscript. As Onfray said, such doodles are highly suggestive of a patient who in the early stages of an attack of migraine idly sketches the teichopsia he is experiencing. Such a practice is not unknown to migrainologists. In far more elaborate form it is to be found in the illuminated text of the mystical works of the Abbess Hildegaard of Bingen, a powerful and intelligent woman widely regarded as having been a victim of migraine. Is this particular page of the manuscript, then, to be regarded as additional evidence for migraine?

So rests the case for the diagnosis of migraine in Blaise Pascal. No one had proffered this explanation before Onfray in 1949. Is the evidence weighty enough?

Without doubt Pascal was a man of supernormal intellect but one obsessed with a complicated theistic philosophy. He was a highly sensitive individual whose childhood showed abundant signs of emotional disturbance. His sudden paraparesis—the precise duration of which we are not told—has yet to be explained. With the data available, it is impossible to exclude an organic problem. Multiple sclerosis comes to mind, but if that were so, Pascal's case would be the first to be recorded by a century and a half. One's instinct is to look upon that particular episode as hysterical.

Some would not hesitate to read into this record a migrainous diathesis. Pascal was admittedly a life-long victim of headache. There is, however, no evidence of periodicity, unilateral distribution, or accompanying nausea or vomiting. At no time is there any verbal, as opposed to pictorial, indication of teichopsia.

The notorious *abîme* which Pascal experienced is certainly suggestive of an hemianopia. One would have welcomed information as to how often this experience befell Pascal and how long each episode would last. Incidentally, how often do migrainous patients show such alarm when their visual field is disturbed? In a long experience I have never encountered or heard of such an excessive reaction.

Lastly, is the graphological documentation, interesting though it is, enough to warrant a confident diagnosis of ophthalmic migraine? Suggestive, I would say, but nonproven.

"Hemicrania" by Carolus Piso: A Seventeenth Century Personal Account of Migraine

Early in the sixteenth century there lived in Nancy, France, an apothecary named Le Pois or Lepois. In 1525 a son, Antoine, was born who later, after studying medicine in Paris, returned to his home town where he became court physician to Charles III, Duke of Lorraine, and his wife Princess Claude. Antoine's principal interest was, however, in numismatics.

His younger brother Nicolas, born in 1527, also qualified in Paris and practised in Nancy. When Antoine died in 1578, Nicholas succeeded him as medical adviser to the Duke of Lorraine. His researches into medical history were much admired by Boerhaave in Leyden.

Nicolas's youngest child was Charles, born in 1563. He studied medicine first in Paris and later at the University of Padua. In 1590 he too returned to Nancy where he succeeded his father, first as physician to Charles III and later to his successor Henri II. Moreover, he was appointed professor of medicine at the newly established University of Pont à Mousson. Among his writings was a monograph on hysteria, wherein he rejected the conventional uterine theory in favour of a cerebral origin. In 1633 he fell victim to typhus, which was raging at the time in and around Nancy.

In 1618 he had written an account of a malady with which he had been afflicted chronically, recognisable today as migraine. All his writings were in Latin, and he referred to himself under the classical sobriquet Carolus Piso.

His monograph, entitled *Hemicrania*, comprised a fairly detailed account of migraine as it affected him personally. The paper is a lengthy one because of a certain amount of repetition. As a clinical document it rates far below the writings of Thomas Willis on the same topic about a half-century later. Nevertheless, it is not by any means devoid of interest. Lepois recorded his observations in 1618 when he was 55 years of age.

We learn that his periodic headaches began when he was a boy, and he was tempted to ascribe them to the posture in which he slept, "leaving the head unprotected." These early headaches were not associated with vomiting or drowsiness, such symptoms appearing later in life.

His headaches increased in both violence and frequency when he was a student, presumably of medicine. This period of exacerbation lasted 4 years. Within the body of the written account we learn that the headaches particularly involved the front of the head, although later in the essay his headaches were said to be always right-sided.

Lepois' essay was both clinical and pathological—perhaps it would be more accurate to say "mythopathological"—the two aspects of hemicrania being considered together. In other words, he did not adopt the recognized technique of first describing the symptomatology in detail, then informing us about the frequency and duration of the attacks, the apparently precipitating factors, the treatments he received, and finally his ideas as to aetiology and pathogenesis. Unfortunately, these points were discussed in no logical order.

The author was a convinced follower of the humoural hypothesis concerning the disorder and also of the *modus operandi* of each attack. Like most of his contemporaries, he was an uncritical exponent of the ideas formulated by Galen, which retarded medical progress for many centuries.

During his adolescence and thereafter, Lepois experienced intense vomiting in association with his headache. He paid close attention to the appearance of the material vomited. Mostly he disgorged "a clear watery humour like the white of an egg." The fluid, he considered, emanated from the head, and he asked: "Why do we not acknowledge a head to be the source of the humour vomited in hemi-crania?" At other times, however, the watery humour contained some bile, and Lepois wondered whether or not in such cases there is "belly trouble arising from the liver and the fluid from the liver and the fluid from the head flows down to it."

Lepois commented that his headache was often assuaged after he had been sick. Migrainologists today would agree that this is often the case although by no means always so.

The author believed that in an attack of hemicrania the membranes of the head were "drawn together," a condition which disturbs the abdomen equally in all its parts, so "it is inevitable that the disordered gallbladder should overflow and pour out bile into the stomach." It must be remembered that until the outbreak of the Second World War migraine was confidently ascribed to a dysfunction of the gallbladder and, moreover, that one of the most favoured prophylactic measures consisted in the ingestion of bile salts thrice daily.

The very act of vomiting, as is well known, may intensify the headache for the moment. Lepois mentioned this fact, saying that the head may seem to be splitting in two, with the coronal suture bursting apart of its own accord. This he related to a temporary tightening of the meninges.

Lepois also referred to the sleepiness or stupor that steals over the victim of hemicrania at any hour of the day, "a not unwelcome bewitching or drugging of the pain." The source and origin of the sleep, according to the author, was to be found in the watery humour of the head. It is, of course, well known that at the end of an attack of migraine the patient usually sleeps. However, in protracted attacks lasting 2 to 4 days, sleep is disturbed either by vomiting, pain, or unpleasant dreams featuring pain equivalents.

Interesting remarks appeared in his monograph concerning some of the factors which provoke an attack of hemicrania. He emphasized meteorological causes. His own headaches were more frequent during the autumn, "not merely when the north wind was blowing but even when the atmosphere was calm after rain, or when rain-clouds broke across the sky." Contemporary specialists in migraine are well aware that sufferers are adversely affected by such climatic conditions as the mistral, or *Föhn*, in central Europe or the chinook which comes off the Rocky Mountains in America. Another agent which Lepois found precipitated his own hemicrania was toothache. An "intemperate mode of life" was also invoked as being unpropitious.

Sweating is not a typical symptom of migraine, but Lepois referred to this more than once. Possibly there were occasions when an attack of hemicrania happened to coincide with some independent febrile illness.

Nowadays we realise that attacks of migraine may vary in severity in the same patient. Moreover, the headache may not always be accompanied by either vomiting or drowsiness. Lepois was apparently aware of this fact, for he specifically stated that "it is possible for an individual not to be attacked by all these manifestations at one time, but by some at one time and by others at another."

The occurrence of visual aurae, whether in the way of fortification figures, scotomas, or hemianopia is nowhere mentioned. Presumably Lepois himself did not experience such phenomena; otherwise he could scarcely have refrained from giving them prominence.

Lepois was aware of the association of hemicrania with the menstrual cycle, for he wrote that during the terminal 20 hours of the cycle an attack of hemicrania would abate. Perhaps he realised that the premenstrual days were unfavourable, although he did not say so.

He firmly believed that there was an association between hemicrania and epilepsy, as Tissot was to proclaim later in 1790. This idea was one which died hard among physicians, and even such authorities as Gowers discussed the matter in his *Borderland of Epilepsy* in 1906. Headaches are undoubtedly common in epileptics, especially after a seizure, but the pains are not those of migraine. Again, some rare patients with migraine occasionally faint or otherwise lose consciousness in the course of an attack; Bickerstaff has spoken of this association under the term "basilar migraine." On the whole, however, it can be said that hemicrania and epilepsy are distinct, non-related entities.

Unlike Willis, Lepois was not alive to the common premonitory symptoms of euphoria, excessive appetite, and a feeling of well-being which so often occur during the evening before an attack.

The Case of Professor Max Müller, P.C., M.A. (1823–1900)

Until recently there was a widespread belief, or at least an impression, that a relationship of sorts exists between migraine and lofty intelligence. Thus in 1888 William Gowers, in his *Manual of Diseases of the Nervous System*, wrote: "The disease [migraine] is often associated with high intellectual ability, and many distinguished scientific men have suffered from it and have supplied more careful observations of the subjective symptoms than we possess of any other malady." Gowers drew attention to the monograph written by Edward Liveing, actually his next-door neighbour, who, despite his chronic ill health, eventually published a comprehensive treatise entitled *On Megrim and Sick-headache*.

This appeared in print in 1873, though largely compiled 10 years before. Liveing was more cautious but said: "We are often consulted with those in a somewhat higher social grade . . . where a development or aggravation of the malady has been brought about by excessive brain-work with a deficiency of bodily exercise, short restless nights, and insufficient sleep." In other words, it was not so much the commanding intellectual power which he felt to be at fault as the life style that *la vie spirituelle* engenders. Liveing went on to say: "the influence of these conditions . . . may often be seen among ambitious students, the candidates for University distinction or professional qualifications; and later in life as an effect of the struggle for competence or professional position." He spoke of "a latent neurosal disposition" and also of its more homespun equivalent, "brain-fag." "It is remarkable," Liveing continued, "how many distinguished literary and scientific men have suffered severely from megrim, and it would seem that some of them have succeeded in ridding themselves of the malady by the adoption of some simple hygienic measures." Liveing, too, had his own list of famed *migraineurs*, but neither he nor

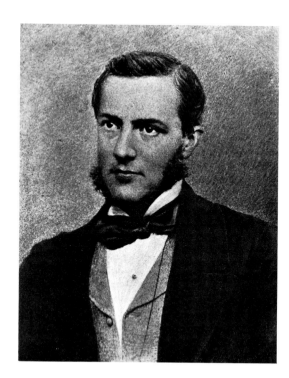

FIG. 3. Professor F. Max Müller at age 30.

Gowers made mention of an academic of whose erudition they must have been well aware, even if they had not been acquainted with him socially or professionally. I refer to that mastermind Professor Max Müller, Fellow of All Souls and holder of the Corpus Chair of Comparative Philology at Oxford (Fig. 3).

Max Müller was a German, born in 1823 in the town of Dessau within the Duchy of Anhalt, a region now lying within the Eastern bloc. We know little or nothing of the medical history of his parents (except that his paternal grandfather died at 61, prematurely senile), but both were of exceptional erudition and artistry. On the maternal side, there was a family history of deafness. His father, a teacher by profession but by predilection a poet, later became librarian to the Duke Leopold of Anhalt-Dessau. He wrote verses that were put to music by Schubert. His poem "Die schöne Mullerin" was a favourite of the singer Jenny Lind. His mother, also of high scholarship, came from an illustrious family. Her father had been the chief minister of the Duchy, and her mother was a musician and a descendant of von Basedow.

From quite an early age Max became devoted to music. He was a close friend of Mendelssohn and was known to Weber and Liszt.

He first attended the Nicolai School at Leipzig, where he excelled in Greek and especially in Latin. He also found time to write some verse and to continue his musical studies. However, at the age of 18 he gave up all ideas of a career in music and entered the local university to read literature and poetry. This was an important period of his life, for here he began his enduring preoccupation with Sanskrit and

Hinduism. At this juncture, too, he rejected an offer from a wealthy cousin of a post within the Austrian diplomatic service. Instead, he went on to the University of Berlin to pursue his Sanskrit studies. He also read philology under the aegis of Professor Franz Bopp, the first to study the comparative grammar of the Indo-European languages. Max Müller furthermore embarked upon a study of Arabic and Persian (now commonly spoken of as Farsi). His academic life in Berlin brought him in contact with von Humboldt, Rückert, and Schilling.

Max Müller's knowledge of Sanskrit induced the directors of the East Indian Company to offer him a grant to undertake the formidable task of translating, editing, and publishing the *Rig-Vedas*. He left Berlin in 1845 for Paris to study certain Sanskrit manuscripts in the Bibliothèque Nationale. He did not remain long enough in that city to attain real proficiency in French. His work next took him to London, where he was befriended by the wealthy Prussian diplomat Baron von Bunsen, a famed scholar in the fields of theology and philology.

Max Müller's engrossment in his Oriental researches caused him to reject the offer of a post as tutor and later the appointment as assistant librarian at the British Museum. It became necessary for him to consult certain manuscripts in the Bodleian Library, and this visit was the start of a life-long enchantment with Oxford. His academic prestige was furthered in 1847 when he read a paper at the British Association on the relationship between the Aryan and the aboriginal languages of India.

At the age of 25 Max Müller settled in Oxford where he remained until he died at age 77. While at Oxford he added Hebrew to his word bank. By this time he spoke English fluently, but he never lost his German accent overlaid by the intonation of Dessau. Incidentally, his command of written English became outstanding, his prose style being exceptionally attractive, lucid, and at times arresting. We are reminded of the mastery of English displayed by another foreign philologist, Otto Jespersen of Denmark. Perhaps Müller's prose owed something to his close friend Francis Palgrave, educationalist, later professor of poetry at Oxford and compiler of *The Golden Treasury.*

In 1850 Müller was invited to lecture at the Taylorian Institute on The History of Modern Languages. The Oxford authorities were deeply impressed, except for the Radcliffe librarian, Sir Henry Dyke Acland, who bit his nails and fidgeted throughout, muttering "these lectures frighten me." Müller's success led to his being appointed the Taylorian deputy professor and, later, full professor. His linguistic researches caused him to ponder deeply into the philosophy of language and its possible origins. He came to the realisation that *Ratio* and *Oratio* were one and the same, as implied by the Greek term *logos*. "Language is the autobiography of the human mind" was one of his tenets. Another of his statements was to the effect that the Liguria-Karinthia region of Europe was a veritable "linguistic rookery in which all the lost daughters of the European family of languages had taken refuge."

In 1854 Lord Macaulay visited Müller to seek advice about the languages appropriate for candidates seeking a career in the Indian Civil Service. Characteristically,

Macaulay did all the talking throughout the interview, giving Müller no opportunity to speak.

In 1861 he delivered at the Royal Institute a course of lectures which he published as a two-volume monograph entitled *The Science of Language*. This important work attracted considerable attention and also some controversy, as it conflicted in some ways with the views of Charles Darwin. By 1877 the book had run into nine editions.

Max Müller hoped that in due course he might succeed to the Boden professorship of Sanskrit. However, it was not to be. Instead, the University in 1868 founded for him a personal chair in comparative philology.

His chief loves were the philosophy and languages of ancient India. Although he never actually visited the Far East, he became a world-famed orientalist maintaining written contact with many contemporary Hindi scholars.

The nature of his life in Oxford is well told in his book *Auld Lang Syne*, published in two volumes in 1898 and 1899, respectively. Even in his terminal illness he dictated fragments of his autobiography, which was edited by his son and published posthumously in 1901. Throughout the whole of his life Müller dedicated himself to his work but was privileged to meet a host of notables in the arts, literature, science, politics, even royalty—a serious Chips Channon among the *cognoscenti* in fact. Some of those he met became intimate friends, including Dean Stanley, Matthew Arnold, Ruskin, Froude, Thackeray, Charles Kingsley, Tennyson, Browning, Emerson, and Oliver Wendell Holmes. Most of his time at Oxford he lived at No. 7 Norham Gardens, where in 1905 Osler and his wife came to live.

Within the pages of the autobiography we learn that Müller was a chronic migrainous sufferer. His own words may be quoted.

> As far back as I can remember I was a martyr to headache. No doctor could help me, no one seemed to know the cause. It was a migraine, and though I watched it carefully I could not trace it to any fault of mine. The idea that it came from overwork was certainly untrue. It came and went, and if it was one day on the right side it was always the next time on the left, even though I was free from it sometimes for a week or a fortnight, or even longer.
>
> It was also strange that it seldom lasted beyond one day, and that I always felt particularly strong and well the day after I had been prostrate. For prostrate I was and generally quite unable to do anything. I had to lie down and try to sleep. After a good sleep I was well, but when the pain had been very bad I found that sometimes the very skin of my forehead had peeled off. In this way I often lost two or three days in a week, and as my work had to be done somehow, it was often done anyhow, and I was scolded and punished, really without any fault of my own.
>
> After all remedies had failed which the doctor and nurses prescribed (and I well remember my grandmother using massage on my neck, which must have been about 1833 to 1835), I was handed over to Hahnemann....
> I swallowed a number of his silver and gold globules, but the migraine

kept its regular course, right to left and left to right and this went on till about the year 1860. Then my doctor...told me that he would cure me, if I would go on taking some medicine regularly for six months or a year. He told me that he and his brother had made a special study of headaches, and that there were so many kinds of headache, each requiring its own peculiar treatment....I was not a little abashed on being told that my headache was what they called the Alderman's headache...the doctor, seeing my surprise, comforted me by telling me that it was the nerves of the head which affected the stomach, and thus produced indirectly the same disturbance in my digestion as an aldermanic diet...what I do know is, that by taking the medicine regularly for about half a year, the frequency and violence of my headaches were considerably reduced, while after about a year they vanished completely. I was a new being and my working time doubled.

In his autobiography, Müller mentioned three doctors whom he had consulted at various periods: S. C. F. Hahnemann, Sir Andrew Clarke, and Dr. Symonds of Oxford.

S. C. F. Hahnemann (1755–1843) was, of course, a local physician in Germany. Born in nearby Meissen, he studied at Leipzig University and in 1789 settled in practice in that city. It was there that he advanced his famous "law of similars." In 1800 he was putting into practice his ideas of minimal doses, and in 1810 his principal work entitled *Organon der nationale Heilkunde*, or what he called homoeopathy, was published. This aroused so much hostility, especially among the apothecaries in the city, that in 1820 he was banished from Leipzig. However, he was befriended by the Grand Duke of Anhalt-Köthen, who permitted him to practise in the nearby town of Coethen.

From time to time he would visit Dessau in order to see patients, and it was then that the young Max Müller came under his care. Müller recalled him as a powerfully built man of imposing personality. Later in life, Hahnemann moved on to Paris where he pursued a lucrative practice, and where at the age of 80 he married a young lady, Melanie d'Hervilly. He continued to see patients, eventually dying at the age of 88.

Müller also later sought the advice of Sir Andrew Clarke...the "beloved physician"...but not for migraine. He had been suffering from one of his periodic attacks of hypochondriacal depression, insomnia, and anorexia. Sir Andrew examined him minutely and then assured him "with a bright look and a most convincing voice that he had never seen a man of my age so perfectly sound in every organ." The effect was dramatic. Feeling vigorous again and elated, he left Harley Street, where he unexpectedly bumped into a friend. The two of them dined together and shared dozens of oysters and some pints of porter with no ill effects.

Max Müller had much to say about the merits of a doctor who always instils confidence in his patients, an art which he realized as something more potent than physic. We are reminded of what Lord Conway wrote in 1651 to his migrainous daughter-in-law, the Viscountess Anne: "To have a good opinion of the Physitian doth contribute mutche to the case."

While living in Oxford Müller consulted a Dr. Symonds who was probably the brother of the famous Dr. John Addington Symonds of Bristol. The latter was the son of an Oxford general practitioner and hence the seventh doctor in direct succession. After qualification he went to Bristol where, along with a group of fellow Quakers, he established the General Hospital and became its founding physician. He rapidly attained a lucrative practice and took up residence in a beautiful mansion known as Clifton Hill House. His son, who bore the same name, became the famed historian of renaissance art. In 1858 Dr. J. Addington Symonds had delivered the Goulstonian lectures on the topic of headache, and many of his sagacious observations were subsequently quoted by Liveing.

The medication prescribed for Müller by the Symonds of Oxford proved successful; its nature we can only surmise. Probably Symonds followed his brother's advice and used as a prophylactic either muriate of ammonia or zinc valerianate, relying on strong coffee to alleviate an actual attack. Müller stated that he showed Dr. Symonds' prescription to a doctor friend in Germany who proclaimed he would not give it to a horse!...a comment which appears to be neither here nor there.

One is in some doubt as to what Dr. Symonds meant when in discussing Professor Müller's symptoms he referred to the "alderman's headache." Possibly he was implying an overindulgence in turtle soup and port, neither of which were applicable in Müller's case. Neuroanatomists are of course familiar with the alderman's nerve, which supplies the skin over the mastoid processes and which at a banquet one ceremoniously dabs with water to rekindle the appetite. By the term alderman's headache, Dr. Symonds might have meant a neuralgia of the superficial petrosal nerve.

Lastly, one is intrigued by Müller's statement that after an attack of headache the skin over the site of the pain might desquamate, a phenomenon first described by Dr. John Fordyce in 1758. This may represent that rare, but well-known symptom of herpetic vesiculation accompanying an attack of migraine. More likely the peeling of the skin was the result of a local application of a rubefacient. Symonds often recommended aconite ointment for the relief of any localized pain.

Professor Müller's accolade came in 1896 when Queen Victoria appointed him a member of her Privy Council. He died in 1900 at the age of 77. He had been ill for the 2 years previously from what appears to have been cerebrovascular insufficiency which, however, spared his great intellect.

Enough has been said to indicate the manifold accomplishments of Professor Müller. In itself polyglottism is not an index of superior intelligence, nor yet musicianship. Over and above these endowments Müller's intellectual status was such as is granted to few. Many would say no wonder he was a victim of migraine. Yet sapiency does not necessarily bring migraine in its train. Francis Galton was a near-genius but no *migraineur*. Hughlings Jackson never had a headache in his life.

Some writers have also described a "migraine personality." Mental rigidity, perfectionism, and obsessional modes of thought and behaviour have all been invoked. Professor Müller seems to have been free of such habits. His was a warm,

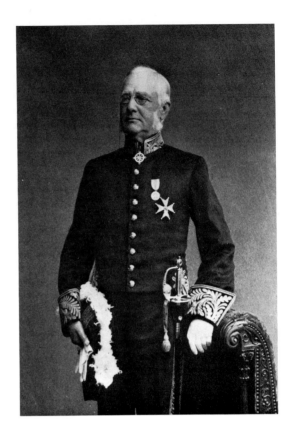

FIG. 4. Professor F. Max Müller later in life, in the uniform of a privy councillor.

high-minded disposition. He loved his work and his friends, and particularly his life in Oxford, though not its politics.

In his own words: "I take all the blame and shame on myself as a useless member of Congregation and Convocation, and of society at large. I was wrong in supposing that the walls of Jericho would fall before the blast of reason, and wrong in abstaining from joining in the braying of rams' horns and the shouts of the people. I was fortunate, however, in counting among my most intimate friends some of the most active and influential reformers in University, Church and State, and it is quite possible I may often have influenced them in the hours of sweet converse; nay, that standing in the second rank, I may have helped to load the guns which they fired with much effect afterwards."

Oscar Wilde and His Associations with the West Country

Oscar Wilde was associated with the West Country at two very different periods of his life: the commencement of his adult career and towards its end. It was while an undergraduate at Oxford that Wilde first began to visit Bristol and the surrounding countryside. In contrast, the city of Reading is unforgettably and tragically bound up with his days in prison.

Wilde's connection with Bristol primarily came about through his friendship with William Welsford Ward, a fellow student at Magdalen but a year senior. The two young men occupied rooms on the same kitchen staircase overlooking the Cherwell, and when Ward went down Wilde moved in. William Ward was the son of a well-known solicitor in Bristol. After attending school at Radley he went to Oxford, where he was for some reason or other widely known as "the Bouncer" or "little Mr. Bouncer" after a character in the popular Victorian novel by Cuthbert Bede, *Mr. Verdant Green.*

Several times Ward invited Wilde to stay with him in Bristol, at Cliff Court on Frenchay Common. This house (Fig. 1), which stood unaltered until quite recently, passed into the possession of a Dr. Elliott in 1898 and was lately the residence of Mr. Gordon Paul, F.R.C.S., a surgeon on the staff of the Bristol Royal Hospital.

On going down with a double first—like Wilde the following year—William Welsford Ward returned to Bristol and joined the family law firm. He became deeply immersed in local charities and activities, and was a keen supporter of the Gloucestershire Cricket Club in the days of Dr. W. G. Grace. In 1886 he married Charlotte Rogers of Carwinion, Cornwall. He died in February 1932, survived by a daughter, his only son having been killed in the First World War.

Many letters from Wilde to Ward are available, covering the period March 1876 until the summer of 1881. They are not of any great intrinsic interest or importance, being mainly chatty notes retailing the gossip of academic Oxford and the doings of mutual friends such as Reginald Harding, who was always referred to as "the Kitten" and who later became a member of the London Stock Exchange. In his letters Wilde often referred to visits to High Anglican or Roman Catholic churches and described how he had heard Cardinal Manning preach. The writings of Pusey and Liddon and the promulgation by the Pope of the doctrine of the Immaculate Conception were other matters which intrigued him, and he continued to comment on theological and ecclesiastical themes. He had just read Elizabeth Browning's

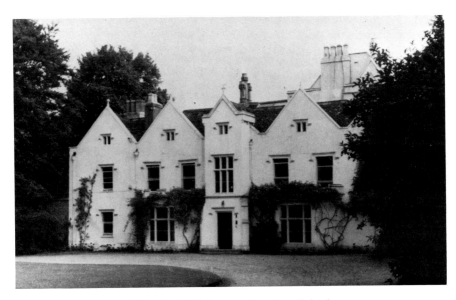

FIG. 1.   Cliff Court in Frenchay, Bristol.

Aurora Leigh, which with characteristic overenthusiasm he ranked with *Hamlet* and *In Memoriam*. In a faintly shocked fashion he mentioned having espied Charles Todd (destined to become chaplain general to the Royal Navy) seated in a private box in a theatre with a choirboy. Todd was probably only "mentally spooning" with the boy, he wrote, but it was foolish of him. He urged William Ward not to disclose this to anyone, as "it would do neither us nor Todd any good." Later he referred to a great friend of his mother, Aubrey de Vere, as a cultured but sexless poet and a convert to Catholicity (as he called it).

Oscar Wilde usually prefaced his letters to Ward by "My dear Bouncer" or "My dear boy." At first he signed himself "Your affectionate friend Oscar O'F. W. Wilde"—later, "Ever yours." That his cumbersome name was becoming to him a somewhat self-conscious thing is shown in a letter from Dublin which ended "Ever yours Oscar F. O'F. Wills Wilde", and as postscript "I like signing my name as if it was to some document of great importance as 'Send two bags of gold by bearer,' or 'Let the Duke be slain tomorrow and the Duchess await me at the hostelry.'"

Hints of a light-hearted turn of fine phrase and of literary banter now began to creep into his letters to Ward. He spoke of Elizabeth Browning "overstraining her metaphors till they snap." He wrote that he considered "that man's reason is the most misleading and thwarting guide that the sun looks upon—except perhaps the reason of woman."

When William Ward went down, Oscar Wilde and their mutual friend the Kitten gave him a heavy gold ring in the form of a buckled strap inscribed with the Greek words *Nmenósunon philiasantiphiloūnti philoi*, meaning "a token of friendship from two friends to a third." Inside were the initials "O.F.F.W. and R.R.H. to W.W.W. 1876." Today this ring lies among the treasures of Magdalen College.

Wilde continued to write after Ward had left Oxford and was travelling in Italy, and gossiped about the freshmen newcomers. He took up Masonry, which he hoped would not be an embarrassment to him if he finally decided to secede from what he called the "Protestant heresy," and he wrote about breakfasts with the Jesuit Father Parkinson of St. Aloysius'. He complained of his "Protestant jumps" and confessed he was "altogether caught in the fowler's snare, in the wiles of the Scarlet Woman," and he dreamed of paying a visit to Cardinal Newman. He did nothing of the sort, however, for he was shrewd enough to realise that to go over to Rome would be to sacrifice and give up his two great gods, "Money and Ambition." The tone of his correspondence grew more intimate. "Your letters," he wrote, "are charming, and the one from Sicily came with a scent of olive-gardens, blue skies and orange trees, that was like reading Theocritus in this grey climate. Ever, dear boy, your affectionate friend, Oscar Wilde."

In succeeding letters, more and more contrived phrases would creep in, faintly homosexual in hue. He referred to Robert Armitage (later a high dignitary of the Church of England) as having the most Greek face he had ever encountered. Regarding the varsity sports, he said: "Bullock-Webster's running was the most beautiful thing I have ever seen: . . . like a beautiful horse trotting."

As Wilde's finals drew near, he began to apply himself to study. Ward was now "My dear Willie" and Wilde was signing himself "Very truly yours, Oscar."

Wilde's last letter to Ward was from Tite Street, Chelsea, in June or July 1881. When Bogue published his collected poems, he wrote: "Dear Will, My volume is out: I wish you could review it: no one is more qualified to be a critic than you with your kind insight and exquisite taste. I wish in any case you would let me know what you think of it. But I am very anxious to be read, and a review in a Bristol paper might cause a sale in that lovely old town. Ever affectionately yours, Oscar."

The Wilde–Ward friendship seems to have gradually petered out. After Ward's death, his daughter Miss Cecil Ward handed over the letters to Magdalen College. Subsequently the president showed them to Wilde's son, Vyvyan Holland, who reproduced them in his book entitled Son of Oscar Wilde. An appendix to this volume contained an essay on Wilde at Oxford written by W. W. Ward.

There were still other reasons why Wilde was fond of Bristol and enjoyed his visits. One attraction was Clevedon Court (Fig. 2) with its remarkable collection of family portraits—still to be seen there. Wilde was familiar with the fact that Thackeray had been a frequent visitor to the house. He had depicted Clevedon Court in Henry Esmond under the pseudonym "Castlewood" and had written much of this novel while staying there. Thackeray had been emotionally involved with one of the family, Jane Octavia Elton (Fig. 3), who was then married to the Reverend Brookfield (Fig. 4), curate of St. James's, Piccadilly. These were the parents of the actor Charles Brookfield (Fig. 5), whose malice did so much to bring about Wilde's downfall in 1895. Here then is dramatic irony indeed. Wilde probably knew, too, about the association of Clevedon and Clevedon Court with Arthur Henry Hallam, to whom Tennyson dedicated his In Memoriam.

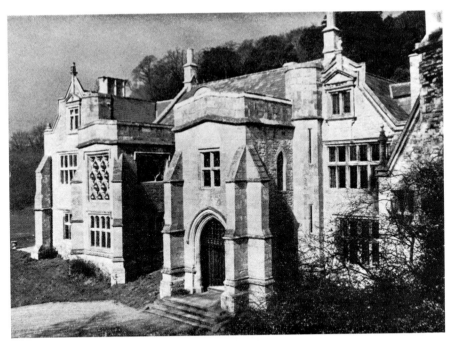

FIG. 2. Clevedon Court in Somerset, near Bristol. The South Front.

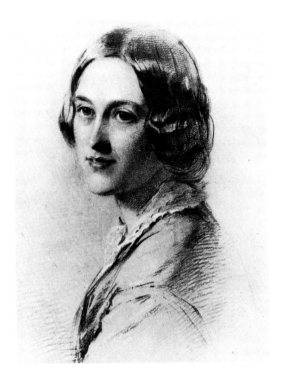

FIG. 3. Jane Octavia Brook-field at age 30.

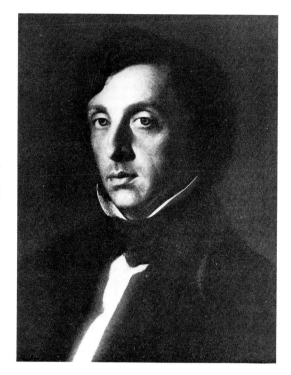

FIG. 4. The Reverend William Henry Brookfield at age 40. From the painting by Samuel Laurence.

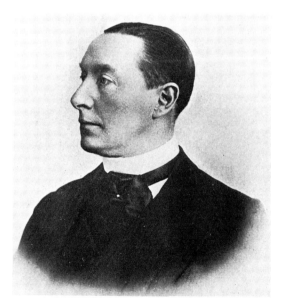

FIG. 5. Charles H. E. Brookfield.

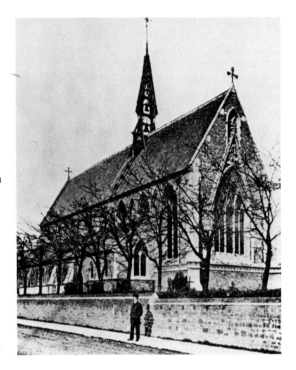

FIG. 6. St. Raphael's Church in Bristol.

In 1884 Sir Edmund Harry Elton, the owner of Clevedon Court, was much interested in applied art and instigated the local Sunflower Pottery. It is possible that Wilde's interest in Clevedon Court was focused more upon the so-called Elton ware than upon the family portraits.

Another reason for Wilde's interest in Bristol was the notorious St. Raphael's Church on the Cut (Cumberland Road). The chaplain, the Reverend A. H. Ward, was in all probability a relation of William W. Ward, the Bouncer. For more than one reason St. Raphael's was a very unusual church (Fig. 6). It had been founded by the Reverend Robert Miles, the rector of Bingham, Notts, and Prebendary of Lincoln Cathedral, with whom the undergraduate Wilde used to stay. The rector was a member of the wealthy Miles family of Bristol. Another relative was Frank Miles, the artist, also a close friend of Wilde's when they were both at Oxford. Later they shared rooms in Keats' house in Chelsea, but afterwards they fell out, parted company, and Miles died later in a Bristol mental hospital. The Miles's had endowed an almshouse for the widows of seamen, in addition to St. Raphael's Church. The latter, which became known as the "Sailors' College," was opened in May 1859. The Chapel was unusually beautiful, with fine gothic entrances and interesting corbels depicting a friar and a nun. St. Raphael's soon became a source of scandal throughout the country because of its high church practices. The ornate and elaborate ceremonial provoked wide comment, even scandal, with its stations of the cross and ornate statuary, and the church attracted many fashionable ritualists. Complaints were made, and throughout 1877 the bishop of Gloucester repeatedly urged the Reverend Ward to abandon his illegal ceremonial. The chaplain replied that he could not conscientiously do so, and in March 1878 the bishop revoked Ward's licence. The church, which as a matter of fact had never been consecrated, was closed, and it remained so until 1893. Thereafter it was reestablished under the auspices of clerics who were more conforming in their practices. In 1940 a German bomb caused much damage, though short of total destruction. In 1946 the church was declared redundant and was demolished.

Yet another attraction in Bristol was the romantic associations with the ill-fated boy-poet Thomas Chatterton. Wilde felt strongly that a memorial should be erected, and perhaps a museum as well, somewhere in Bristol, preferably within the precincts of Colston's School, Chatterton's *alma mater*. This never came about, but an official collection of Chattertoneana was opened on the occasion of the poet's bicentenary within his original dwelling opposite Redcliffe Church. It contains a life-size statuette of a boy dressed in the uniform of a Colston scholar of that time. The collected letters of Oscar Wilde, so ably edited by Rupert Hart-Davis, contain several references to Thomas Chatterton, and we learn that Wilde lectured at Birkbeck College on the subject of Chatterton—the writings which he had bogusly ascribed to a nonexistent medieval poet—and his suicide.

Finally, one may mention two other indirect associations between Wilde and Bristol: One is Oscar's elder brother William (an intelligent but alcoholic ne'er-do-well, usually spoken of as "Wuffalo Will"), who was engaged at one time to the composer Ethel Smythe, then living in Bristol. Secondly, Edward William Godwin (who was born in Bristol and was Ellen Terry's husband) happened to be his friend and also the architect who decorated his house in Tite Street, Chelsea.

Aside from the foregoing associations, the most obvious activity which drew Wilde to the West Country was his capacity as a lecturer, discussing *art nouveau* and the aesthetic movement. The opening of *Patience* at the Savoy Theatre on 23 April 1881 was topical indeed, for contemporary taste in applied arts was undergoing a revolution. In September *Patience* also opened in New York. Wilde has often been regarded as the prototype of Bunthorne, but it is more likely that Gilbert and Sullivan had Rossetti in mind. Nonetheless, Wilde and his eccentricities were now so notorious that they offered a wonderful opportunity for theatrical publicity. To launch Wilde on an American lecture tour was almost certainly a calculated act, either to advertise the latest of the Gilbert and Sullivan operettas or to cash in on its success.

Wilde (Fig. 7) therefore embarked upon an American lecture tour, arriving in New York in January 1882 and leaving in December that same year. An account of Wilde's transatlantic adventures, his quips and wisecracks, and the response of his American audiences would occupy a lecture in itself. Returning to England, Wilde was sent off on a hectic provincial tour which occupied most of his next 2 years.

On Monday, 3 March 1884, we find Wilde visiting Bristol. Staying at the Royal Hotel, he lectured in the afternoon and again in the evening at the Victoria Rooms (Fig. 8). The topic of the first talk was The House Beautiful, and the second concerned his personal impressions of America. Both lectures were said to have

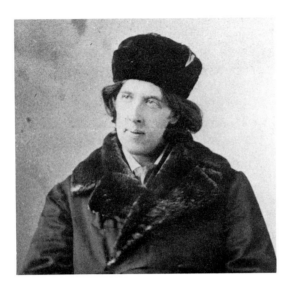

FIG. 7.   Oscar Wilde in America.

been "tolerably well" attended despite bad weather, and the audiences were attentive and appreciative. The orchestra pit in front of the stage had been arranged by a local furnishing store so as to resemble a drawing room, with exquisite curtained screens and oak cabinet work. Another local firm was responsible for a selection of art wall decorations, Wilde himself having chosen the furniture and supervised the layout.

Both lectures were admirably reported in the local papers of that time. It would be interesting to discover the identity of these anonymous journalists, for their comments were refreshing and at times witty.

Wilde's attire naturally came in for comment. All the reporters agreed that his clothes were "surprisingly inconspicuous." He wore morning dress. The trousers were a vivid plaid, of a broad check material such as one might expect to see in a

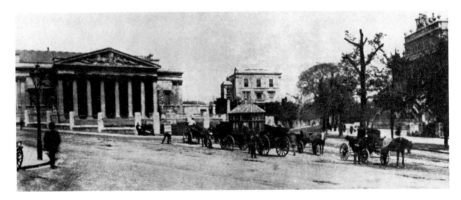

FIG. 8.   Victoria Rooms in Bristol.

cartoon in *Punch*. His necktie and breast-pocket handkerchief were of a matching tint described as "a compromise between pink and terra-cotta," and his collar was low and down-turned. Wilde himself was said to be striking in appearance, being tall and well built, with a fine curly head of hair, admirably regular features, fine eyes, and a clean-shaven face. His voice was fine and ringing, melodious and pleasant, and skilfully employed. After making his bow, he deposited upon the table his light-yellow gloves and white handkerchief, caressing them alternately with his reversed linen cuffs. The lecture was the exposition of an enthusiast, delivered in admirable style. The speaker possessed high elocutionary and histrionic powers, "with no more affectation than one might expect in the average curate." His gestures were "animated and appropriate"; "not infrequently his eyes would be fixed in rapt contemplation on the ceiling," though whether in silent disapproval of its design was not clear to the reporter. Each paper made mention of Wilde's wit and his sense of humour. Every now and again he would give an anticipatory and irrepressible smile, which heralded a clever bit of ridicule directed against some horror of nineteenth-century house furnishing or decoration which met with his condemnation or dislike.

In October of the same year Wilde revisited Bristol to lecture on the subject of Dress. This lecture makes faintly amusing reading today. It is sadly dated, of course, but to the historian interested in social Victoriana it is an important document. The more florid period of Wilde's dress was after all an anticipation of the contemporary sartorial extravagances of Carnaby Street. We recall Whistler's caustic letter to the Committee of the Natural Art Exhibition of November 1886: "What has Oscar in common with Art? Nothing except that he dines at our tables and picks from our platters the plums for the puddings he peddles in the provinces..."

Let us turn over the pages of history a dozen years. Wilde had by now become famous, successful, and tolerably rich. Whether his fame rested upon merely a second-rate modicum of talent is still a matter of debate. St. John Ervine, a stern critic, called Wilde a minimum poet, bloated and vain, who bragged and boasted of success, and sneered at rivals. This may be a little harsh. But like most hysterical psychopaths, Wilde certainly came to regard himself as outside and above the law, one to whom the common rules of behaviour did not apply. Yet another deviation had developed. The fastidious artist in words and ideas began deliberately to plunge into the depths and dregs of experience. As Ervine, again, has said, the florid life was no longer the whole of his existence; there were also the pseudo-aesthetic, heavily curtained rooms smelling of stale incense in the back streets of Westminster, where mincing stable-boys were waiting to be visited. As Wilde wrote years later, "I went down the primrose path to the sound of flutes. But...I had to pass on. The other half of the garden had its secrets for me also." During these heady years of achievement, the stage was being set with great care for the performance of a strange tragedy in which there was not a single noble character, in which comedians were suddenly called upon to take tragic parts for which they were unfitted both by temperament and appearance. The words are again those of St. John Ervine, but in the climate of extreme biographical tolerance which exists today they surely need saying. As inevitable as in a Greek tragedy, events caught up with Wilde. When the showdown came he behaved with such blind folly, making one false move after another, that he almost literally broke into Reading Gaol.

On 25 May 1895 he was sentenced to 2 years' hard labour for gross indecency. From Pentonville he went to Wandsworth, and on 13 November 1895 he was transferred to Reading Goal to serve out the rest of his term.

It is often stated that the circumstances of his imprisonment constituted a brutal psychic trauma. The authority is Wilde, but the story has been taken up with embellishments by one commentator after another. It is alleged that a change of trains took place at Clapham Junction and that for 30 minutes Wilde shivered on the station platform in handcuffs (or chained with other convicts; or manacled between two warders—the accounts differ), during which time he was the cynosure of flocks of gaping travellers who recognised him, tittered, and made uncouth comments. One man actually spat in Wilde's face. The sheer improbability of these allegations and the stark inconsistency of the details are only too often overlooked. Let us not gloss over the fact that Wilde was an unreliable and overimaginative witness who lied when it suited him and whose friends were even less scrupulous in their testimonies.

Whatever the truth of this episode, we may recall the verse written by James Agate (*Ego 4*, p. 124. Harrap, London, 1940) on the opening night of the revival in 1938 of *The Importance of Being Earnest*:

> *Volte-Face*
>
> He spat and passed.
> The pederast
> Nor bowed, nor shook his head;
> The world unkind
> Drew down the blind
> On one it deemed was dead.
>
> The man who hissed,
> The moralist,
> Now laughs to split his side;
> The world uncertain
> Rings up the curtain
> On one who has not died.

The abrupt translation to the shame and rigors of imprisonment naturally provoked a severe reaction in one who had for so long lived a life of pampered ease. Wilde's luxuriant hair was cropped, and he was made to wear coarse canvas suits marked with broad arrows. He slept on a plank bed devoid of mattress or pillow. His hard labour entailed the teasing-out of ship's rope. Cannonballs had to be carried from one pile in the courtyard to another in the opposite corner, and then back again. Finally, he was made to work the heavy treadmill for 15 minutes on end, with a 5-minute break; and then another spell, and so on. Conversation, reading, and writing were not allowed. For months visitors were forbidden. At mealtimes, Wilde, whose table had always been red with wine and roses, was given meat, black bread, and water.

Undoubtedly Wilde developed a severe depression with insomnia and loss in weight; there is some indication too of delusions and nocturnal hallucinations. Robert Ross visited Wilde in Reading Gaol and described how thin he had become. His face was a dull brick colour and his eyes horribly vacant. Throughout the interview he wept and proclaimed he had nothing to say: He feared he was losing his reason.

As a prisoner, Wilde must have come in touch with criminals from all classes of society and of every psychological and antisocial type. Unfortunately, we know little of what Wilde thought of his fellows and nothing at all of what they made of him. However, Wilde was brought into contact with three important individuals where the relationship is known.

First was the prison governor, Colonel Isaacson. Although never afforded the opportunity of defending himself, the governor has been written off as a harsh, small-minded, and bigoted administrator. The very nature of Wilde's offence seemingly provoked a violent reaction within his prejudiced system of moral standards. Wilde was no cunning old lag and as a bewildered first offender often was in trouble. For these infringements the governor handed out oppressive and uncomprehending punishment. Isaacson carried out the penal system with the greatest harshness and stupidity. Redress of a kind came eventually, however. Wilde petitioned the Home Secretary not only for a reduction of sentence but also for mitigation of the austerities which fell so heavily on him. Outside the prison there were influential friends who were not inactive. Wilde complained of the total lack of humane or humanising circumstances; the absence of books and of writing materials; of his increasing deafness and failure of sight. He feared he was going out of his mind.

In due course some alleviation followed, after Colonel Isaacson left to take up another appointment.

The second contact was the prison doctor, Dr. Oliver Calley Maurice (Fig. 9), a worthy practitioner of Reading, a Justice of the Peace, and surgeon to the Royal Berkshire Hospital. He was also medical officer to the local police, to Reading School, and the Blue Coat School. Furthermore, he was an original member of the select Aston Key dining club, which unfortunately no longer exists. He was the president of the Reading Pathological Society in 1897. Born in 1837 in Marlborough, he qualified at St. Thomas' Hospital. He was the founder of a distinguished family dynasty of highly respected doctors who settled in Marlborough and district but who had been trained at St. Mary's.

Dr. Maurice and Oscar Wilde did not hit it off. Wilde found him unsympathetic; the doctor regarded the prisoner as shamming. Robert Ross interviewed both the governor and the medical officer at Reading Gaol and took a dislike to both. Ross found the doctor "snuffling and shuffling about, making impatient gestures." Wilde wrote of a horrible duel between a half-witted prisoner and the doctor. The doctor was fighting for a theory; the man was fighting for his life.

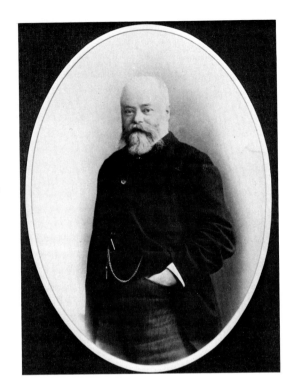

FIG. 9. Dr. Oliver Calley Maurice.

There can be no two opinions, however, about the third person who influenced Wilde in gaol. I am referring to Isaacson's successor, Major Nelson. The new governor went out of his way to temper the wind as far as Wilde was concerned. Because of directives from the Home Office and the recommendations of visiting Justices, made up of such local notables as Alex Cogham, Charles Hay, Munter, Thursby, and George Palmer, the prisoner was seen by an aurist and an oculist; appropriate treatment was afforded for his otitis, and glasses were furnished. His mental state was also reported upon by Dr. Nicholson from Broadmoor Criminal Lunatic Asylum. Most important of all, Wilde was permitted to write in his cell, and books were provided according to his own choosing. It is of interest to observe the volumes which Wilde requested. They included a Greek testament; Milman's *History of the Jews*; works of Tennyson, Marlowe, Carlyle, Dante, Keats, Chaucer, and Spenser; Renan's *Vie de Jesus*; Ranke's *History of the Popes*; and essays by Cardinal Newman and by Emerson. Major Nelson had censored some other requested items, including Lecky, Huysmans, Dickens, and Walter Pater. The Home Office approved the amended list, provided the total cost was not more than £10.

When further books were permitted, Wilde asked for language texts. He decided to tackle German, saying that prison seemed to be the proper place for such a study. Italian grammars and dictionaries were also requested, as well as the works of Wordsworth, Matthew Arnold, Hallam, Dryden, Burns; the *Morte d'Arthur*, and Froissart's *Chronicles*.

A third gift of books included works by Meredith, Hardy, R. L. Stevenson, Rossetti, the Goncourts, Goldoni, and Filon. On this occasion, Huysmans slipped past the governor's ban, probably because this author had been recently commended by W. E. Gladstone. The line was drawn, however, at current issues of the monthly review *Nineteenth Century.*

The foregoing books were apparently regarded as part of the prison library and were not taken out by Wilde on his release. It would be interesting indeed to learn the present whereabouts of these volumes, which are no longer within the precincts of the gaol.

Richest gift of all, however, was the privilege of ink and pen and four foolscap sheets of prison paper daily. Wilde now applied himself to the composition of his *De Profundis*, which, like Dostoevski's *Memoirs from the House of the Dead*, ranks among such powerful *Gefängnisschriftssum* as St. Paul's *Prison Epistles*, Bunyan's *Pilgrim's Progress*, and Hitler's *Mein Kampf*. Each night the four written sheets were collected, and each day saw the maturation of one of the most curious pieces of prose in the English language. In essence it was a bitter invective against his protegé, Lord Alfred Douglas. The impression he leaves upon the reader is that of an insincere, self-pitying poseur. After his release from prison, Wilde handed the manuscript to Robert Ross, who had copies typed and then locked away in the British Museum for 60 years. Ten years after Wilde's death an expurgated version was published, the bitterest diatribes being suppressed. However, 3 years after that, the High Court ordered the full text to be produced, and Douglas for the very first time became aware of the full savagery of Wilde's philippic from gaol and his strange duplicity after his release.

Despite the overall artificiality of *De Profundis*, here and there one stumbles upon instances of magnificent writing. For example:

> If after I am free a friend of mine gave a feast, and did not invite me to it, I should not mind a bit. I can be perfectly happy by myself. With freedom, flowers, books, and the moon, who could not be perfectly happy? Besides, feasts are not for me any more. That side of life is over for me, very fortunately, I daresay. But if after I am free a friend of mine had a sorrow and refused to allow me to share it, I should feel most bitterly. If he shut the doors of the house of mourning against me, I would come back again and again and beg to be admitted, so that I might share in what I was entitled to share in. If he thought me unworthy, unfit to weep with him, I should feel it as the most poignant humiliation, as the most terrible mode in which disgrace could be inflicted on me. But that could not be. I have a right to share in sorrow, and he who can look at the loveliness of the world and share its sorrow, and realise something of the wonder of both, is in immediate contact with divine things, and has got as near to God's secret as anyone can get....

What of the famous *Ballad of Reading Gaol*? Wilde had been greatly moved when a fellow prisoner was executed for the murder of his young sweetheart. After his release, he composed this piece of versification, virtually his last major literary effort. Though pregnant with feeling, the ballad is mawkish, contrived, unconvincing, and of minimal artistic worth. It does not approach the standard to which Wilde had aspired when as a prisoner he had written: "if I can produce only one beautiful work of art, I shall be able to rob malice of its venom, and cowardice of its roots."

Let us not leave with any too bitter memory of the poet Wilde, the playwright and scintillating wit, as one who had been victimised at the hands of harsh Victorian prudery. May we perhaps forget the sordid incarceration, the treadmill, the solitary confinement, the oakum-picking, the bread and water. Wilde himself mellowed. He wrote that he would go out of gaol remembering the great kindness that he had received here from almost everybody, and on the day of his release he would give thanks to many people and ask to be remembered by them in turn. This indeed was so. Free once again, he corresponded with some of the prison officers and with Major Nelson, to whom he sent a signed copy of the *Ballad*. In a letter to the *Daily Chronicle*, he described the governor as a man of gentle and humane character, greatly liked and respected by all the prisoners. Though he could not alter the rules of the prison system, he had altered the spirit with which they had been carried out under his predecessor. Popular with prisoners and warders, he had quite elevated the whole tone of prison life. Of Martin, one of the warders, Wilde wrote how struck he had been by the singular kindness and humanity with which he spoke to him and to the other prisoners. "Kind words are much in prison, and a pleasant 'Good morning' or 'Good evening' will make one as happy as one can be in solitary confinement. Martin was always gentle and considerate." In Wilde's case the immediate shock of prison life had been catastrophic: the subsequent reaction, gentle. For the first year of his imprisonment he could only wring his hands and cry: "What an ending, what an appalling ending!" But towards the end of his time he would often exclaim: "What a beginning, what a wonderful beginning!"

Finally, let us play a literary feedback and recall the glorious sonnet written by Lord Alfred Douglas, whose life with that of Wilde had for years intermingled in a tragic saraband:

> I dreamed of him last night, I saw his face
> All radiant and unshadowed of distress
> And as of old, in music measureless
> I heard his golden voice and marked him trace
> Under the common thing the hidden grace,
> And conjure wonder out of emptiness,
> Till mean things put on beauty like a dress
> And all the world was an enchanted place.
>
> And then methought outside a fast locked gate
> I mourned the loss of unrecorded words
> Forgotten tales, and mysteries half said
> Wonders that might have been articulate,
> And voiceless thoughts like murdered singing birds;
> And so I woke, and knew...that he was dead.

Arteriosclerotic Pseudo-Parkinsonism

In 1929 my paper on arteriosclerotic parkinsonism appeared in *Brain*. It attracted no little attention, and this expression passed smoothly into the currency of neurology. However, since the significance of dopamine began to unfold, coupled with the dramatic effect of the ingestion of L-dopa, doubts accumulated as to the status of arteriosclerotic varieties. Some went so far as to express the view that it was an imaginary disorder, wholly unrelated to the condition known as paralysis agitans or Parkinson's disease. I am well aware that there are mythical maladies of the nervous system, a topic which I have described elsewhere, but arteriosclerotic parkinsonism, I strongly submit, does not belong to that category.

Let it be stated emphatically that the essential nature of Parkinson's disease was not established 25 years ago with the discovery that certain transmitter substances in the palaeostriatum was deficient. The story of parkinsonism is older, more complex, and more interesting.

Few neurologists today can realise that during the second decade of this century their senior colleagues were seeing actually more cases of postencephalitic parkinsonism than of conventional paralysis agitans. The appearance of this striking extrapyramidal disorder in young adults had something dramatic about it, for scarcely ever before, since 1817 when James Parkinson published his monograph on "the shaking palsy," had this syndrome been observed except in the middle-aged. The excitement aroused was considerable, just as widespread and profound as the resurgence of interest sparked off by the advent of L-dopa.

Neurologists of the last generation also became alive to the fact that a chronic encephalitis was not the only aetiological factor which might provoke the onset of a syndrome emulating the shaking palsy. My senior colleague Kinnier Wilson, who devoted most of his professional life to uncovering the mysteries of what he called "the old motor system," isolated a clinical variant associated with neurosyphilis—then quite a common disorder. He spoke of "mesencephalitis syphilitica," preferring it to the alternative terms "syphilitic parkinsonism" or "paralysis agitans with tabes," and there was an extensive literature on the subject.

At about the same time it was also realised and never disputed that parkinsonism could appear as an industrial disease in those who worked with crude manganese. Here again there was no argument: The evidence was too great.

Occasional references also appeared in the literature suggesting that a parkinsonian-like state could arise in patients with deep-seated, infiltrating brain tumours. Admittedly this was a great rarity, and many neurologists would probably be sceptical about this association.

Then, too, arose the suggestion that sometimes a parkinsonian-like picture could develop after head injury. This important medicolegal conception became, as can be imagined, a source of heated argument, with flushed and angry clinicians maintaining an attitude either strongly for or violently against. Sometimes their viewpoint actually varied as chance took them from one high court to another. However shaky the scientific basis for such a hypothesis, no neurologist who has had experience of punch-drunk boxers, as I have, can deny that extrapyramidal signs are often so prominent in some patients with dementia pugilistica, as to raise difficulties in the differential diagnosis.

Thus arose the conception that parkinsonism was a syndrome with multiple aetiologies, and that idiopathic paralysis agitans was merely the clinical model where the causation was obscure, possibly abiotrophic.

Then came World War II, and interest waned. However, the idea of symptomatic parkinsonism became resuscitated during the 1940s, when our psychiatric colleagues found themselves furnished with pharmacological weapons, the nature of which they only dimly understood. We now began to witness iatrogenic parkinsonian states consequent upon the prodigal employment of such drugs as phenothiazine, reserpine, and many others.

It was against the background of the realisation that there was something inherently vulnerable about the extrapyramidal system that arteriosclerotic parkinsonism saw the light. There was nothing novel about it, and it was no rarity: anything but. Those conversant with the rich European literature of that time were aware that the Germans were familiar with a syndrome they called *"arteriosklerotische Muskelstarre"* that was liable to affect hypertensive, middle-aged arteriopaths. A comparable picture was also familiar to the pioneer neurogeriatricians, and Jakob had described a syndrome of dementia, advanced age, and a parkinsonian-like state. Those who were acquainted with this picture in nonagenarians called it Jakob's disease, not to be confused with the Jakob-Creutzfeldt syndrome.

That illustrous group of French neurologists was likewise aware that a disability reminiscent of Parkinson's disease could arise in arteriosclerotics. Pierre Marie in particular was eloquent on this subject. He demonstrated a pathological condition where the basal ganglia and adjacent white matter were riddled with minute perforations like a sieve, an appearance he called the *état criblé*. This worm-eaten state was partly due to multiple small infarctions, but partly also to shrinkage of the white matter in the posterior perforated zone, away from the tiny blood vessels coming up from below. Pierre Marie described this entity as a "progressive lacunar degeneration," and it became customary to refer to an individual patient as a *"lacunaire."* It is of interest that this particular pathology can at times be visualized in a brain scan.

There is no real difference between the arteriosclerotic parkinsonism that I described, the arteriosclerotic muscle rigidity of the Germans, and the French conception of progressive lacunar degeneration.

Far from being a rarity, it is commonplace, and, as I have repeatedly emphasized, one is perhaps more likely to meet with such cases socially than professionally.

Indeed, on one occasion when I was speaking of this condition before a distinguished if sceptical audience of my colleagues, there was seated in the front row a most striking and unmistakeable example of the syndrome, a friend whom I viewed with mixed feelings of sadness, embarrassment, but clinical understanding.

I have stressed the similarities between the arteriosclerotic and the idiopathic types of parkinsonism. Are there any differences? There are.

1. Tremor does not occur.

2. Additional focal manifestations may complicate the arteriosclerotic cases, depending upon the presence and site of other ischaemic foci. Hence pyramidal, cerebellar, or pseudobulbar pictures may coexist.

3. The psychical state may differ. Emotivity is common and mild dementia not rare, especially in the later stages.

4. The course of the disability is not the same. Rarely is there a steady downhill progression. The descent may be step-like, as in a shopper who prefers to walk downstairs rather than use an escalator. The prognosis really turns upon cardiovascular and cerebrovascular considerations.

5. Arteriosclerotic parkinsonians are not helped by L-dopa, and presumably there is no cellular deficiency in dopamine. Consequently, studies on Parkinson's disease which are epidemiological, genetic, and pharmacological in nature should be strictly confined to the idiopathic cases of paralysis agitans and exclude all symptomatic types, whatever their aetiology. Otherwise, statistics become hopelessly disarrayed and meaningless.

It can therefore be argued that all the symptomatic cases of parkinsonism—syphilitic, postencephalitic, arteriosclerotic, etc.—are states which are merely mirrors of the picture painted by Parkinson 160 years ago. In retrospect, I will admit that it would have been more appropriate to have spoken of arteriosclerotic *pseudo*-parkinsonism, but no other disclaimer will I make.

Suspension Treatment of Patients with Tabes Dorsalis

Tabes dorsalis is such a rare disease these days that it is hard to imagine the long, drawn-out misery of such patients with their intractable lightning pains and their unsteady gait. The symptoms were resistant to stock palliative measures especially as the syphilitic aetiology was for a long time not proved, although suspected, and the modern specific treatment had yet to be discovered.

Little wonder that Romberg in his *Manual of Nervous Diseases* wrote: "If in any case the busy activity of the physician increases the sufferings of the patient, it is in tabes dorsalis. When one of these unfortunate individuals presents himself to us, we generally find his back seamed with cicatrices; he brings us a heap of prescriptions; and gives a long list of the watering places he has visited in search of health.... Incurable patients should be allowed to spend their lives quietly in their family circle, that their last moments may be soothed by the fond cares of those whom they love."

It was in such a climate of ineptitude that a form of treatment was devised which purported to stretch mechanically the spinal roots and even the cord itself. That such a drastic measure could conceivably be of service in reducing pain was suggested by the practice of treating sciatica with forced extensor movements of the lower limb.

Gowers referred to this stretching procedure in his *Manual* of 1886. The first to adopt this technique, he said, was Langenbach. (Gowers gave no reference.) From the text it is uncertain whether the case in question was one of sciatica or locomotor ataxia. Stretching of the nerve trunk in the leg under general anaesthesia was followed by "remarkable and mysterious lessening both of pain and of incoordination." Later the patient underwent stretching of the upper limb in an effort to relieve pain in that situation. The patient died under the anaesthetic, and Westphal, who carried out a postmortem examination, reported that the spinal cord was healthy, but he did not explore the peripheral nerves or the brachial plexus.

It seems that suspension at the neck level as a remedy for tabetics was the idea of Professor Moczutkorski of Odessa, based no doubt on the experience of peripheral nerve traction in cases of sciatica. According to Gowers, this suspension manoeuvre had since been carried out many times in tabetics. In some, the pains were temporarily relieved; in a few instances the ataxia became for a time less marked. In many cases no improvement followed. Obviously sceptical, Gowers proclaimed that suspension was justifiable only as a last resort and only in patients in whom the pains were intense, and where the principal site of pain was in the distribution of the sciatic nerve. He warned against promises that were too sanguine, and he mentioned the risks of death under chloroform, of erysipelas, and of spinal haemorrhage. His conclusion was that suspension was a form of therapy that was "passing into merited disuse," and that "it will probably before long be forgotten."

When Moczutkorski's contrivance reached the ears of Charcot, he deputed his assistant Gilles de la Tourette to put this form of therapy to the test. In collaboration with Chipault he studied a series of cases, and the treatment—far from dying away, as Gowers had expected—passed into common usage not only in France and Russia but also in England. The apparatus employed was devised by Sayre of the United States. It consisted of straps passing underneath the chin and both armpits, the attached cords going up to a stout cross bar (Fig. 1). By means of a pulley, the patient would be bodily lifted off the ground, and kept in this attitude for a matter of minutes. The belief that the roots of the spinal roots and also the cord itself were temporarily elongated was not confirmed. Gilles de la Tourette proved by research on cadavers that such an effect did not occur, but he found that forced anterior flexion of the trunk actually did stretch the cord to some extent.

Oppenheim (*Textbook of Nervous Disorders*, 1894 [English translation, 1911]) was also cautious in his evaluation, though less critical than Gowers. He asserted that patients with advanced tabes were unsuitable, as were those whose disease was complicated by arteriosclerosis or bulbar symptoms. Peripheral palsies and syncope may complicate the treatment, and he quoted a case reported by Fischer where softening of the spinal cord resulted. Beneficial effects of the suspension included lessening of the pain and the ataxia, and an improvement in potency and even in visual acuity. Oppenheim also referred to modifications of Sayre's apparatus so that the suspension treatment became gentler. Thus the patient might be suspended while seated or while lying on an inclined plane.

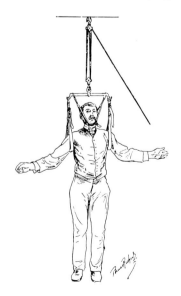

FIG. 1. Sayre's apparatus. (Courtesy of Dr. F. Clifford Rose.)

Reports as to the immediate effects of suspension upon a known tabetic are available to us. The French writer Alphonse Daudet (1840–1897), who was afflicted with locomotor ataxia, kept a diary of his symptoms *La Doulou* (Pasquelle, Paris, 1931). But first we may observe the comments of those contemporary gossip-mongers the Goncourt brothers who were friends of his.* On Sunday 27 January 1889, one of them met Daudet in the street who told him about his "hanging," a new treatment imported from Russia by Charcot. For this mysterious operation the patient had to wait at the baths until everyone had gone and then furtively proceed to a dimly lit room full of shadows. There in the presence of Killier and another doctor, the hanging takes place: "... a long, long minute, a minute made up of 60 seconds. Then they unhook you and you find yourself on the ground with a dreadful pain in the neck." "That hanging in the half-light is something quite indescribable," said Daudet. "A real Goya!" I said. "Yes, that's it. A Goya!"

Let Daudet himself elaborate on this experience. In his diary we read: "In the evening at Killiers' the suspension of the poor ataxia patients is sinister. There is the Russian, hung up seated in a chair. Two brothers and the little man of dark complexion, kicking his legs about. ... I remain as long as four minutes in the air and for two am held up only by my jaws. Pain in my teeth. Then, when I am let down and unfastened, there is a horrible uncomfortable sensation in the region of my back and neck, as if my whole spine were melting. I am obliged to crouch down and straighten up gradually as—it seems to me—the spine which has been stretched goes back into place. ... No perceptible curative effect. ... Thirteen suspensions. Then spitting blood which I attribute to the congestive fatigue of the treatment."

Whatever the effect of suspension upon the central nervous system, it must have caused irreparable damage to the ligamentous structures around the vertebrae.

Although in 1890 Risien Russell and James Taylor reported that suspension, as carried out on a large number of tabetics at Queen Square, had no real influence on the disease, the practice continued. Certainly it was in use 45 years later when I was a house officer at that hospital. The ritual was carried out in the "exercise room," where the original type of Sayre's apparatus was installed. The resident doctors had their evening meal at 7:00 o'clock and at 8:00 o'clock they began the supervision of the patients selected for suspension. No drastic ill effects were observed and, for that matter, no benefit either. The principal effect of the suspension treatment was an interference with the social life of the residents, who found themselves unable to study or, worse still, to participate in the night life of London's West End. Finally, two of them were bold enough to publish in the *Lancet* a short but unequivocal paper entitled "On the Futility of the Suspension Treatment of Tabetics." The point was taken: The article did not pass unnoticed by the physicians to the hospital, and no more hangings took place. The apparatus, however, continued to clutter up the exercise room like stocks outside a village graveyard, a token of byegone gullibility.

---

*Edmond Goncourt (1822–1896) and Jules Goncourt (1830–1870) *Les Journaux.*

The Secret World of the Singer

While listening to music, some sensitive sophisticates are capable of perceptual extremes especially when the stimulus is massive. V. Gollancz touched upon this matter when he wrote that there are various pleasures to be had from listening to music, and he proceeded to specify the intellectual and the sensuous. He went on to write: "But there are moments, and not only in listening to the works of the few supreme masters, when it is no longer a question of mere pleasure or even of happiness; it is a question of joy inexpressible."

It is precisely this "joy inexpressible" which I have described under the term ecstasy.* Ordinarily, "ecstasy" is something pertaining to the disciplines of both theology and psychology, but it also applies to musical appreciation. What is meant is a sense of merger of self with external reality, reality being seemingly endowed with a peculiarly personal significance, linked perhaps with the illusion of self-oblivion. There is something well-nigh ineffable or transcendental about these experiences, but they may be identified as including what is technically called depersonalisation. One seems to be outside of oneself, looking on, listening per-haps. This state is indeed implied in the etymology of the word ecstasy. There may be an obliteration of the actual environment; a loss of time sense; a subjective shrinkage or, less often, an augmentation of self. Then, too, there is the mysterious, yet by no means uncommon experience of synaesthesia, whereby musical sounds evoke an imagery of colour. This phenomenon of *audition colorée* may be vague or vivid, stationary or mobile, associated perhaps with kaleidoscopic shapes and forms. Many of the great masters have been so endowed—Beethoven, Scriabin, Rimsky-Korsakov, Liszt. Indeed it is possible that most musicians are synaesthetics but take it for granted, even perhaps in the belief that everybody else is similarly privileged. The colours evoked may vary according to the character of the music, the key, the individual instruments, or the composition as a whole. Synaesthetic subjects, musically sophisticated, have at times spoken of Mario's singing as golden, that of Sims Reeves as a rich brown, of Grisi a primrose yellow, and the powerful contralto of Clara Butt has been associated with the colour violet.

To what extent are instrumentalists and singers capable of, or susceptible to, such synaesthetic phenomena and such states of ecstasy? This question is difficult to answer with confidence. An orchestral conductor may be so, while at work, but only to a limited degree, because above all he must never lose control of the actions

From Critchley, M. (1983): In: *The Voice*, edited by K. Faulkner. Macdonald, London, with permission from Macdonald & Co. and Schirmer Books, a division of Macmillan Inc.

*See *Music and the Brain*, edited by M. Critchley and R. A. Henson. Heinemann, London, 1977.

of those under his direction. He must be an ever-watchful commander of the situation like a tennis champion or a pilot performing aerobatics.

The listener, on the other hand, is in a fortunate state of passive inactivity, a receptive vessel. A professional music critic is a little different, for he has to be in a permanent state of vigilant appraisal. The musical executive is still less susceptible because of the technical demands imposed upon him by composer and conductor. Technology transcends aesthetic passivity.

Where does the singer belong? In his *Psychology of Music*, C. E. Seashore observed that a fascinating problem is raised by the question as to whether it is necessary for the singer actually to feel the emotions he is portraying. The author pronounced that a "yes" or a "no" answer has lost its meaning, and he successfully evaded tackling the question.

In general, the singer—like the instrumentalist—is also the slave to technique rather than to enchantment. But there are many grades of both song and singer, and these diversities of circumstances lead to diversities of performance.

What prompts an individual at any particular moment to give voice? In solitude, song probably reflects some mild feeling-tone, mood, or affect, given of course a modicum of vocal proficiency. It may reflect contentment, mental vacuum, a talisman which wards off the task of thinking. Here belongs the solitary whistler. Among underprivileged persons, ululating, intoning, or some other kind of vocalism may accompany and perhaps facilitate hard physical exertion. This phenomenon is probably familiar to anyone who has witnessed a team of lascars coaling a steamship in an Oriental port.

The niche occupied by the solitary singer differs from the more usual state of affairs whereby there are others within earshot. At times the audience may comprise merely one other person, not necessarily attentive, as when a mother croons a lullaby. The serenade may also belong here.

More commonly the audience is large, even though all who are present may be participants rather than listeners, as in the choirs of the Welsh valleys. Here it matters little whether other onlookers and listeners are present. In this category belong the ecclesiastical choristers, members of Bach choral societies, and the singers participating in the *Messiah* or *Elijah*. Without doubt in such circumstances, expertise is linked with a shared aesthetic pleasure. The Welsh term *hwyl* exemplifies this state.

To adopt an *argumentum ad absurdum* we can assert that when a number of persons break into song musical ability may be irrelevant. In hilarious assemblies, in vaudeville audience participation, the louder the noise the greater the applause. This may perhaps represent the basest possible level of ecstasy, but an experience outside the world of the professional singer.

When it comes to the concert or operatic singer, constant awareness is paramount regarding voice control, the ordinances of the composer, the conductor's beat, the performance of fellow singers with whom he must accurately coordinate. The singer cannot afford to relax the dictates of virtuosity and technique.

Nonetheless, some elements of the listeners' ecstatic-synaesthetic feelings may invade the world of the singer. Thus most accomplished singers are temporarily oblivious of the passage of time. Many, too, lose awareness of the audience before them. This is not always so, for some sensitive singers make great efforts to transmit to their hearers something of the emotions which he or she is feeling. This represents a heightened sense of sharing as between executant and recipient. At times the emotional as opposed to the technical faculties reach great intensity. Especially so when a climate of religious exaltation is concerned. Although an unlikely event in Gregorian chants or in the cathedrals of the Eastern Orthodox Church, it may, however, be conspicuous among revivalists and the *chazzanim* of the synagogue. Here, the earlier cantorial display singing with its tonal embroidery has given way to fewer embellishments, ornaments, and trills to become disciplined by a hard apprenticeship as a *meshorer*. Nevertheless, the *chazzan* is always an advocate, the defending counsel of his fellow worshippers. To quote Nathan Ausubel, "He tries hard—sometimes even too strenuously—to evoke by means of his singing all the multitudinous moods and nuances of liturgical piety. These run through the entire emotional spectrum of pathos, contrition, repentance, compassion, God's anger, lamentation, despair, tenderness, humility, fidelity, sweet reasonableness, exhortation, laudation, invocation, thanksgiving, adoration, and many other tonalities of faith, self-revelation, and petition."

Here then is ecstasy both experienced and transmitted by a singer.

The operatic singer is in a different category, but some professional artistes in their work at times experience to a lesser degree something of this "joy inexpressible." An example may be quoted in the case of Giudetta Negri, better known as Pasta. According to a critic who attended her performance of Paisiello's *Nina*, "Not only did this enchantress hold her listeners spellbound; she was herself so seized and carried away that she collapsed before the end. She was recalled, and duly appeared; but what a sight! Too weak to walk alone, supported by helping hands, more carried than walking, tears streaming down her pale cheeks, every muscle of her expressive face in movement, and reflecting as touchingly as her singing, the depth of her emotions! The appearance rose to the highest conceivable pitch—and she fainted!" It must be confessed that the pure gold of her exultation seems to have been tainted by the dross of hysteria in this case.

De Musset appears to have taken it for granted that the great singer is the servant of the feelings. Referring to Pauline Viardot, he said that: "Before expressing something, she feels it. She does not listen to her voice but to her heart."

When Malibran was at her peak, she used to describe her voice as something separate from herself, almost as an enemy. A psychologist would read into this remark evidence of a depersonalization coupled with a malefic type of dissociation.

A clear example of *audition colorée* is to be found in Duprez who, when referring to his rival Nourrit, spoke of his voice as slightly guttural, and "white."

Regarding Adelina Patti, Clara Louise Kellogg said that she knew the extent to which emotions would exhaust and injure the voice, and she sang accordingly. Later, the same view was held by Melba.

If then some controlled degree of emotivity has been felt by singers belonging to the golden age of music and the grand operatic era, the same cannot, in all probability, be said of the earlier exponents during the seventeenth and eighteenth centuries. This was the heyday of *bel canto*, when *castrati* and falsettists were in vogue. The *martellato*, trill, turn, *appogiatura*, *canto figurato*, and fantastic volume control marked the acme of cold technical brilliance. However much the listeners may have been enraptured, the singer probably concentrated entirely upon his vocal gymnastics.

So far we have been dealing with the harmonic music of the West. What is the situation as regards the purely mensural type of music of the East with its lack of musical notation? Although in the Islamic world, as also in India, instruments are employed, greater store is set upon song, with its complicated *iqa* or rhythm, its quarter-tone decorations, and its repetitiousness. In the *Arabian Nights* we read that "to some people music is meat, and to others medicine." Indeed the Persian philosopher and mystic Al-Ghazālī (d. AD 1111) discussed the state of heightened auditory and visual power engendered by listening to music. In his treatise *Music and Ecstasy*, Al-Ghazālī set out seven reasons for maintaining that singing is more potent than the *Qur'ān* in producing pure ecstasy.

How far does the Islamic singer share these transcendental states produced by his complicated art? To a considerable extent possibly, more so than applies to his Occidental counterpart. Whoever has heard the singing of Um Khaltoum, the Melba of the Islamic world, would find it hard not to believe that she was as entranced in her own way as was her appreciative audience.

Passing from one extreme to another, there is the question of whether "joy inexpressible" ever comes within the experience of the contemporary "pop" singer. In the first place, what constitutes the line of severance between the noble and the ignoble in the world of song? Perhaps this is to be found in the "microphone-in-hand" technique of the performer who is unable to liberate himself from the shackles of an electric life-line. And yet without doubt the modern scene is one where the pop singer, alone or one of a group, is capable of rousing a most abandoned spectacle of frenzy in his audience. How far is he, too, sensuously involved? The picture is one of mass hysteria wherein the singer may find himself prisoner as well as instigator. Hysteria represents the basest example of emotional upsurge, for which the word ecstasy is far from appropriate. As to the artiste himself, the frenetic state may all too often be complicated by chemical corruption in the way of alcohol, pot, and various other psychedelic drugs. The pattern conforms more with the Voodoo orgies of the Caribbean.

The subject is potentially an ugly one, but it cannot be overlooked or brushed aside in any serious attempt to explore the psychology of musical expression and perception.

Two or One?

When a boy I lived in the Somersetshire town of Weston-super-Mare. Not far from the High Street was an intriguing complex of arcades similar to the covered-in bazaars of Istanbul but on a smaller scale. To explore them held for me a fascination because they were dark and mysterious and contained many curious little shops selling books and junk. One day—the date was 1911—I chanced upon a closed door with a notice-board "Visit *Kap Dwa*, the two-headed Patagonian giant. Admission one penny." Within was a huge glass case at floor level, and inside it I beheld an awesome figure stretched out, brown and wrinkled, 12 feet in length. One fist clutched a club, while upon the shoulders sprouted two sinister-looking heads (Fig. 1).

The brochure, which set me back another penny, informed me that the monster was *Kap Dwa* of Patagonia, who had been captured alive by marauding Spaniards. Like Gulliver in Lilliput, he was overpowered, trussed up, dragged on board their vessel, and brought to England in 1673. Although he had been tightly bound to the main mast, he managed to break loose and slay four of the crew. He was quelled only when a boarding spike was plunged into his heart.

Was it genuine or was it a fake? Just 20 years later the same dilemma confronted me when I visited Lenin's tomb.

An enterprising showman purchased the mummified *Kap Dwa* and took it on display from one town to another. Today, I am informed, the specimen belongs to the Scott Enterprises and is based, when not on tour, in Lanoka Harbour, New Jersey.*

The memory of *Kap Dwa* came back to me 10 years after my boyhood experience. I was then a medical student doing my clinical work in hospital. One day a terrified woman "on the district" gave birth to a full-term infant complete with two heads. Fortunately it was dead. The specimen was taken to the mortuary, photographed, and x-rayed, but regrettably it was not dissected with the thoroughness appropriate to a once-in-a-lifetime experience. There were two heads, normal looking, and two necks. Fusion of the cervical spines took place at C6–Th1 to form a single vertebral column.

Excitement at the hospital soon waned, as attention was focused upon impending final examinations. But years later the memory of this bicephalic stillbirth and also of *Kap Dwa* revived. In 1949 I was immersed in a consideration of the body image, then a theme that was dimly understood, realising how important a role the conception of corporeal awareness plays in neurology. Suppose that the stillborn

---

*For news of its present whereabouts I am indebted to Mrs. Lyn Morgan.

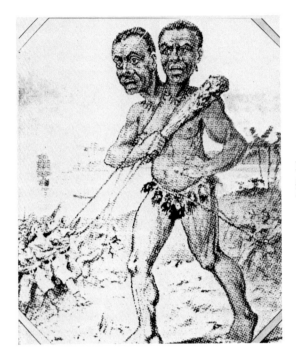

FIG. 1. *Kap Dwa*, the Patagonian giant. (Courtesy of Lyn Morgan.)

infant had survived—there seemed no obvious reason why it should not have lived and attained adulthood. (That *Kap Dwa* could have been anything but bogus was not credible.) If the skimpy literature on the subject could stand up to scrutiny, there were certainly precedents on record—few in number, however, and anecdotal rather than trustworthy.

In my paper of 1950, "The Body-Image in Neurology," I gave vein to my flights of fancy about adult bicephalics, speculating upon some of the problems—anatomophysiological, philosophical, moral, and legal—which such a situation might bring about. This was breaking new ground, though Eccardus was said to have touched upon such whimsies in the case of the Hungarian twins (1701–1723) quoted by Pope and by Buffon. But these were not bicephali, being conjoined twins sharing a common bladder, anus, and vulva.

Let us consider some of the quandaries, predicaments, repercussions, handicaps, and problems which might befall a two-headed adult. In the first place should one use the singular or the plural in our citations? Are we dealing with one person saddled with a supernumerary and unwanted organ, or with two persons sharing the burden of a common body? Surely the latter, for the situation involves two separate brains and all that that implies, and two sets of special senses.

Each of the four cerebral hemispheres would doubtless possess the mechanisms whereby a faculty of language can be developed. In that event the two heads can be expected to be able to talk, and not even simultaneously. The content of the speech need not be the same. There seems to be no ostensible reason why the two heads should not hold a conversation with each other. Expression of thoughts on paper is another matter. Assuming that in youth they had received conventional instruction, they will have acquired the skill of writing. But with which hand? If a pen is held with the right hand, is it guided by the *caput dexter* or the *caput sinister*? Both perhaps, though the principal impulse probably comes from the right head. Indeed the *caput sinister* might well be predominantly left-handed. If so, it is possible that bilateral synchronous writing could take place, the subject matter, however, being different.

If talking is possible, so must be singing. The two heads might perform independently, or in unison, or in harmony. The pygopagous twins Millie–Christine are said to have sung duets, but there is no good reason why they should not have done so, for they were two well-formed females united by a common sacrum.

In all likelihood the facial contours would be somewhat similar, even identical, although from the available literature we read that in Besse's case they were not, nor were they in the case of Martha and Mary. Voluntary movements of the face, jaws, tongue, and eyes would, no doubt, take place independently. This is in contrast with the case described by Sutton, where the teratological defects comprised a small supernumerary head, with its own brain, attached to the side of the subject's head. In this instance all voluntary movements of the parent's eyes and face were mirrored by simultaneous, similar, synkinetic movements in the parasitic organ.

The two crania of a bicephalic creature would participate in the same circulatory system. Consequently the host would have to manage a double cerebral circulation; the heart would necessarily be both hypertrophic and malformed, with supernumerary carotids.

Personality is the product of activity of the brain, influenced by the circulating hormones of the endocrine orchestra. In the context we are considering, this orchestra would be askew, for despite common sex organs and suprarenals there would in addition be independent hypophyseal-thyroid-parathyroid complements. The effect might prove lopsided. Would, then, the two heads have been endowed each with its own individual personality, its innermost likes and dislikes? For example, while appetite would be mutual, the sense of taste might not. One head might have a liking for something that revolts the other. That would not matter so long as what is ingested does not upset the stomach they share. A dispute between *Dexter* and *Sinister* might arise as to what should and what should not be fed into that stomach. This difference might extend to habits of smoking and alcoholic drinks. What is a pleasure to one head might be anathema to the other.

The question of the sleep cycle promises to be interesting. Do both heads drop off to sleep synchronously and wake at the same time? What of their dreams— shared or not? Unless an understanding exists between *Dexter* and *Sinister*, one of them might want to relax and doze at a time when the other prefers to be active. Supposing one elected to stay in bed while the other one importuned the common body to get up and dress. . . .

Because the blood circulation is communal, so would be the blood chemistry. This would tend to bring about a certain psychosomatic harmony. Thus they would experience the same visceral sensations including those of bladder and bowel movements. Sensory stimuli to the trunk and limbs would be perceived in both brains, although there is a possible inequality of sense perception. Much depends upon what happens when the spinothalamic tract reaches the point of unnatural bifurcation at C7–Th1. Beyond that point their routes may not necessarily be symmetrical.

Relationships with the outside world need to be considered. As in the case of monozygotic twins, the two personalities are not necessarily identical, despite the *corpus commune* which complicates the issue in bicephalics. One head, indeed, might be attracted by some member of the other sex who arouses dislike in the other.

Sociological complications are bound to arise. Would the state regard them as two citizens or one? At once we can detect a medicolegal bone of contention. The church would probably have no doubts whatsoever: in the case of Martha and Mary, both heads received baptism, dying after a few days of life. The situation might well be a source of perplexity to the government. Are *Dexter* and *Sinister* to be taxed as two individuals? If so, they would surely claim the privilege of double pension rights and social assistance.

A more down-to-earth question concerns the voluntary motor control of the arms and the legs. The integrity and formation of the pyramidal tracts is all important. In the case of the lower limbs the corticospinal pathways from both heads might be expected to merge somewhere in the upper dorsal region of the cord. No abnormality of the lumbosacral plexuses is visualized. Hence both heads independently would be capable of moving either leg. To perfect such coordinated activities as walking, running, jumping, kneeling, the four existing motor cortices must contrive to act in a synchronous and exquisitely regulated fashion. This harmony may develop only slowly, and hence the bicephalic creature might be relatively late in learning to walk.

Voluntary movement of the upper limbs is a far more complex matter. If spinal fusion does not take place until the level C7–Th1, there will be only two brachial plexuses instead of four that are operative. That means movements of the right arm are effected by impulses originating in the motor cortex of the left hemisphere of the right brain, proceeding by the pyramidal path and the right brachial plexus. Hence the left *caput* plays little if any part in moving the right arm, being entirely concerned with movements of the left upper limb.

The structure of the roots emerging from the right side of the left neck and the left side of the right neck at the levels C4, C5, and C6, is obscure. Probably the structure is vestigial and functionless. With the Tocci bicephalic brothers Giovanni and Giacomo (b. 1877), the anatomical problem was a little different. Fusion had taken place in the midthoracic region, and consequently there were four arms.

Finally, one comes to the problem of ill health. Aches and pains arising from lesions within the trunk and extremities would be perceived by both *capita*. Not necessarily to an equal degree, however, for sensitivity, tolerance, and vulnerability to pain are facets of one's personality. The brain of one of the heads might be more pain-reactive than the other. With troubles arising from structures in the head or neck, the situation is different. One can readily imagine headaches, toothaches, or shingles limited to one side only.

Migraine raises its own set of questions. During an attack, would fortification figures and unilateral throbbing pain be experienced simultaneously in both *capita* or only in one? Bicipital hemicrania would certainly please some pharmacologists and some allergists with their own personal theories about the cause of migrainous attacks. Epilepsy is an even more baffling eventuality to consider. During a seizure, would both brains of necessity lose consciousness? To conceive of one head looking on at widespread convulsive movements while itself remains conscious and uninvolved is a macabre thought. In the case of epileptiform attacks due to a metabolic dyscrasia such as uraemia, the effects would perforce be universal, and consciousness would be lost.

Death, whatever its cause, will liquidate all cerebral activity of the two heads synchronously. Such was so with the Sassari bicephalus (b. 1829) (Fig. 2). One head, which had been named Ritta, fell victim to an illness, the nature of which was not stated. At the moment of her demise, Christine, the other and "healthy" head, which was feeding at its mother's breast, suddenly relaxed hold and perished.

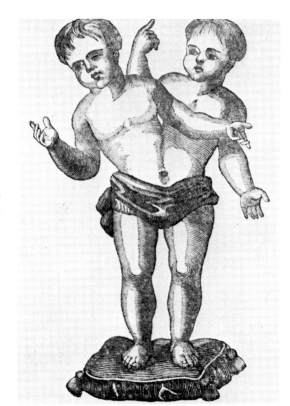

FIG. 2. Ritta and Christina, the Sassari twins, born in 1829. (From an old print.)

In the case of conjoined twins, death does not necessarily occur at the same time, though both Eng and Chang, the notorious Siamese twins, died on the same day in 1874, one of them having been hemiplegic for some time before. The survivor may, for a limited matter of days, remain chained to a cold and stiffened corpse, a plight that cannot be endured for long. If ancient records can be accepted in evidence, the twins described by Roger of Wendover died within 3 years of each other. We are reminded of Mezentius, the savage King of the Etruscans, who securely fastened the bodies of his captives to corpses, leaving them to their fate.

A boost to the understanding of the problems which would beset a bicephalic has come from an unexpected source: a study of animal behaviour. Thirty or so years ago a giant two-headed terrapin came to light somewhere in the United States. The creature was active, and it thrived and attained maturity. Observation in the laboratory made it evident that the situation was one of two turtles united by a single trunk. For example, one head might avidly feed itself while the other head was drinking or perhaps doing nothing. At those times when the terrapin was ambulant, one head might seek to go this way and the other that. This lack of concordance was emphasized if a piece of cardboard was inserted between the two heads. When this barrier was removed, the two heads might turn inwards so that each caught sight of the other. Conflict was the usual result. The animal psychologists were in no doubt that this two-headed tortoise possessed two separate personalities.

Whether this particular species is more than ordinarily liable to freakish errors of development is not known, but in 1981 another two-headed terrapin turned up in a Nottinghamshire pet shop. As the proprietor remarked: "I have named the heads Terry and Pin because they are so different. I think they often try to swim in different directions" (Fig. 3).* So rests the case.

More points than one are at issue. In the first place, is bicephaly compatible with survival? Is physical and mental development feasible? Is there on record unmistakable evidence of bicephalic adults? If so, would such a creature possess a single persona, or would there be two? If the latter, is the state of affairs supportable or one to be deplored? Can any advantages be visualized?

When considering these questions the dictum of the jurist Baron Lubbock should be remembered: "Our duty is to believe that for which we have sufficient evidence, and to suspend our judgement when we have not."

Regarding any incertitude as to whether bicephaly has ever been witnessed, I am in no doubt. "What mine eyes hath seen I can proclaim." During my professional career I have witnessed two such cases, one of which was x-rayed and photographed. Both, however, were neonates, and neither was living. The cause of

---

*In a letter the manager kindly informed me that Terry–Pin came to him in a batch of 50 terrapins and was approximately 1 year old at the time. It lived another 7 months, an object of great admiration, having made an appearance on television. Many visitors came to see him and debated whether the creature was a single or a double entity. An x-ray examination was therefore carried out that demonstrated one body and two heads. During life the two heads acted independently as regards feeding (evidenced by their fighting over a piece of meat) and sleeping.

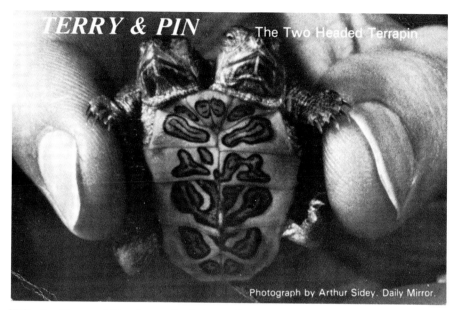

FIG. 3.   Terry and Pin, the two-headed terrapin. (From Syndication International—Photo Trends, with permission.)

death I do not know: Whether modern intensive care could have saved them I cannot answer.

Over the past 500 years a small handful of cases can be cited where a bicephalic infant has survived and lived for a matter of years. Is the evidence of these few cases credible? How weighty are such precedents, or are they fables belonging to the legends of mythological medicine? The Tocci brothers date from the last century. There is pictorial evidence of their existence, and they were said to be well and active at the age of five; how much longer they lived is not recorded.* Mary and Martha, who lived only a couple of days, date from the seventeenth century. Such a distinguished authority as Ambroise Paré (1510–1590) asserted that he had seen an infant with two heads (Fig. 4). Besse's bicephalic was a woman of 26 years, but the report also dates from the sixteenth century and is too exiguous to be acceptable (Fig. 5).

The ground for accepting survival is questionable, being little more than anecdotal. In this connection the authenticity of the Tocci brothers is crucial. Perhaps the literature of teratology would be fruitful.

The evidence to date is scant, and speculations in this field may be little more than idle pipedreams.

---

*Data concerning the Tocci brothers were obtained secondhand from Gould and Pyle's *Anomalies & Curiosities of Medicine* (Saunders, Philadelphia, 1898). Their chapter on "Major Terata" provides considerable information and many case reports. Unfortunately, the bibliography is often inadequate. See also Thompson, C. J. S. (1930): *History and Lore of Monsters*. Williams & Norgate, London.

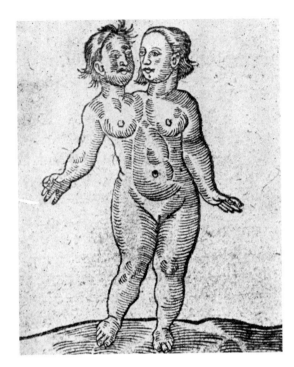

FIG. 4. Girl with two heads. Paré, 1579.

FIG. 5. Monsters seen by Rhodiginus. Boasistuau, 1576.

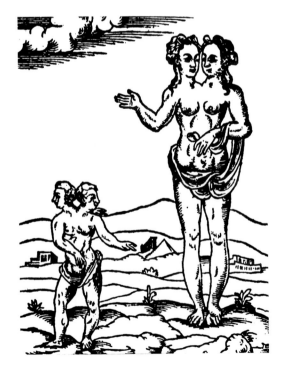

But today genetic engineering is a bold pursuit—some might use the word meddlesome—one which probes deeply into matters of life, growth, and structure. From their juggling with genes, whether deliberate or inadvertent, who knows what to expect? Centuries hence, many monstrosities, including bicephalic twins, may appear too often on the scene to be comfortable.

Supposing the Tocci twins be deemed acceptable as a valid precedent, we are back to the question of whether bicephalic adults should be considered as two persons or one. The answer will doubtless be that they are two separate individuals encumbered with a common body. Is that a plight which is tolerable? Surely the conclusion must be that in such an event two heads are not better than one.

The Inscrutability of Pain

The head pains in migraine offer an opportunity for mulling over the nature and meaning of painful experiences in general. Migraine is a common disorder, afflicting, it is believed, at least 10% of the community. It has been known to medical men longer than any other disorder with the exception of epilepsy. More than 2,000 years ago it was clearly described, and since then there have been scores of brilliant accounts of the symptomatology, many supplied by physicians who were themselves *migraineurs*. During the past 30 years an upsurge in interest has taken place throughout the world in this subject, and yet, despite much physiological and pharmacological research, the advance in basic knowledge has been disappointing. During the past century speculation as to the cause of the migrainous diathesis, and even the actual source of the pain, has roamed far and wide. Within living memory, indeed, the *fons et origo morbi* has shifted from the liver and bile ducts to the cerebrum.

Again, one can seriously question if the power to relieve an attack of migraine has materially improved over the years, and if prophylaxis has become more effective. Our memories do not go back far enough, so that comparisons are not possible. That there is a gap in our ability to shorten the attacks and to reduce their frequency has given support to a considerable hotchpotch of incursions into alternative medicine. This would never be so if we were in firm possession of a panacea.

Migraine is by no means the sole variety of headache. For reasons we do not understand, the head constitutes a *locus minoris resistentiae*, and headache must surely be one of the commonest complaints which induces a person to seek medical advice. Some have ventured to explain this clinical fact by reference to the concept of the body image, pointing out that the focus of personal identity lies, most of the time, somewhere in the forepart of the cranium. This may be so, but the hypothesis is not supported by the realisation that pain in the small of the back is an even commoner complaint than headache.

The cause of headache in a particular patient may prove to be trivial and no threat to the organism; on the other hand, headache may be a warning of such a pathological calamity as meningitis or tumour, or an intractable and enduring condition such as Paget's disease of the skull.

Diagnosis is not helped by any correlation between intensity and gravity. A patient with an intracranial growth may be walking around and working despite his headache.

Reprinted with permission from Critchley, M. (1985): *Psychiatric Aspects of Headache*, edited by C. S. Adler, S. Morrissey Adler, and R. Packard. Williams & Wilkins, Baltimore.

Philosophers have had a great deal to say about the nature of pain and in particular its function. Much of it is nonsense and based upon superstition as sanctimonious as it is cruel. Has pain, irrespective of its site, any teleological meaning, any purpose? In the past, biologists have tended to regard the role of pain as protective, betraying the presence of injurious influences or of disease. Thus Herbert Spencer pronounced: "Pain is the correlation of some species of wrong—some kind of divergence from that course of action which perfectly fills all requirements." Presumably he was trying to say "pain means that something is the matter." Though short, the memory of pain may condition behaviour. Richet said that pain is one of the bases of intelligence, as the existence of pain determines the conduct of all beings above the rank of pure automata. Some have gone further and claimed that suffering has stimulating powers of immense therapeutic value; that it may constitute a positive virtue and in some persons act as a spur to work (St. John Ervine). Charles Bell, who should have known better, said that pain is the companion and the guardian of human life. One hundred and fifty years ago, an eminent surgeon proclaimed that pain was a wise provision of nature, and patients ought to suffer pain while their surgeons were operating—that they were all the better for it and recovered better. Some theologians—like some savages—have proclaimed pain to be a cleansing experience, and that victims undergo a state of spiritual purification.

If pain is a "vigilant sentinel," to use a common cliché, then it must be rated a highly inefficient one, erratic and unreliable. Some deadly disorders, slowly or rapidly advancing, run their sinister course without the victim having suffered a moment's "pain," in the true sense of the word. On the other hand, certain intense and incurable pains serve no ostensible purpose; they are meaningless. As examples we can enumerate tic douloureux, the postherpetic neuralgias, and certain "central" pains, like those occurring in phantom limbs or the hemialgia of thalamic disease.

Surely pain is more malefic than protective; Nietzsche spoke of "the senselessness of suffering." As Sir James Young Simpson, the pioneer of chloroform anaesthesia, put it: "All pain is per se, and especially when in excess, destructive, and even ultimately fatal in its action and effects. It exhausts the principle of life. It exhausts both the system and the part. Mere pain *can* destroy life." Alfred Schweitzer, too, was in no doubt about any alleged atoning effect. "Pain is a more terrible lord of mankind than even death itself."

For that matter, is it conceivable that migraine is an exception, and that it may fulfil some purpose or bring about some cryptic benefit to the victim? The only possible advantage might be in the role of a feedback (in the strict sense of that much abused word). Could it be that when stress of an emotional, mental, or physical kind reaches a critical level, an attack of migraine might intervene and bring a temporary halt to such a potentially nocuous influence? If so, one would expect to find within the community a negative correlation between migraine and the various ailments we currently regard as stress disorders, e.g., peptic ulcer, coronary disease, rheumatoid arthritis, ulcerative colitis. At present, we simply do not know how to answer this quite straightforward question. Surely this would be a rewarding investigation well within the scope of community physicians, general practitioners, and immunologists. I have often thrown out the suggestion, but so far no one has taken it up.

Still within the ambit of the philosophy of pain is the matter of the intensity and character of headache. When a patient proclaims he is suffering from a head pain, the doctor must accept the statement as a subjective truth. There are no physical signs specific for pain. When, however, the headache is migrainous, subtle objective signs may be present. A localized area of the scalp is tender as is one eyeball. Tenderness is a subjective symptom, but it is confirmed if the patient winces or recoils when the allegedly tender area is stimulated, as by pressure. As a rule the eyelids droop. The artery in the temple may be more conspicuous on the side that aches. Pulsations are more bounding, and the vessel is sensitive to the touch. Local applications, either ice-cold or hot, bring temporary relief.

When one seeks to ascertain the severity of any pain and its character, the physician relies upon two factors: the behaviour of the victim and his description of the symptom.

During an intense bout of migraine the patient seeks to stay immobile, either flat in bed or sitting propped up. Patients differ in their choice of posture, but always they avoid movement. They do not toss or turn the head if they can avoid so doing. Never do they thump the skull or bang it against the wall, like some headache victims. Möbius spoke of an "akinesia algera." When an intense restlessness is coupled with a complaint of severe pains in the head, one can usually exclude the principal states characterized by intense pain, viz., subarachnoid bleeding, acute meningitis, the headache that follows air encephalography or even lumbar puncture, and some cases of migraine. The suspicion of underlying psychological disorder becomes uppermost.

The patient's statements are our only clue to the character of the pain (whether pressing, pounding, throbbing) and its force. It is within the latter category that the physician is in most doubt. Not only do degrees of severity exist in the case of migrainous headaches, but, more particularly, the choice of language complicates the issue. Some patients habitually employ superlatives and describe as agonizing or excruciating a headache which, from the patient's ability to carry on as usual, can scarcely be very severe.

A serious language problem may complicate an interview with a patient from some underprivileged racial community. The word "pain" is rarely employed there, and odd metaphors may be used which bewilder the English-speaking doctor. Thus patients from the Caribbean may speak of a "weakness" in the head (or on the "top-flat," "noggin," "dome," or "biscuit"). Again, among some primitive peoples, one can elicit no information in reply to a straightforward question such as: "Do you ever get headaches?" To a Zulu, such a direct enquiry would be offensive, and no reply would be forthcoming. A highly unorthodox clinical approach must be employed by a physician experienced in the verbal taboos of such a patient and he would adopt a roundabout method of interrogation.

One has only to cross the Tweed to realize that a "sore head" represents what is conventionally called a "headache" elsewhere.

Quite apart from the choice of words to describe severity, there probably exists a true continuum of sensitivity to pain. At one extreme are the hypersensitives who react severely to actual pain, who suffer greatly from even the mere anticipation of pain. By contrast, there are those who seem to possess a relative indifference to pain and for whom it holds no dread. The physical and mental correlates of this continuum are obscure. Certainly race is an important factor. Another is the intellectual level as well as certain psychotic factors. Although long-continued pain is often followed by feelings of despondency, deep melancholy may lie outside the picture. As Hippocrates taught, physical and moral pain are in some ways antagonistic. Few take their lives because of sheer agony. Furthermore, many depressives elect to destroy themselves by methods that are potentially most unpleasant. Interviews with a number of failed suicides have indicated to me that slashing of the wrists or incompetent cutting of the throat was not attended by physical pain at the time.

Physicians in charge of pain clinics might learn much from stepping outside their profession for a moment and questioning those sinister beings whose odious job it is to inflict pain deliberately on others. The period 1930 to 1950 has probably witnessed more proficient torturers than at any time since the Middle Ages.

Physicians realise, of course, that there is a clinical curiosity known as "congenital insensitivity to pain." It is, however, a rarity, mysterious in nature. By the time adolescence is reached, there are numerous scars of cuts, burns, and old fractures, all of which occurred at an earlier date outside the awareness of the subject.

There also exists a limited form of nonsensitivity, however, probably not an uncommon occurrence, the explanation of which is unknown. In some ways it represents the antithesis of migraine. I refer to those otherwise normal persons who admit, or even boast, that they have never "known what it is to have a headache." Severe blows to the head may produce dizziness or syncope, but not pain. And yet their tissues are not analgesic. Aftermath of alcoholic excess is marked by a hangover in which headache plays no part. Febrile illness, even such commonly painful ailments as sandfly fever and dengue, run their courses without headache.

This headache immunity usually comes to light socially, in the course of conversation. No objective features offer any clue to this lack of pain experience. Although we commonly associate "rank in nature," including high intelligence, with hypersensitivity, I can straightway quote as individuals belonging to this headache-free class three such erudite academics as Hughlings Jackson, Kinnier Wilson, and C. P. Snow.

The study of an obscure clinical phenomenon or function can surely be furthered by observing the effect of the absence of that function. This is a physiological axiom.

It is difficult to conceive any anatomical explanation, such as an absence of nerve fibres around the intra- and extracranial blood vessels, for we know of no precedent in human morphology that is relevant. Although I have repeatedly called attention to this anomalous condition and urged that the subject be seriously investigated, we remain in the dark.

Patients with various psychological disorders not infrequently complain of pain, especially headache. It is then that one hears bizarre descriptions of pain, sometimes associated with odd similes. Probing on the part of the physician often leads to the conclusion that the patient is really referring to a cephalic sensation not quite identical with what is generally understood by "pain." The sensation may prove to be more in the nature of an uncomfortable pressure on top of the head, or a tight band around the cranium, or a sense of fullness or tension within the skull. Feelings of such types are usually not assuaged by even heavy doses of the ordinary analgesic drugs. On the other hand, they may respond to antidepressants or tranquillisers. A therapeutic test of this kind is often a useful aid to differential diagnosis.

A true hypochondriac may employ extravagant terminology and speak of a distressing sensation "as though the scalp or even the cortex were being eroded by acid or by insects." The use of the term "as if" renders unlikely the existence of a hallucinatory state.

Then there is the vexed question as to whether psychogenic pain has any existence at all. In essence, this is something of a quibble. It is dangerous to speak of, or to visualize, any such entity as an imaginary pain. Pain is a subjective experience; and although one might well challenge the patient's evaluation of its intensity, it would be unsafe to question its actual existence. At one time, my colleague F. M. R. Walshe expressed serious doubts as to the bona fide of hysterical or psychogenic pain. In characteristic language he said that a patient whose pains were psychologically determined "may continue for months as fat as a partridge, as rosy as an apple, and in a state of beatific calm."

Yet pain, either focal or generalized, may be induced by suggestion as, for example, by hypnosis. Similarly powerful emotion may inhibit, if only temporarily, the pains due to injury in the excitement of sport or battle. During states of ecstasy pain may be swamped or even replaced by a pleasurable experience, as evidenced by the martyrology of religion or the self-immolation of fakirs.

Suffering brings in its train a number of mental concomitants, especially if protracted and severe. Oddly enough, depression, as we have seen, is not profound. A state of pleasure through pain is suggestive of a psychotic state. It has been well stated that pain suffered for a cause glorifies it and provides gratification (Louis Nizer).

René Leriche, whose contributions to our ideas about the nature of pain were both original and stimulating, wrote: "Physical pain is not a simple affair of an impulse travelling at a fixed rate along a nerve. It is the resultant of a conflict between a stimulus and a whole individual." How does that conflict show itself? Much depends upon whether the pain is a frequent visitant, in which event the sufferer is at least spared the dread as to its possible significance. A sudden, unexpected pain brings with it considerable anxiety as to its nature, its import; and a sense of impending death may arise. Blissful calm is a myth, for irritability is an understandable accompaniment. Severe pain is demoralizing; it swamps the whole sensorium and concentrates thought to the exclusion of all other feeling. The sense of time is prolonged to an unconscionable degree. The somatic symptoms associated with enduring pain comprise anorexia, constipation, loss of weight, and sleeplessness.

The more complex psychological side effects of abiding pain arouse the most interest. Complicating and nonspecific in essence, they differ from one victim to another. Often they are very difficult to describe. Hence the truth of the saying: "If you wish to probe the secrets of nature, read what poets and novelists have had to say." As professionals in manipulating words, nonmedical writers are in a strong position to elucidate what is almost ineluctable, that is, the transcendental pain experiences which may baffle the linguistic capacity of less literate sufferers.

It would not be appropriate to quote passage after passage, though this would be easy. One description at least may be taken as exemplifying the intricacy of the matter. Regarding the birth of her second child, Nina Van Pallandt wrote:

> I had two breaths of gas. As the pain grew less I seemed to look into an incredible warm yellow light which became whiter and brighter as I was lifted and floated, slowly spinning, upwards. My body stretched, expanded and dissolved into this now unbearable but beautiful blinding white light. An explosion—a death. It was as if, in one split second, I was totally part of the universe. In the next instant I heard a cry. *"Es una nina,"* the doctor said.

The colour imagery with the use of the words "yellow" and "white" is particularly interesting, for it suggests that the writer might have been a potential synaesthetic. It is by no means unknown for patients in the throes of an agony to become aware of shapes and particularly colours. The phenomenon is one which lies midway between a vivid image and an actual hallucination. I have described it as experienced by mechanics who have sustained powerful electric shocks. Perhaps the earliest reference to this "synalgia" was made by Homer when in the *Iliad* he wrote about "arrows, the harbingers of black pains."

For impressive accounts of the distress experienced in a severe attack of migraine, Pamela Hansford Johnson (herself a victim) was unsurpassed. Other extraordinary descriptions of pain are to be found in the writings of Jack London (subjected to torture); Hugh Walpole, who betrayed a veritable and almost masochistic preoccupation with pain; Moritz Jokai, who wrote convincingly about a psychogenic topalgia arising as a manifestation of guilt; Leonhard Frank, also a synalgesic; Marcel Proust (who dealt with pain in states of sleep); Emma Goldman (with her description of a transmission of pain from the victim to a sympathiser as in the case of the martyred Perpetua); and Brenda Dean Paul (finding that surgical pain brought gratifying relief to the intolerable apathy of her drug withdrawal).

Special mention is deserving of the incredible diary of torment kept by Alphonse Daudet, incapacitated by locomotor ataxia. His volume, entitled *La Doulou*, which is a Provençal word meaning pain, described incomparably the generalized pains that he endured over the last years of his life. This work is probably unique as a personal account of tabetic pains.

Whether there is any limit to the sensation of pain is a question raised by H. G. Wells. Does a steady increase in the violence of the stimulus automatically evoke a parallel heightening in the intensity of the pain? Or is there a limit or plateau of feeling? Wells suggested that if pushed beyond a certain point nociceptive agencies may even prove pleasurable. This is rather borne out in the case of a naval officer who managed to escape death from drowning. After his rescue he told me that as he tried to inhale while submerged, he had felt an intense vice-like pain in the chest, increasing with each breath. Later, however, his anguish abated. "I appeared to be in a pleasant dream, although I had enough will-power to think of friends at home and still retain vivid recollections of the clearness of the sight of the Grampians, familiar to me in boyhood, which was brought to my view. Before finally losing consciousness, the chest pain had completely disappeared, and the sensation was actually pleasant" (Critchley, M., *Shipwreck Survivors*. Churchill, London 1943).

Some pains in neurological practice baffle understanding as well as all attempts at mitigation. Take, for example, the following account of a patient of mine seen in 1935:

> A male, aged 57, at the age of 35 had sustained a crushing injury to the right foot. Though no bones were broken, the resulting pain was severe. Twelve months later, after months of hospital treatment, the foot was amputated just above the ankle joint on account of the persisting pain. The pain, however, continued not only in the stump but also in the phantom. Two months later a second amputation was carried out in the upper third of the thigh, but with no effect on the pain. A year after that, the stump was explored and the ends of the severed nerves freed and sectioned at a higher level. As this measure was ineffectual, the sciatic nerve was then exposed and divided in two places. No benefit followed. Nine years after the original trauma, a posterior rhizotomy of the lumbosacral plexus was performed, and as this operation did not help a chordotomy was next conducted in the upper dorsal region. Even this measure failed to assuage the pain. The last therapeutic intervention was an injection of alcohol into the stump, but this too was unavailing. When seen 22 years after the original accident, the patient was still complaining of severe and immutable pain in the stump. The pain in the phantom foot had ceased a year or two previously.

Here then was a patient whose intractable suffering could possibly be in the nature of "central" pain, although the injury had been remote both in place and in time. Alternatively it might be dismissed as hysterical. In such a case a therapeutic test might have been considered as helpful in differential diagnosis, but the effect proved to be ambiguous. An injection of morphia (0.5 gr or 0.03 mg) was consequently given and the effect observed. An hour later, the patient said the pain was "a trifle less," but very soon afterwards it was as severe as ever.

The "Gross and Scope" of a Migraine Clinic

Long experience in conducting two migraine and headache clinics has shown me the value of this type of specialized medical provision. Benefit accrues to both migraineurs and migrainologists.

Sufferers from chronic headaches have the advantage of detailed clinical study, followed, if need be, by advanced investigative techniques. Not surprisingly, differential diagnosis every now and again discloses an unsuspected brain tumour, a state of malignant hypertension, or a problem that is of purely emotional origin.

Such a clinic also affords the opportunity for drug trials of various remedies in an endeavour to find something a little more effective and a little less toxic than available hitherto. This function, I suggest, ranks lowermost in the role of the clinic. Incidentally, in some such clinics there are opportunities for occasionally treating a patient in the throes of an unexpected acute attack. The victim is allowed to rest and relax in quietude, to be mildly sedated while studies are perhaps carried out on the clinical state and its chemistry.

However, the importance of an adequately staffed migraine and headache clinic is potentially much greater to the well-being of the community. As a matter of experience it can be asserted that the bulk of those attending suffer from some variant of migraine complicated by an overlay of a nonorganic character. Hence the evaluation of each clinical quandary may be far from simple. In the same way, management and treatment are complicated matters. Migraine, one finds, is a way of life and all too often a veritable *via dolorosa*. Diagnosis must not only be shrewd but be seen by the patient to be shrewd and penetrating. The platitudinous term "diagnosis," let us remember, does not entail merely the act of attaching a label to someone's symptoms. By definition, the Greek expression "to diagnose" is to attain knowledge permeating right through the patient and his problem, and of necessity implies the understanding not only of the nature of the trouble but also its essence, cause, probable outcome, and means for its alleviation.

Having ruled out the likelihood of grave intracranial mischief, the doctor must discuss with the patient sympathetically, searchingly, and at length the clinical niceties of the case. As Dr. Samuel Johnson said: "Questioning is not the mode of conversation among gentlemen." Nor among doctors for that matter, but at the same time the interview should not be a monologue on the part of the patient. Now and again the doctor must pose a question, for patients do not always realise the relative significance of the individual symptoms. Otherwise some key points may be glossed over, some totally forgotten. Occasional interventions on the part of the doctor also demonstrate that he is still alert and interested. They even manifest warmth and serve to oil the wheels of the consultation.

The personal history must be traced back, and every detail needs to be elicited, not only as regards the present disorder but also the sufferer himself. This will mean close enquiry into innermost social, dietetic, domestic, familial, and environmental circumstances. One fact which will probably emerge is the elucidation of the factors that provoke an attack, and what it is that determines whether a patient is in a good patch or a bad one at a particular period.

There is no substance in the objection that such a manner of working is grossly time-consuming. It is not a question of how long can be spared for an individual patient, but how many patients in such circumstances can be adequately dealt with in a single session. The answer may well be "only very few." This means more doctors on hand at the clinic, for this kind of approach may be required during follow-up visits after the initial consultation.

Such, I submit, is the master plan for coping with a forbearing clientèle, victims of a recurring torment which, without shortening one's days, racks one with pain and threatens to disrupt domestic happiness, professional advancement, and social enjoyment. Thank heaven we avoid the faceless horror of officialdom, where "your name is a number: your story a 'case'; your need a 'Request. Your hopes 'will be filed... fill up this form... come back next week'" (Carlo Menotti *The Consul*).

Haptics, or the World of Touch

Let us revert to the year 1923, when the name Henry Head was paramount, even though before him various neurologists, physiologists, even philosophers had written a great deal about what they called haptics, or the world of touch. Among the more important recent contributors was the brilliant René Leriche (b. 1879). He thought deeply and contributed much that was original to our ideas on touch— painful or painless—its detection, its mode of transmission, and the mechanism of appreciation at the highest level (Fig. 1). Today Leriche seems to be well-nigh forgotten, and the crumbs of his genius have largely been swept under the carpet of modern thinking. I look forward to the day when at least some of his exciting ideas will be retrieved.

During that same period it was Henry Head who was suzerain among those who explored the mysteries of touch. His personality made this come about. Head was a man of great intelligence, endowed with much erudition, a polyglot, and a humourless obsessional. Over the years 1905 to 1918 he had dedicated himself almost exclusively to an analysis of disorders of the various sensory modalities, their transmission and perception (Fig. 2). Day after day would be spent in the most scrupulous, even meticulous testing of the human subject, using the patient as a touchstone or indicator. Soon he came to realise the shortcomings of this particular technique, depending as it did upon the reliability of the subject and the inadequacies of communication. Head endeavoured to overcome or bypass these faults by eliminating the testee altogether. This was possible only by using himself as a human guinea pig and severing one of his own peripheral nerves. Probably never before had such auto-observation been carried out so thoroughly and so repeatedly.

But there was another side to his personality. Coupled with the exactitude of his self-survey was a speculative cast of mind which was apt to tempt his thinking far beyond permissible limits. A notorious instance was the conception of a two-stage anatomical hierarchy of peripheral sensation, one older and cruder, and the other younger and more discriminative. This was the well-known epicritic-protopathic dichotomy. The allure of such creative thought was considerable. Acclaimed on all sides, it soon became part of established neurophysiological thinking.

This honeymoon period did not endure, however. In 1909 and again in 1913 that neurosurgical philosopher Wilfred Trotter, in collaboration with Morriston Davies, repeated the autoptic experiment even more exhaustively. Not one, but several of

---

Reprinted from Critchley, M. (1983): *Centenario de la Neurologia en España (1882–1982)*, edited by D. L. Barraquer Bordas, Servei de Neurologia del Hospital de la Santa Creu i Sant Pau, Barcelona.

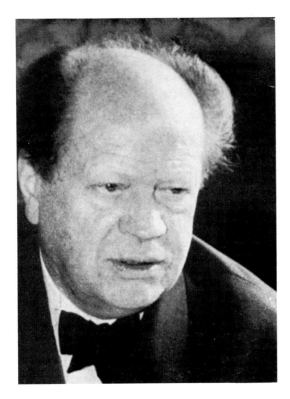

FIG. 1. Professor René Leriche.

FIG. 2. Dr. Henry Head, ca. 1914.

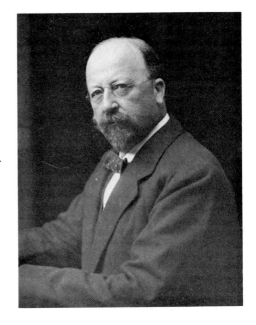

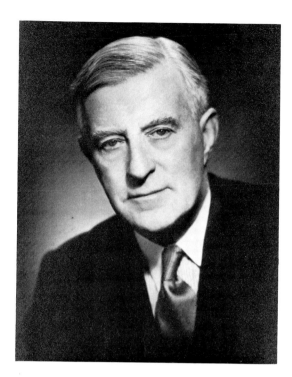

FIG. 3. F. M. R. Walshe.

their cutaneous nerves were cut, and at different times. Their findings were similar to, but not identical with, those of Head and his co-worker Rivers, but in explanation of their clinical data they did not find it necessary to invoke any mythical pathways. In 1916 the Swedish psychologist Boring came up with comparable findings which led him, too, to views contrary to those of Head. Twenty years later came Thomas Lewis's hypothesis of a "nocifensor system of nerves," but again unsupported by any anatomically demonstrable evidence.

The *coup de grace* to Head's speculative ideas was delivered by F. M. R. Walshe in 1942 (Fig. 3). As he wrote:

> No hypothesis largely dependent upon phylogenetic considerations can ever be capable of scientific proof, yet it may well have the compensating attraction of being equally incapable of disproof, and there are always some who are ready to accept a hypothesis upon these equivocal terms.

He quoted Karl Pearson, who writing in his *Grammar of Science* made a statement which is just as relevant today as it was in 1902. What he wrote was this:

> It is easy to replace ignorance by hypothesis, and because only the attainment of real knowledge can in many cases demonstrate the falseness of hypothesis, it has come about that many worthy and otherwise excellent persons assert an hypothesis to be true because science has not yet by positive knowledge demonstrated its falsehood.

The existence of Head and Rivers's "protopathic animal" was laughed out of court by Walshe.

> Such a creature, even if it could take the steps necessary to propagate its bewildered kind, which appears doubtful, could have no survival value for on receipt of a stimulus which it could not localize, from a stimulating agent whose nature it had no means of discovering, it could respond only by curling up and micturating. Yet this is the animal that Head and Rivers present to us as our common ancestor.

But we must press on, and I will omit all references to Head's work on the sensory pathways in the spinal cord, the role of the thalamus, and the fascinating thalamic syndrome.

More important and more enduring was the study which Head pursued in 1912 on sensory disturbances from cortical lesions. This research was carried out in association with Gordon Holmes, a man of greater calibre than some of Head's previous collaborators. Head and Holmes had certain qualities in common. Both were almost fanatically obsessional. Both were punctilious observers. Both were tireless. There the resemblances ended. Nothing intrigued Head more than to weave webs of speculative thinking. To Holmes this was anathema. His dictum was: "Observe and describe: That's all." Scrupulous accuracy was paramount. He had no time whatsoever for woolly, creative thinking (Fig. 4). At the bedside, the joint clinical sessions of Head with Holmes often appeared like a noisy altercation. The end results were all the richer because of the stormy alliance of two masterminds. Perhaps this explains why this particular study has endured—supplemented, complemented, augmented, but never assailed.

This work of Head and Holmes represents the scaffolding of what we now regard as the syndrome of the parietal or sensory cortex and subcortex.

Research of this kind unfortunately did not lend itself to auto-experiment. The intervention of an intelligent and cooperative patient was essential, combined with the testing techniques of highly experienced clinicians. Gordon Holmes once told me that he and Head found they had to reject as unsuitable subjects for sensory testing two classes of patients. First, schoolteachers, who being prolix and unduly introspective, would talk too much during a test situation; and secondly, all Scotsmen, because when touched with a stimulus, would never give a straightforward "yes" or "no" response—being overcautious and highly suspicious.

Time does not permit me to do more than recapitulate briefly the principal manifestations as we now recognize them:

1. Over the contralateral side there is a patchy and minimal alteration in the threshold for light touch, pain, and temperature. This "hypaesthesia" exists *unbeknown to the patient*. He does not complain of numbness. It is a surprise finding, and even after its demonstration it does not endure in the patient's awareness. The alteration in feeling cannot be expressed in the quantitative terms of a plus or a minus. To the patient, the stimuli feel "different," rather than dulled or diminished. If the patient is blindfolded, some touches with a feather or a pin are noted to be

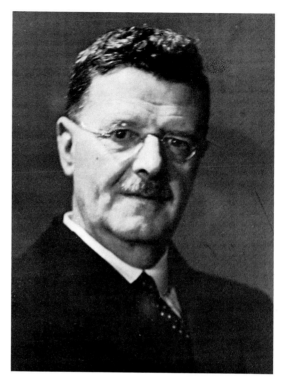

FIG. 4. Gordon Holmes.

missed altogether, whereas others are felt. Increasing the force of the stimulus does not necessarily increase the frequency of positive responses.

2. Bilateral simultaneous stimulation is almost always felt only on the normal side. This is the phenomenon of *tactile inattention* (or extinction). After repeated testing, this phenomenon may break down (the "extinguishing of extinction"). A faint stimulus to the normal side, e.g., a feather, may take precedence over a much stronger and painful stimulus applied to the affected side. Even an auditory stimulus in one ear may "extinguish" a tactile stimulus to the opposite side. As a rule, a proximal stimulus outweighs a peripheral stimulus, even on the same side of the body (the *"face–hand" phenomenon*).

3. The chronogenic, or time, quality may be altered. A sensation may linger on unduly *(tactile perseveration)*. Other changes may occur in the timing or rate of adaptation. The precise moment of stimulation may be unsure and, still more so, the moment of removal of the stimulus. The duration of the sensation may be either shortened or lengthened.

4. Localization of touch is always faulty. The stimulus is usually referred to a more proximal point. The longer the stimulus is maintained, the more accurate the localization gradually becomes. Occasionally, the stimulus is referred to an anatomically mirror-opposite point *(alloaesthesia)*. Very occasionally the patient refers the source of the stimulus to some point in outer space *(exosomaesthesia)*.

5. Of particular value are the various tests for the differentiation of sensibility. One is the compass test of *tactile discrimination*. The ability to appreciate the duality of two points simultaneously applied is most sensitive and accurate over the tip of the tongue, then the lips, and after that the fingertips. Two points of a compass applied elsewhere are felt as one, unless the distance of separation is considerable. In clinical circumstances it is sufficient to concentrate on the finger-tips and to compare one hand with the other. This discriminative test can be elaborated to the simultaneous application of three, four, five, or even six points, the last being the limit that can be detected when the stimulus is applied to a nonmoving fingertip.

6. An important property of the sensory cortex is identification, through the medium of touch only, of an object placed in the hand. As a research project, rather than a diagnostic aid, the patient may be asked to describe the physical properties of the object, its size, shape, weight, consistency, and surface details. Very occasionally the patient can do this quite well and yet fail to recognise the identity of the object (*hylognosis with astereognosis*). When the diagnosis is doubt-ful, it may be useful to complicate the test by asking the patient to identify two, three, or four objects placed in the palm simultaneously. The test can also be made more difficult by asking the patient to wear a pair of gloves and then test for stereognosis. Gloves may bring to the fore a one-sided defect which previously had not been obvious. Consequently, this is a test of the utmost clinical importance. Most astereognosic patients have no insight into their handicap even though they constantly fail to identify the contents of their trouser pocket.

7. *Graphaesthesia*, or the recognition of numerals traced on the skin with a blunt object, is a test which I used to consider too complex to be of clinical value. However, having watched the technique practised by my late friend, Morris Bender, I am now satisfied that this testing procedure can prove to be of diagnostic importance.

I have by no means exhausted an account of the fascinating and unexpected signs of sensory cortical dysfunction, but time is running out. I want to turn the coin from the obverse to the reverse and consider not what happens when disease processes are at work, but *what peaks of attainment are possible in the normal*. What is the acme of sensory skill?

In *Homo sapiens* the hand, freed from the dingy duties of ambulation, blossoms as a most delicate and dextrous organ of sensibility and manipulation. Not only is it the most deft of instruments, it constitutes the chief implement for exploratory touch. Nor is that all. As the principal contrivance for *gesture*, it also fulfils a communicative role, thus participating in that essentially human endowment, lan-guage.

It is only with the sensory functions that we will deal here. Learning and practice perfect the perceptual skill of the hand without necessarily lowering the threshold for touch. Watch a silk mercer at work or a wholesale tobacco merchant. In the latter case, the buyer plunges his hand into a "skip," or container, and allows the slivers of cut leaf to slip between the fingers, as he gently and caressingly rubs the grains between the pulp of the thumb and fingers, in this way assessing the size, weight, brittleness, and moisture of the tobacco.

May I quote this little piece which I lately came across in a magazine, for it does have a bearing on our theme?

> On his rare trips to London, he would be expected to escort his lady wife around the West End dress-shops. His aching back is relieved only on those blessed occasions when he espies an unoccupied chair tucked away among the racks of frocks, fineries, fripperies and Lord knows what. This whistle-stop is a relaxing and even entertaining lull, for he can watch cohorts of females of all ages, sizes and shapes, scurrying like birds of prey among the fruits of the rag-trade. Their gimlet eyes are focused upon the distance, darting this way and that. But one and all perform the same lightning-like ritual. Each harpy, as she hurries from A to B, grabs a piece of material, and without looking, and oblivious of colour, shape, size, or price, with greedy fingers hoists in at fantastic speed the nature of the fabric. Is it cotton, or a man-made fibre? Durable? Drip-dry? Tumble-dry? Linen or silk? Non-crease? Will it dry-clean? Does it stretch? All this information and much more is gathered, transmitted from finger-tips to be stored and evaluated in some pearly cell in the brain. The onlooker notes that not one fumbler in forty pauses to linger and actually hold up the garment for inspection.

Perhaps not one fumbler in a thousand realises the sheer miracle-play of sensory skills which her fingertips have been effortlessly enacting.

Yet another example where tactile mastery can be achieved is met with in China. Han Suyin wrote: "That night . . . we played mahjong the Szechuan way, a very fast game, for the generation above us had played so much that they no longer looked at the carved ivory dice, but felt them with the pulp of the third finger as they picked them up, and did not bother to turn them for inspection before tossing away the unwanted ones. It made the game so quick that I could not follow" (*A Many-Splendoured Thing*. Jonathan Cape, London, 1952).

In our study of the apogee of digital sensitivity, we naturally turn to the experience of the blind, especially those who have at no time known what it is to see. The hands take over from the eyes the art of exploration, and through the sense of touch they are able to judge the physical properties of objects which lie within their digital and manual "space-shells." Distant vistas are unattainable, being beyond "the touch horizon," as are massive or lofty structures and buildings. And yet there is a way around this dilemma. A 6-inch model of the Eiffel Tower conveys to the blind man's touch most if not all of the information needed.

It may not be realised that the threshold for touch, including two-point tactile discrimination and stereognosis, is by no means lower in the blind than in the sighted. Indeed often a little less sensitive, for some who are blind are not of high intelligence. Nevertheless, to a blind subject some activities are possible which would baffle others. They excel in extracting information from minimal sensorial clues. The mental associations linked with tactile data are richer, and the memory of these impressions is more keen. For example, some blind persons are known to have been connoisseurs of ancient coins and medallions, and with their fingers can identify specimens, appraise their quality, and distinguish fakes from originals. Just like any Chinese artist, Helen Keller used to take pleasure in fondling a piece of jade, taking a sybarite pleasure in its texture, shape, and patterning. The blind Gayan has told us that even though colour cannot be distinguished the sense of touch gives him a notion that the eye cannot and which has a considerable aesthetic value, namely, the notion of softness, silkiness, polish. What characterises the beauty of velvet is its softness to the touch no less than its brilliance.

Words such as these would naturally lead to the topic of the aesthetics of touch. This is a fascinating subject which I wish I had time to develop, although scientific readers would perhaps find it inappropriate.

While tactile imagery is still in our mind we can mention the role of the "critical detail," to use Birkmayer's phrase. An intelligent blind man may enter his study and by touching the corner of a piece of furniture can in a flash conjure up a mental picture of the whole room, with its mahogany desk, silverware, Oriental rugs, and easy chairs.

Leaving aside the so-called "sixth sense" which gives warning of obstacles, many sightless individuals are endowed with what is popularly called "facial vision" which alerts them to any obstruction looming ahead. This largely comprises a subtle sense of warmth upon the cheek though the subject himself may describe it as a queer feeling, a shadow, or a pressure.

Are blind subjects endowed with perceptual structures foreign to the normal person? Despite occasional reports to this effect, the idea appears untenable. From time to time we hear, usually from Russia, of blind persons such as Rosa Kuleshova who have the miraculous ability to read print, describe pictures, and recognise colours purely by way of touch. It is said that at the Moscow Institute of Biophysics thorough investigation of this girl led to the conclusion that the skin of her fingertips actually contained rods and cones and other light perceptors, 10 to each square millimeter in fact.

Such claims are, to say the least, implausible. The sensory equipment of the blind does not differ in the sighted, but their striking achievements bear witness to the heights to which human potential can be exalted.

This is well illustrated in the wondrous system of communication devised by Louis Braille. As one might have guessed, Braille himself was blind, having lost his sight when he was 3 years of age. The braille system is made up of 63 symbols comprising one or more bosses constituting a "cell," or cluster, of up to six. As I have already mentioned, six contacts constitute the maximum number of separate contacts which can be "subitized," that is, wholly recognised by a single, immobile, or synthetic touch. The embossed dots are set apart at a distance of either 2.5 or 3.0 mm; it so happens that the threshold for tactile discrimination at the fingertips is 2.0 mm.

What happens if an ordinary, sighted person runs his fingertip lightly across a page of braille? He feels merely a jumble of dots, like so many goose-pimples. Let a blind braillist do the same, and he will interpret the symbolic meaning of these

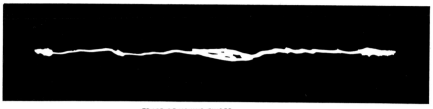

TRACE OF MOVING FINGER.

'PROVE BENEFICIAL TO DR. HEWLETT JOHNSON (BRAILLE TRANSLATION)

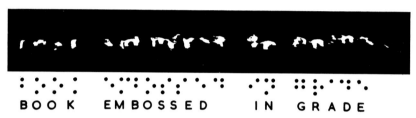

BOOK EMBOSSED IN GRADE

FIG. 5. Top: Tracing of the touch movements of the left index finger, of a male patient of 31 years, blind since the age of five. He is reading the braille symbols depicted and is slowed up when the finger reaches the rather unexpected term "Dr. Hewlett." The circumductory movements of exploration are well shown, but there is no record of the speed of the tracing or of the varying degrees of pressure exerted by the reading finger. The patient was a particularly skilled and rapid braillist, who always used the left hand for reading. **Bottom:** The touch movements of a normal-sighted person who is not a braille reader but who has memorized the visual form of the punctographic alphabet. Large braille type is used. There is no record of the varying pressures or of the very many errors made in trying to identify each symbol in turn. The time taken to read this line was 2 to 3 minutes.

dots at the rate of 60 to 120 words a minute. That is, he is extracting meaning from something like 2,500 dots every 60 seconds.

When reading braille the blind person employs a *master finger*, usually the index of one hand, sometimes of both hands. In three out of four blind persons the left forefinger is the preferred one. Ordinarily the other fingertips do not possess this interpretative skill, although they can quickly be trained. The sightless one can soon acquire the knack of also reading braille with his thumbs, or his toes, or the tip of his nose. A skilled braillist can also read even when a cloth is interposed between his fingers and the sheet of print; or even after he has put on gloves; or he can wear gloves and still read through a piece of material.

As the blind reader studies the page of embossed dots, the tips of several fingers may happen simultaneously to brush the braille type, but actually only one fingertip acts as an interpreter. The stimuli from the other fingers are simply neglected, ignored, or repressed.

Just as the rapid reader in the sighted community does not merely hoist in one letter after another as he peruses a book, so an experienced braillist eventually dispenses with the task of interpreting one punctographic cell after another, for he learns to deal with a string of symbols as a whole, a sort of tactile *Gestalt*.

Again, the finger movements of an experienced braillist resemble the eye movements of a good reader who is not blind. Similarly in the beginning, the smooth and sweeping track whether of the finger or of the eye is interrupted by frequent fixations, even regressions and exploratory movements of search in the case of unusual or unexpected words (Fig. 5).

Braille reading is tiring, and in states of fatigue the threshold of sensitivity of the tactile rosettes in the pulp of the finger may temporarily rise to a slight extent. Diderot located a blind man's soul within his fingertips and considered that the fingers, being the *theatre of thought*, would become as exhausted as the brain of a sighted person.

It should not surprise us to learn that, as an aspect of metalanguage, braille reading is vulnerable to cerebral disease. Braille aphasia, or more precisely alexia in a braillist, is as a matter of fact a well-recognised though exquisitely rare disorder. The loss of skill is not, let me emphasize, the result of any loss of the peripheral sense of touch but is a high-level disorder of linguistic interpretation.

I believe I have said enough to indicate something of man's potential within the world of touch. Lessons gleaned from the acquisition of sensory skills may prove one day to be as revealing as those we learn from studying the effects of disease.

Our knowledge of the touch world of the blind began with the French philosopher Diderot in 1749. We have also learned much from Charles Féré, Révész, Burklen, and Villey, the blind professor of philosophy. Subsequent writers include Manfield, Javal, Nolan, Kederis, and others, but their contributions have been pragmatic, piecemeal pieces of work. We sadly lack the grand strategy of a Henry Head or a Gordon Holmes.

What a wonderful opportunity lies open to a contemporary neurologist blessed with inner vision!

Aurae and Prodromes in Migraine

The most conspicuous and most distressing aspect of migraine is, of course, unilateral headache. This is reflected, in fact, in the name "hemicrania," which we owe to Galen. This particular symptom has given rise to most of the research into the morbid physiology of this disorder. Other symptoms may, however, occur in anticipation of an attack, immediate or remote. These may be subtle or striking, short-lived or protracted. Chief among these are the well-known visual aurae. Although superficially uniform in character, on closer scrutiny they prove to be diverse. Their importance stems from the bearing they may have upon our understanding of the mechanism of migraine. Do our conclusions support or contradict current views as to the causation of the headache?

More intriguing and less uniform are the objective and subjective *precursors* of an attack. Some of these are psychovisual in nature; others anything but. Sometimes these premonitory features antedate an attack over a matter of hours. Others appear only some minutes beforehand and gradually merge into the characteristic aura. Can they be explained purely on the basis of a disordered cerebral vasculature?

These two types of anticipatory phenomena are discussed separately, tracing first the history of our knowledge of the migrainous aura.

I am well aware of the old horse-and-buggy practitioner in the hillbilly backwoods who warned the visiting lecturer to avoid referring to Hippocrates and "all them other Latin fogies." But I cannot in all honesty take this advice, for the visual aura of migraine was well known to Hippocrates and was indeed first described by him 300 or 400 years before Christ, and also long before Aretaeus. In his own words: "He seemed to see something shining before him like a light, usually in part of the right eye; at the end of a moment, a violent pain supervened in the right temple, then in all the head and neck. . . . Vomiting, when it became possible, was able to divert the pain and render it more moderate."

Over the succeeding centuries there were numerous accounts of photisms or spectral phenomena of manifold complexity. Of particular value have been the personal descriptions written by a long succession of intelligent, introspective observers, some of them artists who have been able to reproduce realistically their personal phantasmagoria, others being medical men.

Let us take as an example the words uttered by Charcot at one of his Tuesday clinics. "*Mon Dieu!* It is not surprising that one cannot describe the shock of the scintillating scotoma. Many times have I experienced it. The first occasion when it happened I had, or thought I had, a firework display in front of me. Only later, from closer scrutiny, did I make out a sort of circle like one of Marshal Vauban's fortifications* with its salients and recesses." From such pioneer descriptions, coupled with the weighty clinical experience of migrainologists, we can extract a pattern of events, by no means uniform, which constitute the visual aura.

In the first place, how common are such aurae? Edward Liveing, in his classic monograph written over a century ago, said that an aura was "a tolerably frequent symptom in the more severe forms of migraine." Actually it occurred in 37 of his series of 60 patients, that is, in 61.6%. Subsequent writers have observed a far lower incidence, varying from 1.4% (Flatau) to 17% (Moebius).

The usual pattern is of the sudden appearance of "a germ" or area of blurred vision, centric or eccentric in location. The former type obscures the word or object occupying the focal point of the gaze. Dr. Hyde Wollaston (1824) spoke of a new *punctum caecum*, or blind spot, obliterating the discerning vision.

But the initial manifestation may not be negative in character; it may take the form of a glistening, flickering light, as noted by Hippocrates.

Whether the visual symptom be positive or negative, it soon expands. Sometimes the enlargement is circumferential; at other times the extension is to one side only so as to develop into a hemianopia, as first described by two Dutch physicians, Vater and Hennicke (1723), under the term *visus demidiatus*. Less often the defect is quadrantic. In Christiansen's patient the hemianopia was altitudinal, a symptom, incidentally, not easy to explain.

At other times the disturbance of vision is, to begin with, widely eccentric and then spreads inwards towards the fixation point. Occasionally it forms an arc above the midpoint; rarely below it.

Whether the spread be centripetal or centrifugal, there typically develops a central obfuscation surrounded by positive phenomena. The former is rarely dense but something more like a cloud, the hot air above a chimney-stack, or a "shaded darkness" like the after-image which follows an unwary gazing at the sun. Rarely, it constitutes an area of sheer nothingness—a sort of hole or lacune in the visual field. The edges of the *punctum caecum* form a brilliant, luminous, coruscating border endowed with certain important physical properties. The edge is not smooth, but jagged, like the teeth of a saw. One commonly refers to these phenomena as "fortification figures," a simile first employed by Dr. John Fothergill (1712–1780), or as *teichopsia*, from the Greek *teichos*, a wall. The latter term we owe to Dr. Hubert Airy (1870), who described the recurring spectral illusions experienced by himself and also by his father, Sir George Airy, the Astronomer Royal. They were the first to depict them in colour.

This spiky, castellated border is usually glistening and sometimes polychromatic. Hence the spectral figure is most conspicuous against the black background of the closed eyelids, and appropriate testing makes it obvious that the phenomenon is a binocular one.

---

*Vauban was responsible for the defence of Paris in the Franco-Prussian War of 1870.

The spectral appearance is not static. It exhibits small-range oscillations, or what Liveing called "rapid molecular movements." Lashley (1941) judged the rate of shimmer to be about 10 per second. Hare (1966) put it at 10 to 15 per second to start with, later falling to 3 to 4 per second. Some have described the phenomenon as being "all alive" and have likened it to "the rapid gyrations of small water-beetles." Nor is that all. The castellated wall expands and the individual components broaden. Sometimes a second or even a third teichopsic arc develops within the original outline, so as to form a duplex or triplex arc of scintillation. There is a steady spread of 3 mm per minute, until ultimately either one-half, or the whole, of the field of vision is invaded.

After a matter of minutes, the teichopsia begins to fade. The pattern of its disappearance is less well established. This process embraces not only a universal dimming or waning in brilliance but also a shrinkage, from without in, or perhaps the reverse. At the same time there is a reduction in the speed of the oscillations. As the teichopsia abates, vision returns. The duration of the whole optic experience is usually about 20 to 30 minutes.

John Graham (1970) has compared the visual events preceding an attack to the onset and spread of a grass fire in a prairie or meadow. First comes a sparkling blaze of burning, dazzling light in one visual field or the other. The blaze spreads over 5, 15, to 30 minutes in an ever-growing semicircle, burning black the field of vision in its wake until it reaches the periphery where it scintillates in a zigzag circle. Then it subsides, and the green grass of vision begins to grow back into the charred area, as the headache begins.

The disappearance of the teichopsia typically ushers in the onset of a one-sided increasing headache. But in the later years of a life-long *migraineur*, no headache develops. Just why this clinical difference should be is still not satisfactorily explained. Yet it constitutes an important challenge to any neuroscientist seeking to understand the mechanism of an attack of migraine.

May I now draw attention to a striking and unusual case of some antiquity, where the diagnosis of migraine is probable?

Turning back the pages of history, we come to the life and writings of the Abbess Hildegard (1098–1179). Having founded a Benedictine nunnery at Bingen in the German Rhineland, she proved to be an intelligent, but domineering, politically minded visionary, who spent long hours writing mystical books that were theological, ethical, metaphysical, and semiscientific in scope. Here and there are obscure references to periodic episodes of a glittering, blinding light, explaining that "the light which I see is not located, but yet is more brilliant than the sun....I name it 'the cloud of the living light.'" In another place she wrote: "I saw a great star, most splendid and beautiful, and with it an exceeding multitude of falling sparks with which the star followed southward...and suddenly they were all annihilated, being turned into black coals...and cast into the abyss so that I could see them no more."

Two of her most important writings, *Scivias* and the *Liber Divinorum Operum Simplicis Hominis*, were beautifully illuminated by plates, some of which are, or were, preserved in the Wiesbaden Museum, and others at Lucca in Italy. Their content is obviously hagiographic, but they are embellished by juxtaposed, non-coordinated fragments, often adorned with zigzag figures resembling fortification spectra. Could it be that the Abbess Hildegard suffered from migraine?

Let us now deal with that other important aspect of the migraine problem, namely, the prodromal symptoms, so subtle and varied in nature. During this prodromal period the patient is in a state of vulnerability, and an attack of migraine is liable to be precipitated by relatively minor causes such as would be ineffectual at other times. When vivid visual aurae are the rule, it is interesting, and incidentally not easy to explain, how often visual stimuli, e.g., glare, bright colours, kaleidoscopic displays, or close work at a microscope, quickly provoke first an aura and then a fully fledged attack. May I also emphasize that these prodromes may occur in isolation, constituting a sort of migrainous equivalent, a "migrainous metastasis" as Tissot would have said. Let me at least enumerate them in descending order of frequency.

A period of bienaise with enhanced activity, increased appetite, and euphoria may precede the headache over a period of many hours, sometimes up to a couple of days. During this phase, there is a risk that overindulgence in food, drink, or work may hasten the onset of the migraine. Our knowledge of these prodromes derives from Thomas Willis, who wrote in 1683:

> A beautiful young woman...being obnoxious to an hereditary Headach, was wont to be afflicted with frequent fits of it. On the day before the coming of the spontaneous fit of this Disease, growing very hungry in the Evening, she eat a most plentiful Supper, with a hungry, I may say greedy appetite; presaging by this sign, that the pain of the Head would most certainly follow the next Morning; and the event never failed this Augury. For as soon as she awaked, being afflicted by a most sharp torment, thorow the whole fore part of her Head, she was troubled also with Vomiting....

Almost as common among the prodromes is the antithesis of the foregoing, namely a spell of depression with irritability and mental and physical lassitude. A less common prodrome consists in a rather ill-defined state. It is ushered in by a sense of well-being leading gradually to a feeling of unease, particularly in the visuospatial sphere. Distances of surrounding objects are misjudged, often seeming to be too close and looming up. The speed of moving objects appears to increase, even the vehicle which the patient is driving (*Zeitraffer* phenomenon). Bright lights are enhanced so as to be distressing. Likewise, sounds seem too loud, and there may be a lack of relish for food.

Next in rank are curious distortions of the body image, or as I prefer to call it "corporeal awareness." Such disorders are common but never commonplace. Often they are so bizarre as to be frightening. Many persons are reluctant to divulge these complicated illusory states for fear of being misunderstood or even deemed crazy. As symptoms of migraine, they have received special attention at the hands of Lippman (1952) and Lukianowicz (1967). Here are some of the statements made by victims of migraine:

> I feel that my head shrinks until it becomes no bigger than a small orange.

> Suddenly I get the feeling that I have two bodies and two heads.... I have four legs instead of two, and I wonder how I'm going to walk.... I don't know which of my two right arms or legs to use, the "real" one or the "imaginery" one.

> My head suddenly splits into two parts, right in the middle. Then a miniature image of myself emerges from the fissure, which rapidly expands to the size of my real body. They are both "me" and "I." They are about a foot apart, the "new" body being always on the right side. Yet I've never seen him with my eyes, though I feel his presence very intensely.

> When walking it seems as though from my hips downwards the walking continued, but with no volition or direction. The control was in the upper self, way up above, totally indifferent to the legs' direction.

Disorders of the body image also include such symptoms as an illusory enlargement of the head; hands and feet apparently at a distance from the trunk; or shrinkage of the whole body into dwarf-like proportions. Three of Lippman's patients described a sensation as though the neck was considerably elongated, with the head almost touching the ceiling.

One finds this in *Alice in Wonderland*. Alice sometimes grew to a gargantuan stature and at other times dwindled in a lilliputian fashion. Perhaps it is significant that the author, Lewis Carroll, was himself a severe migrainous sufferer and may well have experienced illusory perversions of his own body image. Dr. J. Todd (1955) went so far as to refer to the "syndrome of Alice in Wonderland."

The same hypothesis may apply to the anatomical aberrations characteristic of the paintings of Modigliani. He was a life-long invalid and died in his thirties from tubercle and alcoholism. Perhaps he too was a migraine sufferer or a victim of the syndrome referred to by Todd.

Lastly, may I mention three patients with bizarre visual aberrations preceding the onset of migraine?

1. *Optic alloaesthesia.* Dr. Beyer, a victim of chronic migraine, was strolling in the streets of his home town in Germany, when he was astonished to see a bright blue rectangular shape outlined against the grey sky, above and to his left. A moment later he was startled to discern a little dog, also above and to the left. He stopped in his tracks, looked around, and then realised that what he had seen was a real dog on the pavement to the right of him, and that the blue object was in reality a letter box of the German *Postamt*. An hour or so later came the typical crashing headache of his migraine. Professor Pötzl used the expression "the migrainous Fata Morgana" in reference to this particular case.

2. *Heautoscopic hallucinations.* Linnaeus, the pioneer of botany, was a life-long victim of migraine. We learn that prior to an attack he would often observe someone walking alongside him, stopping perhaps to examine a flower. It was a little while before he realised that the man he saw was his *Doppelgänger*. Once he entered the lecture theatre prepared to take his class, when he saw someone standing at the

lectern. Thinking that he had arrived before the previous lecturer had finished, he turned away, only to realise he had been looking at a specular hallucination of himself.

Lippmann has also described similar cases of illusory doubling of the personality occurring either just before or during an attack of migraine. One patient said: "I felt as if I were standing on an inclined plane looking at my husband and my children from a height of a few feet, watching myself serve breakfast...There was 'I,' and then there was 'me.'"

The other patient of his also had a distinct impression of being two people—the other one suspended above and to one side—perceiving or contemplating herself in a detached way.

3. *Visual perseveration.* A migrainous patient of mine would experience before her eyes flashes like lightning. Sometimes when at home she would notice yellow blobs all around her. Eventually she realised that these were, in fact, an extension of the yellow checkered tiles on the floor of her kitchen. These visual phenomena would accompany her as she went from room to room. Thirty minutes later, a severe headache would develop accompanied by nausea. Here the visual persever-ation was an aura rather than a prodrome, and the checkered flooring acted as a provocative factor, first of the perseveration and then of the attack of migraine.

May I finish my purely descriptive efforts by voicing my doubts whether these prodromes and these visual aurae lend any real support to the hypothesis of preliminary vasoconstriction of the vessels of the occipital cortex? Surely they favour a process whereby a neuronic spread of excitation is followed by depression, as conceived by Lorente de No, Leão, Lashley, and others. This possibility has been raised by Milner (1958). It was discussed by Goldensohn in 1970 during the admirable conference held in Boston at the Faulkner Hospital. Since then it has been touched upon by Whitman Richards (1971) of MIT and by Baumgartner (1977) of Zürich.

Disorders of Speech in Parkinson's Disease and after Thalamotomy

That certain affections of articulate utterance may follow deep-seated as well as cortical lesions of the brain has been by no means unfamiliar for over a century. Emphasis on this fact has fluctuated considerably, however. One may take Parkinson's disease as a model, where the responsible pathology, although not firmly determined until 50 years ago, had been associated with a lesion either of the medulla oblongata or of some other structure not too remote therefrom. Although disorders of speech do not stand in the forefront of the many symptoms of that disorder, they were well recognised and described as long as 160 years ago.

For example, in his *Essay on the Shaking Palsy* (1817), James Parkinson stated that in the later stages the patient's words might become scarcely intelligible. He quoted some of his own case histories. Thus in No. 2, "the speech was very much interrupted." In No. 6, "convulsive movements began to interrupt the speech," and he mentioned Gaubius who had commented on festination of the muscles, including those responsible for speech. From a search of the literature Parkinson found an account written by a Dr. Maty of a steadily advancing malady—in all probability identical with the "shaking palsy"—that had afflicted the Comte de Lordat. The earliest symptom was a slight impediment in talking. A few months later it had worsened so that only with considerable difficulty could he utter a few words. Three years after that, his predicament was pathetic: "What words he still could utter were monosyllables, and these came out, after much struggle, in a violent articulation, as hardly to be understood but by those who were constantly with him." Happily he was able to read, and he remained as capable as ever of writing upon quite abstruse topics.

From Parkinson's description it appears likely that the disordered speech he had observed was not, strictly speaking, an affection of language but, rather, a dysarthria due to labiolaryngeal involvement of central origin.

The early literature contains instances where deep lesions of the cerebrum were held responsible for disorders of the function of language as opposed to speech. Thus in 1866 Hughlings Jackson wrote: "In some cases of disease of the hemisphere (always, in my experience, near to and involving the left corpus striatum), intel-

Reprinted with permission from Critchley, M. (1983): *Stereotaxy of the Human Brain*, edited by G. Schaltenbrand and E. Walker. Georg Thieme Verlag, Stuttgart.

lectual expression is wanting, and emotional expression is well preserved." It should be remembered that at that early date and for some time later Jackson shunned the term "aphasia," which was infiltrating from France into universal usage; he preferred to speak of "disorders of expression," and he discriminated, moreover, between a loss of superior as opposed to inferior speech or, alternatively, "propositionizing" in contrast to emotional utterance. Jackson went on to assert in this same article: "I believe it will be found that the nearer the disease is to the corpus striatum, the more likely is the defect of articulation to be the striking thing, and the farther off the more likely is it to be one of mistakes of words." In 1874 Jackson returned to the subject. His paper "On the Nature of the Duality of the Brain" contained the opinion that "in the majority of cases, extensive damage to the brain in the region of the corpus striatum on the left destroys speech, and that equally extensive damage in the corresponding region on the right does not affect speech at all." At this point a footnote was added: "In this article I illustrate by cases of *loss* of speech, not because of *defect* of speech. I do this for the sake of simplicity. . . . There are numerous varieties and degrees of defect of speech from different degrees of damage to different parts in the region of the corpus striatum." Returning to the body of this paper, Jackson proclaimed: "I do not believe in abrupt geographical localizations. Thus, very sudden and very extensive damage to *any part* of the left cerebral hemisphere would produce *some* amount of defect of speech, and I believe that similar damage to any part of the right hemisphere might produce *some* defect of recognition."

Over the years, aphasiologists in the main were more impressed by the occurrence of lesions in the cortex of the left cerebral hemisphere—frontal, insular, or temporal—as playing the all-important role in the production of the various types of aphasia. Eponymous terms such as the aphasias of Broca and of Wernicke assumed a status which was perhaps unwarranted. Nonetheless, it should be realised that most neurologists did not imply that aphasia-producing lesions were limited to strictly cortical areas. The conventional belief was that the white matter subjacent to the diseased cortex was always affected as well, playing an essential role in the production of speech loss. Thus the lesion in every case of aphasia was regarded as corticosubcortical, if not indeed transcortical or conductive, in site.

Jackson's belief in the importance of the striatum in this connection remained unnoticed for a considerable time, until indeed the pendulum began to swing back. Comparatively recent work has once more aroused interest in the deeper structures of the brain—the basal ganglia including the thalamus, as constituting supplementary or accessory organs of speech. To some extent this innovation was iatrogenic. The deliberate production of such brain lesions as cortical excisions, stereotactic attacks upon the pallidum and the thalamus, as well as electrical stimulation of exposed areas of the brain or by way of implanted electrodes, sometimes brought about phenomena in the domain of vocalization that were unexpected and often grave. The interpretation of their pathophysiology was all the more difficult because the results were often not only unpredictable and inconsistent but at times diametrically antithetic. Sometimes cortical stimulation would evoke vocal utterances (chiefly nonarticulate) or, *per contra*, a temporary arrest of speech.

Thus Penfield and Roberts (1959) were led to study the occurrence of speech and language disorder following man-made lesions of various areas of the brain in conscious human patients. In their own words, "The electric current, when applied to the cortex, produces two effects upon speech: a positive one—stimulation, and a negative one—interference." Their book *Speech and Brain Mechanisms*, taken as a contribution to aphasiology, is a brief and conventional account with a bias towards a materialistic or localizational concept. Quite apart from ethical considerations, it is unfortunate, therefore, that the authors failed to meditate upon this extraordinary ambivalence in the response of a high level function, to a crude and quite artificial type of excitation. Why should it be that an electrical stimulus can produce either a temporary arrest of function or at times the opposite effect? What was it, moreover, that determined the type of positive response? In the authors' experience, the vocalization so induced was of lowly rank in the hierarchy of language, for it consisted in a vocal cry, either sustained or interrupted, which at times might have a consonantal component. Stimulation of either hemisphere could produce this uncouth utterance. The more usual alterations in "language" were made up of arrest, hesitation, slurring, repetition, and distortion of speech; confusion of numbers while counting; inability to name, with retained ability to speak; misnaming, with or without perseveration; difficulty in reading and also in writing. Similar electrical measures applied to the thalamus have also been known to evoke articulate words or phrases [Schaltenbrand (1965); Purpura (1956); Hassler (1966); Schaltenbrand, Spuler, Wahren, and Rimmler (1971)].

Penfield and Roberts also emphasised the nature and distribution of the subcortical connections of the so-called "speech centres." In part, their observations were based upon work by Earl Walker (1938) on the chimpanzee brain (despite the fact that this animal is not endowed with language) and partly upon the special technique of dissection employed by Klingler. The authors hypothesised that the functions of all three cortical "speech areas" in man are connected by projections of each to the thalamus, and that the elaboration of speech is somehow effected by way of these circuits. Penfield and Roberts concluded that both the anterior and the posterior "speech areas" of the cortex are endowed with projection fibres to the thalamus. These anatomical observations, if correct, have an important bearing upon the role of thalamic lesions in aphasia. Their argument was illustrated by elegant drawings of sections of the brain which look impressive but, to many aphasiologists, unconvincing and unnecessary.

The second impetus to this subject arose out of the introduction of stereotactic ablation of small, circumscribed areas within either the globus pallidus or the anterolateral thalamic nuclei as a therapeutic measure. To those with a wide experience of such surgical interventions, particularly in parkinsonian patients, it became evident that the relief of tremor and rigidity might be followed by disorders of communication, mild or severe, temporary or longer-lasting. As already stated, the nature of these disorders was not uniform. Sometimes the disability was obviously one of articulate speech; at other times the problem was different and entailed language, that is, a much higher aspect of communication. Again, there were some cases where it was difficult to determine whether it was speech or language that was at fault, or indeed whether the observer was not witnessing a more complex phenomenon wherein both speech and language were being simultaneously impaired. Extreme instances were rare cases of mutism or total speechlessness following stereotaxy.

Irving Cooper, the pioneer in this field, became quickly aware of this unexpected set of complications. In a series of careful studies over a period of years, he published the results of *ad hoc* investigations into the subject of speech impairment after hemipallidectomy, cryotherapy, thalamectomy, and other stereotactic variants. To these ends he devised research programmes of extreme thoroughness with the help of a multidisciplinary team of co-workers comprising psychologists, speech therapists, neurologists, and neurosurgeons. It became a routine practice to submit every candidate for stereotaxy to an exhaustive battery of tests before surgical intervention as well as at successive intervals after operation. Tape recordings were made of what transpired during each interview, and these were replayed as often as necessary so as to enable a thorough analysis of the nature of any defect. These results were published in a series of remarkably detailed articles [Riklan et al. (1958); Buck and Cooper (1956); Cooper (1961); Levita et al. (1964); Waltz et al. (1966); Cooper et al. (1968); Samra et al. (1969); Riklan et al. (1969)]. Outside Irving Cooper's clinic at St. Barnabas' Hospital, New York, other neurosurgeons had at times witnessed comparable complications after stereotaxy though on a much smaller scale, their cases being submitted to far less profound assessments of the speech faculties [Bonduelle and Guillard (1962); Krayenbühl and Yasargil (1961, 1964); Gillingham (1960–1961); Riechert (1962); Mundinger and Riechert (1963); Svennilson et al. (1960); Allan et al. (1966); Markham and Rand (1963); van Buren (1963); Guist et al. (1961); Bertrand et al. (1964); Schaltenbrand (1965); Ojemann et al. (1958); Hermann et al. (1966)]. These and other workers were exhaustively quoted by Riklan et al. (1969).

From the data which emerged it is possible to discuss—tentatively at any rate—a number of questions:

1. How often do such linguistic complications occur, and how long do they endure?

2. What is the role of the antecedent Parkinson's disease in predisposing to speech disorders after thalamotomy?

3. Is the sidedness of the stereotaxy in its relation to cerebral dominance an important factor?

4. What is the precise nature of the speech disorders?

5. Why is there inconsistency in both the frequency and the nature of these verbal complications?

Some of these questions can be completely answered. Among the earliest of the reports concerning frequency of occurrence was a 1956 paper by Cooper and Buck. Of 49 parkinsonian patients who were treated with either occlusion of the anterior choroidal artery or by chemopallidectomy, about half exhibited speech that was the same after operation as it was before, or it was even better. In the other half, there was a slight falling-off in speech efficiency 6 to 8 weeks after surgery. Indeed,

18 of the patients proclaimed that their speech was worse. The authors concluded that the purpose of surgery in parkinsonians should not be an attempt to alleviate speech impairment.

Krayenbühl and Yasargil (1961) noted a betterment in the speech in 8.4% of 226 patients who underwent unilateral thalamic electrocoagulation. Of the bilateral cases, 24% of those subjected to thalamotomy worsened, as did 48.2% of those treated with pallidothalamotomy.

Gillingham (1960–1961) reported an improvement in the volume of the voice in 10% of 113 cases where unilateral surgery was carried out. In some others, however (the author did not mention how many), the volume was reduced.

Cooper, in association with Levita and Riklan (1964), found that chemothalamectomy had a rather more adverse effect upon speech than cryothalamectomy, the interventions in both cases being carried out on the left side.

In 1969 Cooper, assisted by Samra, Riklan, Levita, Zimmerman, Waltz, and Bergman, made some important observations based upon a pathological study of the brains of 27 parkinsonian patients who had died some time after stereotactic surgery to the thalamus. The authors were at pains to distinguish between defects which concerned speech and those which involved language. Death had occurred 3 days to 5 years after surgery. All 27 patients had been tested in great detail psychologically as well as linguistically. Evaluations had shown that mild changes in language expression had already been present prior to operation in two patients only. On the other hand, all had shown defects in speech abilities—the quality of the voice, the articulation, and the volume of the speech being the aspects most often impaired.

Nineteen patients out of the series of 27 had undergone unilateral surgery, 13 on the left side of the brain and 6 on the right. The remaining 8 patients had been subjected to bilateral or "second side" surgery, the interval between the first and second operations ranging from 6 months to 5 years. In one case, two surgical procedures had been carried out on the same side: chemothalamotomy followed by chemopallidotomy. The target in all cases was the posterior part of the ventrolateral nucleus of the thalamus.

Of the 27 patients, 4 developed mild defects in language after surgery to the left side. Eight patients (6 left side, 2 right side) immediately after operation showed a worsening of their preexisting speech impairment. After "second side" surgery, 4 of 8 patients sustained defects of language, and 6 of the 8 showed deterioration in their articulate speech.

All the patients with dysphasic-type symptoms were only mildly affected, and the defects cleared up within 6 months of the operation. Of those who showed speech disturbances, the impairment was rated as "mild" in eight cases, "moderate" in four, and "severe" in two. The patients with mild disturbances of speech improved spontaneously within a few weeks, whereas in the severe cases intensive speech therapy was required.

As to the postmortem findings in this series of 27 cases, it was found that there was no definite correlation between the size of the lesion and the development of disorders of either language or speech. The authors came to the conclusion that whether a patient will develop deficits either in speech or language after thalamic surgery depends to a great extent upon the preoperative integrity of the brain.

As already hinted, it is sometimes difficult to determine with confidence the precise nature of an advanced parkinsonian's inability to communicate, whether he has been the subject of stereotactic surgery or not.

In some cases, perhaps in most, the trouble seems to entail a failure to articulate clearly coupled with enfeebled power of vocalization. The result is the characteristic mumbling, monotonous, hushed dysarthria which at times may be so extreme as to baffle comprehension. This objective finding must be the product of a severe subjective state of incommunicability, for articulatory defects of this degree usually render the victim severely laconic. It is tempting to correlate the poverty of speech with the typical akinesis which in some patients attains a state of stony immobility. When lack of movement is so grotesque as to preclude manual and gestural activities, a virtual mutism supervenes. Not only does the patient sit or lie in silent impotence, he is unable to convey his wants or ideas by any channel—writing, sign language, or facial mimicry. Ironically, his plight is linked with an integrity of perception and thought. He hears and understands but is a prisoner gagged and bound, immobilised like Daphne, the nymph of the Metamorphoses. Nonetheless, language, *sensu strictu*, is not involved.

But this is not always so. At times there is good reason to believe that verbal expression and perception are impaired over and above any existing dysarthria. This suspicion arises more often in the postoperative cases. The suspicion develops that the patient does not always comprehend to the full the content of what is said to him, and furthermore that he is at times at a loss for a word. His difficulties in communication transcend mere articulatory shortcomings. Maybe he uses a word wrongly, a fact of which he may or may not be aware. Moreover, in his cramped and shaky penmanship, errors can be detected of a dysgraphic sort.

Obviously in such cases there has developed a disorder belonging within the category of language. Is it, however, aphasia? At times it certainly is, but it may well be argued that this is not always correct. Following surgery, with its attendant pre- and postoperative medication, the elderly patient may develop a condition of mental confusion. During this period of obnubilation, fortunately a transient one, the victim may well have difficulty in comprehending speech and in communicating coherently.

Questions of terminology arise. Is it appropriate to apply the term "aphasia" to cases of language disorder which are consequent not upon a focal lesion of the so-called "speech area" of the brain but from a confusion or a dementia? Most purists would say no and would seek some alternative term to categorize speech impairment in such cases. This observance has not always been respected, however, and has sometimes been disregarded, especially by those unversed in aphasiological niceties.

This topic of nomenclature has been specifically raised all too rarely (Critchley, 1937) and awaits firm establishment in neurological teaching.

To return to the question of aphasia or aphasia-like disorders arising as a consequence of focal but deep-seated lesions of the brain, we may refer to the paper written by A. R. Luria (1977) not long before his death. His patient, a woman of 25 years, suffered from a small aneurysm located near the left thalamus. Surgical removal resulted in a number of defects, among them a severe disturbance of spontaneous speech, repetition of words, and naming. For various reasons, Luria rejected the diagnosis of aphasia and regarded his patient as exhibiting "quasi-aphasic speech disturbances." His arguments against the conception of aphasia in his patient are not altogether convincing, but the term he coined is an interesting one and might well be applicable to some of the parkinsonians who have difficulty in communication.

In summary, one may assert that the topic of speech impairment in parkinsonians, whether before or after thalamotomy, is an interesting one which merits more thorough study. There seems to exist a continuum of speech disorders, with pure dysarthria lying at one extreme and dysphasia at the other. Somewhere between are a number of atypical, mixed or complicated cases which are well worthy of study in their own right.

Observations on Volitional Movements

Anaxagoras indeed asserts that it is his possession of hands that makes man the most intelligent of the animals; but surely the reasonable point of view is that it is because he is the most intelligent animal that he has got hands. Hands are an instrument; and Nature, like a sensible human being, always assigns an organ to the animal that can use it. . . . Now the hand would appear to be not one single instrument but many, as it were an instrument that represents many instruments. Thus it is to that animal (viz. man) which has the capability for acquiring the greatest number of crafts that Nature has given that instrument (viz. the hand) whose range of uses is the most extensive.—Aristotle, *De partibus animalium*, IV, X

Our knowledge of volitional movement has been erected upon a tripod of clinical observation, experimental physiology, and psychology. Our present-day nomenclature needs revision; "voluntary," "volitional," "willed," "purposive," "purposeful," and "deliberate" have been inappropriately used as if synonymous, and they have been contrasted with "involuntary," "unwilled," "spontaneous," or "pseudospontaneous" activities. Still more unjustified is a careless reference to volitional movements as though they were mediated specifically along pyramidal pathways, initiated by the cells of the motor cortex, and comparable with the effects of electrical stimulation. The pitfalls of loose thinking upon such topics have been disclosed in great detail during the past 45 years.

Some elements of the problem of volitional movement have at times been forgotten, as, for instance, the fact that there are degrees of volition. We are too apt to assume that the voluntary component of movement is a straightforward mental phenomenon. On the face of it, the attributive "volitional" implies that action has taken place as the result of some operation of the will. This leads us to the question of what is meant by volition, and at once we find ourselves in the deep waters of philosophy. Immediately we see the fallacy of making an artificial antithesis between voluntary and involuntary movement, or between voluntary and nonvoluntary movement. To choose the term "volitional" helps only a little. The phenomenon of volition remains in all its complexity.

William James (1892) believed that the forerunner of a voluntary act lies in a psychic state which comprises an anticipatory image of the sensorial consequences of movements (that is, the motor cue) together with (on certain occasions) what he

Reprinted with permission from Critchley, M. (1954): *Proceedings of the Royal Society of Medicine*, 47:593–601.

called a *fiat*—in other words a decision, express consent, or mandate—that these sensorial consequences should be actualized. Then, too, the act of mental consent necessitates the neutralization of antagonistic, contrary, or inhibitory ideas. Volitional action may comprise action after deliberation, with all its varying types and methods of decision attainment. William James went on to say that at this point the psychology of volition properly stops and that the movements which follow are exclusively physiological phenomena. In his own words: "Volition is a psychic or moral fact pure and simple and is absolutely completed when the stable state of the idea is there. The supervention of motion is a supernumerary phenomenon depending on executive ganglia whose function lies outside the mind. If the ganglia work duly, the act occurs perfectly. If they work, but work wrongly, we have St. Vitus's dance, locomotor ataxy, motor aphasia, or minor degrees of awkwardness. If they don't work at all, the act fails altogether, and we say the man is paralysed. He may make a tremendous effort, and contract the other muscles of the body, but the paralysed limb fails to move."

But in so dismissing the final stage of volition preparatory to movement, William James surely has evaded what to us neurologists are the real issues. Kinnier Wilson (1928) never allowed us to forget the variability of voluntariness. An individual descending a flight of stairs in the dark illustrated, for him, a transition from a very cautious, deliberate motor act to one of facility, speed, and little or no willed effort. Much earlier, Hughlings Jackson (1931) spoke of actions which were "most voluntary" and "least voluntary," "most automatic" and "least automatic," and he even applied these terms to anatomical as well as physiological ideas, segments as well as movements. Indeed he was chary of using the word "voluntary" at all, pointing out that being a psychological term it was not the right word to use when speaking of physical processes.

The experience of paralytic states bears out these points. William James' conception of paralysis was too simple. We neurologists know that an individual muscle may be paralysed in one context but not another. After ablation of the motor cortex, Denny-Brown and Botterell (1948) noticed that any weakness was always most apparent in simple isolated purposive movements when the animal was quiet. The weakness was less obvious when the movement was motivated by desire to escape from its captor. It was still less severe when the animal clutched at objects in falling. Often no paralysis at all was to be noted when the limb was used in behaviour motivated by rage or fright. Gellhorn (1953), too, had found that monkeys paralysed from poliomyelitis performed better under the stress of emotional excitement. It is difficult then to describe these varying sets of circumstances in which some degree of movement occurs either as being volitional or as taking place outside of volition.

An ontogenetic study of willed movements has too long been the perquisite of psychologists rather than neurologists, starting with the spontaneous motor activity of premature, newborn infants. The mass movements of a young baby can scarcely be deemed volitional, for they are amorphous, bilateral, and widespread, irregular in appearance and in rate, uncoordinated and purposeless. Rather, should they be regarded as the precursors of voluntary movements. Later in infancy, a gradual process of increasing economy and efficiency takes place; fragments of this disarray of movement become isolated and gradually achieve a measure of control. Thus a movement becomes capable of being initiated, or inhibited, at will.

According to Ferrier (1886), this is brought about by an organic *nexus* which develops between special sensory centres and motor centres, and so permits the gratification of a specific desire by way of an individual action. Ferrier followed Bain (1864) in associating a factor of attention with centres of inhibition causing acts of volition to lose their impulsive character and acquire an aspect of deliberation. Whether this is a process of aggregating synaptic connexions or one of "individuation" or inhibition of accessory responses is, according to McGraw (1933), not yet known. In Jackson's parlance, this is a process of evolution from the most general to the most special, a continual and gradual "adding on" of new organization—that is, elements which are most special—but at the same time there operates a steady process of "keeping down" of lower nervous arrangements.

Here then are the beginnings of a deliberate volitional movement; all associated muscular activity becomes regulated, though not at a conscious level, so as to form a harmony of movement, of which the prime movers constitute the melody. Thus a synergic unit is achieved. Of this, only the prime movers carry out the deliberate, volitional, conscious part of the act, the other components of the movement taking place at varying levels of unawareness. "The will," as Kinnier Wilson put it, "makes a subjective but not an objective contribution to movement." Our most detailed ontogenetic information concerns the development in a normal infant of the act of reaching for an object, picking it up, and conveying it from one place to another. Using the language of industrial psychology, we can speak of this movement complex as comprising four functional units, or "therbligs," viz.: (1) transport empty; (2) grasp; (3) transport; and (4) release load. In acquiring such a simple motor achievement, the infant passes through many laborious stages, an apprenticeship of trial and error, with gradual, though uneven, progress over a period of some 60 weeks. Should mental development be slow or should states of spasticity exist, these various motor accomplishments are achieved with undue tardiness; the learning process may even be arrested at any stage.

After the normal child has learned to carry out a modest stock of voluntary movements, he continues to acquire adroitness in certain complex movements over the course of the next few decades, depending upon the opportunities afforded by choice and vocation. Some of these skilled movements may reach such a pitch of proficiency as to constitute "expert movements." Although there is now a considerable literature on the psychology of manual skill and on motion-and-time studies, the neurological side has been neglected. This is a pity, because neurologists and psychologists both would benefit from cooperation in this field.

Briefly it can be said that by some process of training—whether this be practice or learning—a particular set of movements, simple or complex, can eventually be carried out with a high degree of efficiency. A skilled movement is not necessarily a delicate one, any more than an unskilled movement is of necessity a coarse movement. On the contrary, some skilled and even expert actions are comparatively coarse, as for instance, in tennis and cricket. What precisely are the criteria, objective and subjective, which distinguish a skilled from an unskilled movement?

1. A skilled movement implies that the particular motor act has probably been performed on many previous occasions. The number of practice efforts probably bears an inverse ratio to the degree of "m" or the alleged factor of innate mechanical aptitude.

2. A skilled movement entails less voluntary effort than a volitional movement. Thus a woman may be able to continue knitting while reading a book; a typist's thoughts may be miles away; a pianist may carry on an animated conversation. Skilled movements, indeed, can often be regarded as automatic movements. But the converse is not true: Automatic movements are not necessarily skilled movements. Some skilled movements never become "automatic," however often repeated. Thus the skills shown by jugglers and acrobats always demand vigilance, perhaps because proximal muscles rather than digital manipulations are concerned and perhaps because the melody of movement is not fixed or predetermined but is impromptu and depends on a play of varying afferent factors. Expressed otherwise, it belongs to the pursuit type of adjustment.

3. Skilled movements are, as a rule, carried out with greater speed than volitional movements, especially when complex in nature. The factors which ordinarily determine the rate of a given volitional movement are obscure. At the command "touch your nose" or "tap the table," a subject will perform these acts at a rate varying between a normal minimum and a normal maximum. This applies when the average inexperienced person first executes a complicated manoeuvre; in this respect, the expert is much faster. In certain disease states, movements, whether simple or skilled, are performed much too slowly, even though the strength is unimpaired. This is a matter which cannot, however, be discussed here.

4. There is far greater economy of movement in the case of the expert, with a more limited range of activity of the prime movers. Skilled movement is restricted to the needs of the situation, but an unskilled voluntary act may occupy a greater spatial extent.

5. Skilled movements tend to dispense with associated movements and with movements of cooperation.

6. Skilled movements are performed with a less forceful contraction of the prime movers than are voluntary unskilled movements, that is, with less expenditure of energy.

7. Skilled movements, like involuntary movements, are less fatiguing.

Dexterity can be transferred to the unpractised hand. Thus a right-handed person who has learned a skill with his preferred hand, finds it possible to perform that act with the left hand more efficiently than a beginner, even though he may never before have attempted that movement with his left hand. Furthermore, a short period of practice will allow an adept to achieve with his left hand the same high degree of skill as with the right. This fact explains the ability of a hemiplegic artist to continue painting with his other hand and still retain his technique. Dexterity can also be consigned from one body segment to another, though with a lesser degree of correlation. Thus an ataxic painter can soon learn to manipulate a brush held between his toes or his teeth. These examples of shifting distribution of the instrumentalities of a learned skill should be of much interest to neurophysiologists.

Whether skilfulness achieved in one complex act can be transmitted to another is less certain and is still argued. Does an ability to play a violin assist in the technique of typewriting or of embroidery? Perhaps the answer depends upon the nature of the training which led up to the original manual skill. Should this have resulted from a matter of practice, i.e., simple prolonged repetition, it is doubtful if dexterity can facilitate the development of other skills. But if the dexterity has stemmed from a process of learning, then it probably can be transferred to other complex movements, as industrial experience shows. Learning (in the strict sense) differs from practice in that it educates the apprentice in the fundamentals of motor efficiency, which stand in good stead whatever new task is concerned. Then, of course, there is Thorndike's (1931) suggestion that practice in one skill may favourably affect practice in another skill because both possess some elements in common.

Knowledge of the difference between dextrous and unskilled accomplishments can be incorporated within the systems of learning and improve industrial output. Various "principles of motion economy" have been enunciated, as by the Gilbreths (1919) and Barnes (1949). Shaw's (1952) five principles are the simplest. According to Shaw, detailed movements should be (1) simultaneous; (2) symmetrical; and (3) natural.* The path of whole movement cycles ought to be (4) rhythmical and (5) habitual. By simultaneity is meant that movements should begin and end together, whereas symmetrical movements are oriented to an imaginary line through the centre of the body. It is important to avoid monotony by breaking up the rhythm of repetitive small-range movements with occasional larger movements. There are many levels of learning up to a study of fundamental principles. Important in apprenticeship is the formation of correct habits of movements and the means of breaking old and inefficient habits. Learning curves illustrate the rate of progress. At first the advance is rapid; then it slows. Indeed progression may halt, and the pupil may even fall back a little. These constitute the plateaux of the learning curve. Whether these plateaux represent periods of increasing integration or indicate the pauses between successive methods of learning is uncertain. How best to allocate the available time into working periods and rest periods is another matter for expert advice.

Are special cerebral structures concerned with the dextrous execution of complicated motor skills? Or are they "represented"—if that term may be excused—in the motor cortex in the same way as other movements? Contradictory statements upon this matter have come not only from different writers but also from the same writer on different occasions. That cerebellar, striatopallidal, and proprioceptive

---

*Aristotle insisted that "natural" movements were less tiring than those which were awkward or associated with faulty posture. Thus in his *Problemata*, Chap. V, we read: "Why is it more difficult to apply prolonged friction oneself to the left leg than to the right? Is it because though our right is the side which is capable of exertion, yet the rubbing of the left leg, since it involves a distorted attitude, is unnatural, and anything which is unnatural is difficult."

influences occur in both kinds of movement cannot be gainsaid. But skilled volitional movements as opposed to unpractised volitional acts possibly entail a wider extent of cortical activity in "elaboration fields" lying both in front of and behind the motor area, and also no doubt in homologous but contralateral parts.

Clinical experience shows that skilled movements (that is, dextrous, practised movements) are highly vulnerable to the brunt of cerebral disease at all levels: pyramidal, cerebellar, pallidal, and proprioceptive. This observation supports the idea that the integrity of all these mechanisms is needed for the correct and effortless execution of acquired skilled movements. In view of what we know about the ontogenetic development of movements, it would be interesting to enquire whether the pattern of dissolution resulting from disease in any way recapitulates the stages of development, especially when the disease is of a steadily progressive order (Figs. 1 and 2).

Neurologists also encounter a dilapidation of skilled movements, apparently in specific and isolated form, in other morbid conditions. We refer, in the first place, to the apraxias. Here, by definition, occurs a defect in the execution of a movement, though motor power, sensibility, and coordination are seemingly intact. Of course, there are many patterns of apraxia, and more orderly thinking upon this subject is much overdue. One difficulty lies in the patient's inconsistencies in performance, for he may do well one moment and fail badly the next. On the whole, the more automatic the movement, the better will it be performed. To some extent then, apraxia is more a disorder of simple volitional movement than of skilled movements insofar as the latter can be regarded as automatic and independent of deliberate and conscious control. (I shun the term "attention" here, as it is still a contentious subject among psychologists.) But if apraxia is not the best example of a specific disorder of skilled movements, we can point to another condition which more adequately applies, namely, the various craft palsies. These essentially constitute a

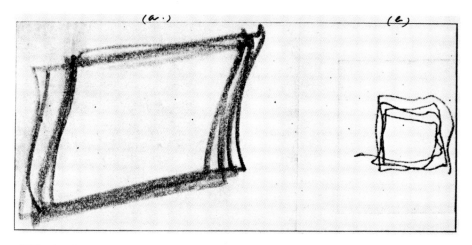

FIG. 1. Drawing squares as rapidly as possible for 8 seconds: **(A)** control; **(B)** patient with primary cerebellar degeneration.

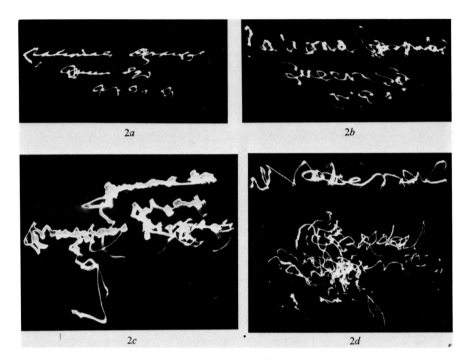

FIG. 2. Cyclegram of the movements of the index finger during the act of writing "National Hospital Queen Sq., W.C.1." **a:** Normal right-handed subject using the right hand. Time taken: 13 seconds. **b:** Normal right-handed subject using the left hand. Time taken: 28 seconds. **c:** Patient with Huntington's chorea using the right hand. Time taken: 54 seconds. **d:** Patient with Huntington's chorea using the left hand. Time taken: >85 seconds.

specific impairment of educated motor skills. The disability cannot be fully overcome either by an effort of deliberate concentration (i.e., by converting them into highly volitional movements) or by downgrading them into "more automatic" movements. Such craft palsies exclusively affect—in the early stages at least—a particular complex movement which has achieved dexterity through tedious practice; they spare all other volitional movements, whether skilled or unskilled, and, furthermore, all movements belonging to Jackson's category of "least voluntary" and "most automatic." To look upon the craft palsies as problems in psychopathology has not proved satisfying even to psychiatrists. On the contrary, the craft palsies are fascinating problems to the physiological psychologist and to the neurologist. The type of error made, for example, by the victim of writer's cramp, is reminiscent of many of the distinctions made between an unpractised complex movement and one which is deft and practised (Figs. 3 and 4).

Brief mention should be made of an unfamiliar type of skilled movement. I refer not to practised movements of extreme complexity but, rather, the reverse. Under the term "skilled minimal movements" one can allude to those unusual tricks of motility whereby a single muscle, or a part of a single muscle, can be made voluntarily to contract. I deliberately avoid speaking of "discrete movement."

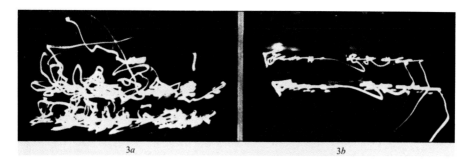

FIG. 3. Writer's cramp. Cyclegrams of the movements of the index, middle, and ring fingers of the right hand during the act of writing. **a:** Patient with writer's cramp. Time taken: 14 seconds. **b:** Normal subject. Time taken: 6 seconds.

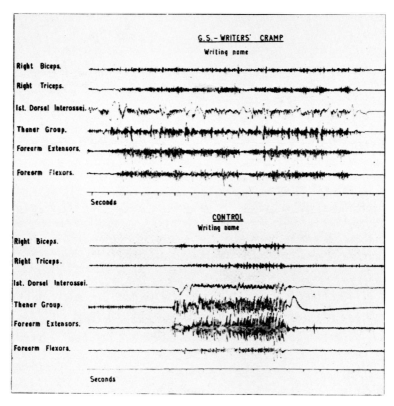

FIG. 4. Electromyograph taken during the act of writing, in the case of a normal subject *(below)* and a patient with writer's cramp *(above)*. (Courtesy of Dr. W. A. Cobb.)

Typically, the muscle concerned is not one which participates in ordinary manipulations but is a proximally situated muscle or, still more characteristic, part of the muscular investment of the trunk. By dint of practice, some few are able at will to contract and relax the muscles attached to the auricle of the ear or to move one-half of the frontalis muscle or a segment of one pectoralis major, deltoid, or rectus abdominis. Students of the Orient will recall the startling repertoire of unexpected minimal muscle movements which can be brought within the category of volitional movements. The mechanism of production of these movements entails a sort of practised fractionation analogous to the infant's increasing power of controlling isolated fragments out of a mass of movements.

One may also mention as another fitting theme for neurological attention the subclinical muscular contraction, or perhaps only action potentials, which can be detected in muscle groups in circumstances of mere imagery of movement or during the mental state of recalling muscular acts or of matters which would involve such a motor concomitant. The importance of these observations, which have been made for nearly a century and which were predicted by Jackson and studied by Lotze, Bain, Ferrier, Golla (1921), and Jacobson (1932), is a fundamental one in psychology, for they throw light upon the nature of thinking processes and suggest that the activities of thought are not confined to closed circuits within the brain. These "shadow movements" do not actually fall within the ranks of volitional movements, though they may be looked upon as the expression of the recollection of volitional movements.

Lastly, in a discussion of volitional activity, a neurologist must decide where mimic movements of gesture precisely belong. And where, too, should we place the tics, especially the more elaborate, quasipurposeful habit spasms? If we subscribe to the doctrine that there are levels of voluntariness, then we cannot rightly exclude either gesticulation or the tics, mindful of the definition made by Meige and Feindel (1907): "A tic is a coordinated purposive act, provoked in the first instance by some external cause or by an idea; repetition leads to its becoming habitual and finally to its involuntary reproduction without cause and for no purpose, at the same time as its form, intensity, and frequency are exaggerated; it thus assumes the characters of a convulsive movement, inopportune and excessive; its suppression associated with malaise. The effect of distraction or of volitional effort is to diminish its activity; in sleep it disappears. It occurs in predisposed individuals, who usually show other indications of mental instability. . . ." Like ordinary volitional movements, tics are fully coordinated actions, preceded by a desire for their execution and succeeded by a feeling of satisfaction. At the same time, a tic is an inapposite and incongruous act which may in certain circumstances even prove harmful. Hence it has been well termed a parasite function. A tic, like a gesture, is a kind of voluntary movement, low in the ladder of volition.

Summary

My purpose has been to stress the fact that volitional movement is a far more complex idea than appears at first sight. Although in the past efforts have been made to align electrically induced motion with volitional movement, one of my objects would be to emphasize the dangers of such an analogy. As to the important contributions of experimental physiology a quotation offers itself as apt:

> Our survey must be circumspect for several reasons. By use of such methods as we are employing, artificial excitation, and so on, and under such observations as these allow, namely the initiation under narcosis of muscular movements or the recording of their immediate defects from normal movement, little light is given in regard to much that goes on in an organ whose chief function is mentality itself. Our expectation must be modest, for modest must be the achievement reached by such means in a problem of such a nature. (Sherrington, 1947)

Prologues to Migraine Congresses: 1980, 1982, 1984

1980

Mr. Chairman, distinguished participants and visitors, ladies and gentlemen, I welcome you heartily on behalf of the Migraine Trust to this its third international symposium. In anticipation of your valuable contributions may I be permitted one or two preliminary remarks, superficially captious perhaps but, believe me, very well intentioned?

Since the days of the Emperor Vespasian, we physicians have been familiar with the lush symptomatology of migraine. And yet, if we are honest with ourselves, we must confess we are still quite in the dark as to the fundamental cause of this tantalising affection, its *fons et origo*, as well as being ignorant as to its logical treatment.

Over the years since I first became interested in this disorder, and the even longer period during which I have suffered its onslaughts, I have witnessed a host of successive hypotheses, each one in turn being advanced with great confidence—even dogmatism—only in due course to vanish into oblivion. Starting with the concept of a hypersensitive cortex liable to detonate periodically, much in the same way as in epilepsy, we proceeded to the notion that migraine was the outcome of eye strain. One of my teachers confidently ascribed migraine to a distension of a lateral ventricle on one side of the brain and said that in the pathological museum of St. George's Hospital there was a specimen that proved this assertion. I pass over the assurances of some psychopathologists who regarded migraine as the product of "baffled rage and humiliation." This psychosomatic doctrine was replaced by the idea that migraine was of alimentary origin, triggered off by a dyskinesis of the gallbladder and its passages. The ductless glands then came under suspicion. In the female, ovaries were implicated, as cynically proclaimed by Balzac in his *Physiologie du Mariage*, while in the male an intermittent swelling of the pituitary was visualized. Then came the idea that migraine was a stress disorder, salutary insofar as it protected the organism from other and more serious consequences of excessive moil and toil. The allergic theory dies hard, for it was very much in vogue 60 years ago, then forgotten, lately to be resuscitated phoenix-like with even greater force. Then came the heyday of biochemical researchers—the philosophers of the furnace, as Francis Bacon called them—seeking to isolate some pain-producing substance, periodically and mysteriously liberated.

Prologues to 1980 and 1984 Migraine Congresses appear with permission from Pitman Medical, London, and Karger, Basel, respectively.

At one time the work of Harold Wolff seemed to provide the answer, by drawing attention to fluctuations in the calibre of the intra- and extracranial arteries and in the cerebral blood flow.

Are we perhaps barking up the wrong tree? Could it be that, after all, migraine is a pure disorder of nervous tissue, the expression of a cyclical upset in cortical activity? Might not migraine turn out to be an authentic and specific neurological disorder, a mysterious dysfunction of those pearly cells of the brain, as Oscar Wilde called them, independent of any chemical dyscrasia or of any anomaly of the circulation?

William Gowers, perhaps the greatest neurological clinician of all time, once proffered this advice: "Cultivate the habit of viewing a chronic clinical problem afresh from time to time; ignore what you *had* thought of it; put yourself in the place of a fresh observer and try and see if it thus bears a new aspect."

Let us face it: Migraine is a 2,000-year-old reproach to our profession. Is it not high time that clinicians and neurophysiologists should shed their modesty and boldly enter the arena and get together to hammer out the problem from an angle that is entirely different from what we have been pursuing up to now?

Let us also bear in mind what Thomas Huxley said: "Sit down before the facts like a little child; be prepared to give up every preconceived notion; follow humbly wherever nature leads, or you'll learn nothing."

And what of treatment? If empiricism fails, and serendipity does not materialize, certainty as to aetiology may in time lead to logical therapy, like alpha and omega, and one day we might be able to respond to Winifred Holtby's plea:

> Constant companion of my wakeful days
> And uninvited bridegroom of my bed,
> Withdraw a little, and thy hand up-raise
> From my tormented head.

1982

Welcome to the fourth international symposium on migraine—that subject which holds us so closely in exasperated fascination. After centuries of empiricism we still cannot envisage confidently the way ahead, and more and more we are turning for assistance to experts in the basic sciences. But as Oscar Wilde said, "Science is limited because it can never grapple with the Irrational." And whatever can be more irrational than migraine, that clinical chaos of immiscible and unconnected particles, "full of vague indispositions and stray miseries and confabulations of the vital juices," to quote Charles Knickerbocker. For we are not dealing with some clinical abstraction or a philosophical concept called "migraine," but with a coterie of migrainous individuals of whom no two are identical. Since the advent of the scientific era in medicine we have made great strides, only to be met with one bafflement after another—metabolic, chemical, vasospastic. Perhaps, as I have said before, we should be looking more closely at the periodic turmoil among those clusters of pearly cells that lie within the tissues of the brain itself.

Like Marc Anthony, "I have neither wit, nor words, nor utterances, nor the power of speech"; nonetheless I venture to emphasize that serendipity is comparatively rare in medicine. Discovery comes to the mind that is already prepared. A more felicitous term for the unexpected innovation is "altamirage," a word we owe to Professor Austin of Denver. The painted caves of El Castillo and Altamira were not a chance outcome of a dog disappearing down a rabbit hole. No. Because of the unusual rock formation, geologists had long predicted that a huge underground cavern must surely lie buried somewhere close by.

I feel confident that somewhere or other there is a little boy or a little girl with a Rubik's cube who one day, in *your* time, will find the key which will unlock the door that is keeping from us the secret of migraine.

But today I make an earnest plea. Do not turn your back on the clinician. The diagnostician still has an important place within the scientific team. I have known promising research founder on the rocks because the protagonists were not aware of the clinical vagaries of migraine and failed to distinguish clearly the sheep from the goats in the pastures of head pain.

Let me finish my remarks by once again offering up a prayer that all migrainologists should observe:

> From an inability to let well alone;
> From too much zeal for what is new and
>   contempt for what is old;
> From putting knowledge before wisdom,
> Science before Art,
> And Cleverness before Commonsense;
> From treating patients as cases;
> And from making the cure of the disease
>   more grievous than its endurance;
> Good Lord, deliver us.

1984

Good morning ladies and gentlemen. A very warm welcome to all who are participating in this, the fifth international symposium upon migraine. In particular I welcome you to London. I imagine everyone in this auditorium knows what Dr. Samuel Johnson said: "To a man whose pleasure is intellectual, London is the place...when a man is tired of London he is tired of life; for there is in London all that life can afford." But how many of my audience recall that Johnson finished his remarks by saying: "The full tide of existence is at Charing Cross."

I have long discovered that the ideal committee is made up of three members, one of whom has sent apologies for absence. Likewise, the perfect discussion group sits around a small table where argument and debate range back and forth like an intellectual ping-pong ball. Larger conferences also have their place, but there are hazards. Ramon y Cajal was not only a histological genius but also an astute philosopher full of wise saws and modern instances. He was sceptical about their value and dubious about that axiom "from discussion comes *light*." "What often transpires," said he, "is the *fire* of exasperation, *smoke* of obscurity, and *ashes* of disillusion." But Cajal did not know that migrainologists are persons of a very special calibre. They may be remote, intellectual types, rather like the Jesuits in the priesthood, but I have always found that they are very friendly and warm-hearted. In fact:

> Celebrated, cultivated, underrated,
> Unaffected, undetected, well-connected,
> Ever-knowing, over-flowing, easy-going.

They are dedicated men and women, united in their quest for an understanding and a cure of this particularly teasing, even tormenting, malady. That is why I thank every one of you for your presence here today.

Migraine is one of those ills when the body has to bear patiently what the soul cannot carry. If to the victim migraine is a recurring calamity of a tomahawk in the skull, it is often a pain in the neck to the general practitioner and a pain in the fundament to the frustrated family.

Having had a personal interest and an acquaintance with this disorder for well over 70 years, I have witnessed the coming and going of overconfident theories and much vaunted remedies. As regards the latter, our only certain cure, I believe, is longevity.

With respect to the tantalising matter of pathogenesis, I am glad to see a growing aversion to theories of vasospastic and even chemical dyscrasias. Please God we will witness the end of food-faddery, and I heartily welcome a revival of pure neurological notions. Once again the idea of Leão's spreading depression is now in the van. Like Marie Lloyd, may I urge that you follow the van and don't dilly-dally on the way?

Mr. Chairman, despite the disappointments from long experience, I am still an optimist. I have a dream, a dream that today our nebulous ideas will become rather more clear and that the crooked pathways will be made more straight. I have a dream that the next couple of days will be an occasion of good fellowship, fine feasting, and fascinating discourse.

Ladies and gentlemen, let us start.

Acromegaly or Paget's Disease?

Two letters from Pierre Marie to Sir James Paget, now in my possession,* mark an interesting point in the early description of acromegaly. Our present knowledge of this disorder dates from September 1885 when Pierre Marie contributed a paper on the subject to the *Revue de Médecine*. This article was followed 3 years later by a longer communication in the *Nouvelle Iconographie de la Salpêtrière*, appearing in serial form. In 1890 Pierre Marie published an article in English on the same topic in *Brain*. The first of these papers was translated into English by Proctor Hutchinson and was issued in book form in 1891 published by the New Sydenham Society, London (Fig. 1). Dr. Souza-Leite's thesis "On Acromegaly (Marie's Malady)" in 1890 was also included in the volume. By this time 38 cases of the disease had been reported. The editor of the New Sydenham Society volume added another 12 examples collected from the British medical literature.

In his papers Pierre Marie drew attention to an unfamiliar syndrome comprising an enlargement of the extremities and of the face, for which he proposed the term *"acro-mégalie."* His original case material consisted in two patients who were in hospital under the care of his chief, Professor Charcot.

One was a woman of 37 years whose menses first became irregular when she was 24. At 33 she began to complain frequently of headache. Her extremities had always been large, but when she was 24 her hands suddenly increased in size, and the appearance of her face altered to such an extent that her relatives scarcely recognised her. Marie carefully described the strange features of the patient and mentioned such symptoms as thirst, excessive secretion of urine, and slight impairment of hearing and vision.

His other patient, also a female, was aged 54 years. Menstruation had ceased abruptly after a shock sustained when she was 29. At 30 she completely lost her eyesight. After 8 months she recovered some vision but only for a matter of 2 years, after which she became permanently blind. When she was 32 she began to experience generalized weakness, and she also noticed that her head was growing larger. Previously she had been referred to as *"la petite,"* but now her waist, hands, and feet were getting bigger. Excessive thirst was another symptom, but only for a time. Marie proceeded to describe her appearance in detail. This patient had also had a long history of "rheumatism," and nodules were present over the hands.

How to identify this strange symptom puzzled Pierre Marie and no doubt his chief, Charcot, as well. An exhaustive search through the world's literature brought to light the records of five other case reports that almost certainly represented the

---

*They were given me by my friend George Riddoch. He, in turn, was probably presented them by his old chief, and patient, Henry Head.

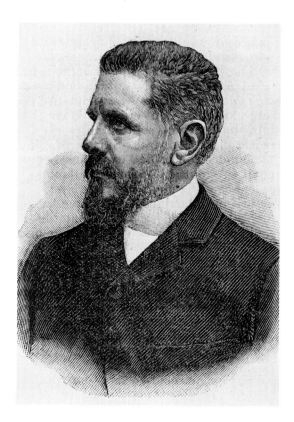

FIG. 1. Pierre Marie. (Courtesy of the Army Institute of Pathology, Washington, D.C.)

same malady [Saucerotte-Noel (1772); Alibert (1822); Friedreich, 2 cases (1868); and Henrot (1877, 1882)]. Later, Pierre Marie changed his mind about the two cases described by Friedreich—the Hagner brothers—on the basis of a later examination of them by Erb. Marie did not commit himself to the diagnosis here, and in particular he would not entertain any such conception as one of "partial acromegaly." Henrot's case was particularly important in that a postmortem examination was made, and an ovoid tumour the size of a hen's egg was found at the base of the brain in the midline, near the pituitary body. Henrot's finding anticipated Minkowski, who associated the acromegalic syndrome with pituitary disorder. This was in 1887. At a later date Marie uncovered a few other cases in the medical literature [Brigidi (1877); Hadden and Ballance (1885); Lombroso (1868); Taruffi (1879); Verga (1864)]. The first example to be described in the United States was Wadsworth's case of "myxoedema with atrophy of the optic nerves" (1885), the patient being subsequently recognised by Hadden and Ballance in 1888.

Marie also dealt with the possibility that his syndrome of acromegaly was somewhat similar to the *leontiasis ossea* as Virchow termed his cases of craniofacial hypertrophy (1867). In all likelihood the cases described by Jadelot (1799), Forcade, Murchinson (1866), Adams (1871), and Le Dentu (1879) belonged to the syndrome described by Virchow. Marie differentiated this syndrome from acromegaly because of the facial appearance, the normal size of the extremities, and the presence of multiple craniofacial exostoses.

Even earlier, in 1876, Sir James Paget had demonstrated at the Medico-Chirurgical Society of London a clinical syndrome characterized by an irregularly distributed skeletal hypertrophy (Fig. 2). Could the cases at the Salpêtrière belong to this category? This was the problem which occurred to Marie and which he was anxious to exclude or confirm before publishing his original case report. At this point we find Marie addressing his first letter to Sir James Paget (translation):

> Faculty of Medicine
> Nervous Disease Clinic
> Salpêtrière
> 30 April 1885

Monsieur et très honoré Maître,
    Professor Charcot has in his service at the present time two patients with enormous hands and an increase in the diameter of the face and skull as well as in the size of the feet. He thinks that it might be due to the osteitis deformans described by you; but he has not got the exact reference of your paper and would be most grateful if you would kindly let him know it or send him a reprint if you still have one available.
    Veuillez agréer Monsieur et très honoré Maître mes salutations respectueuses

> Pierre Marie
> *Chef du Clinique de Professor Charcot*

If any new work has been done on this subject, M. Charcot would be very pleased to know about it.

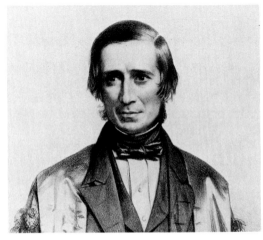

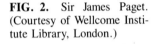

FIG. 2. Sir James Paget. (Courtesy of Wellcome Institute Library, London.)

This letter is of historical interest on two counts. First, it indicates the doubts as to whether the Paris cases were examples of osteitis deformans, better known as Paget's disease; and secondly, it shows the close interest that Charcot, under whose care the patients were, displayed in the clinical problem. The subsequent attachment of Pierre Marie's name to this malady has rather allowed one to lose sight of the fact that Charcot probably identified the original two cases as medical curiosities, recognised the two patients as belonging to the same clinicopathological category, and raised the question of possible identity with Paget's disease. Perhaps it would be most appropriate—so long as eponyms are accepted in neurology—to speak of Charcot-Marie's syndrome rather than the usual *"maladie de Pierre Marie."*

Paget's reply to Marie is not available, but its upshot can be deduced from the content of Marie's second letter (translation):

14 May 1885
Thank you very much for the generosity with which you so kindly put at my disposal all the papers on osteitis deformans; after carefully reading them, I believe that our two patients do not conform to your description; is it a new disease? Is it a variety of osteitis deformans? I think it is difficult to say. The appearance of these patients does not in fact resemble the photographs you were kind enough to send me, as you can infer from those which I take the liberty of sending to you.

In our two patients there is a great increase in the size of the *hands*, the *feet* and the *face*; the skull shows protuberances and depressions but not the hypertrophy you described in osteitis deformans.

I have confirmed these differences all the better since after reading your description I have found in the Hôtel Dieu a patient who could be looked upon as a type of osteitis deformans and who answers your description point for point: He was the subject of a recent thesis (Des *Hyperostoses generalisées primitives* by L. Roger, Thèse de Paris, 1884). Unfortunately the author did not know about osteitis deformans and his article does not mention it.

Veuillez agréer etc.
Pierre Marie

M. Charcot requests me to send you his kind regards.

Charcot, be it recalled, was something of a draughtsman and had always shown interest in disease states as depicted by the world's great artists throughout the centuries. That his visual observation was keenly receptive towards the grotesque and the deformed in medicine cannot be doubted, and we can imagine him halting by the bedside of the two original patients in the Salpêtrière, realising the novelty of the syndrome and at the same time the identity of the two examples. Whether Charcot ever stumbled upon an instance of acromegaly in medieval art is unlikely. Had he been a numismatist as well as an art historian he might also have anticipated Harold Klawans' discovery (1980) that the coins of the Roman Emperor Maximinius I revealed him to have been an acromegalic.

Discoveries come to him who has a mind prepared. It is not surprising to learn that Pierre Marie, with all his excitement over the isolation of acromegaly and already so attuned and mentally receptive was intrigued one November morning in 1889 to find a prognathous, kyphotic Jew sitting opposite him in an omnibus. Marie forced a conversation upon him and found that he was a rather hypochondriacal doctor, complaining of intense thirst, boulimia, and painful enlargement of the hands. No wonder that this case also figured among Marie's final series (as quoted in the New Sydenham Society volume).

An Appraisal of Visual (Object) Agnosia: A Tribute to Professor Otto Pötzl

No more fitting topic than that of occipital lobe dysfunction could be discussed in this fabulous city of Vienna. Still more appropriate is it that we should meet in this historical *aula* or forum. Today our thoughts are necessarily filled with memories of the late Professor Otto Pötzl, who for the 17 years intervening between 1928 and 1945 occupied the exalted University Chair of Neurology and Psychiatry left vacant by the retirement of von Wagner-Jauregg. We can almost sense the presence of these great men in our midst today, and the poignancy of our emotions is enhanced by the chairmanship of Pötzl's assistant, colleague, and worthy successor, Professor Hoff.

The field of neuropsychology—I use that term expressly rather than neuropsychiatry—represents today one of the most exciting expansions of our discipline. It holds abundant promise for the future, for its province is nothing less than the supreme intellectual equipment of *Homo sapiens*. Perception, thinking—abstract, creative, and symbolic—self-awareness, time sense, communication—whether of ideas or of emotions—these are the targets for neuropsychological research, where man in health and disease represents the experimental material, rather than the peripheral neuraxis of the cat or ape.

To this uniquely important subject Pötzl contributed stimulating and original ideas to an extent which must surely be unequalled. From his earliest studies upon imagery and hallucinosis until his monograph upon the world of colour written in his 80th year, his literary output was remarkable. By that term I do not suggest that Pötzl wrote much: He did not; but the range of his questing into man's highest cerebral function was extraordinary. Central blindness; visual agnosia; optic alloaesthesia; palinopsia; hallucinations of sight, polyopia; illusory acceleration of movement; reduplicative agonal illusions; auditory imperception; dysgraphia; juvenile aphasias; conceptions of time and space; inverted vision; the median plane of the body schema—all these were major contributions of his, erudite and exhaustive. Pötzl's writings were unfortunately difficult to follow. He did not possess the happy knack of clear exposition, but we recall that other writers, too, suffered this same demerit—his predecessor at Prague, for example, Arnold Pick, and our

Reprinted with permission from Critchley, M. (1965): *Transactions of the 8th International Congress of Neurology*, vol. 5, edited by J. Konstans. Elsevier, Amsterdam.

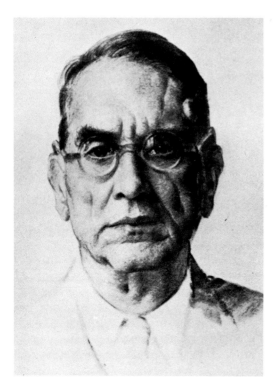

FIG. 1.   Professor Otto Pötzl.

own Hughlings Jackson. Then again, Sherrington's prose was that of a poet and sometimes proved elusive to lesser minds. But Pötzl's obscurity was redeemed by the brilliancy of his creative imagination and the boldness and originality of his thinking (Fig. 1).

I would like to suggest the proposition to Professor Hoff and his team of able co-workers that they would be doing an important service to contemporary neurology were they to assemble the scattered writings, papers, and monographs of Pötzl, and publish one or more volumes representing the collected works of this great man.

As an artist in speculative reasoning Pötzl would probably disapprove strongly of some of the opinions which may be put forward today, 20 years after he relinquished his chair. Certainly he would look askance at many of my own ideas. But to my mind this matters little. Although I have the temerity to disagree with many of Pötzl's hypotheses, I yield to no one in my profound admiration for the sheer scintillation of his mind, and above all his inspired and visionary thinking. But contemporary trends are swinging further and further away from schematic and parcellated notions about brain function, with precise cerebral emplacement and rigid clinical expression.

In approaching our problem of occipital dysfunction, we may with propriety deal first with the most extreme cases. Here naturally belong the instances of total loss of vision due to bilateral posterior polar lesions. These are usually abrupt in onset, for infarction and trauma probably account for most examples. Blindness might be expected to constitute a calamitous blow, bringing dire affects of depression and despair. But, as every neurologist knows, the result is nothing of the sort. The patient usually displays other reactions, all of them unexpected. One patient may be quite unaware that he has lost his sight. This double blindness is usually spoken of as the "Anton syndrome," though it had been described with the utmost lucidity by Seneca centuries ago. Then there is the victim who not only does not realize that he is blind but stoutly denies the fact when it is put to him. I have proposed the term "nosoarnesia" for this total rejection of any suggested dysfunction. Yet another reaction is found when the patient does not repudiate the blindness but merely brushes aside its relevance. This is the "implicit denial" of Weinstein and Kahn. Yet other patients behave still differently. To the tentative suggestion that something might be amiss with the eyesight, the patient may concede grudgingly that perhaps "it's not quite what it should be." He shows no distress, however, for he aligns his symptoms with something quite benign, like presbyopia.

There are still other modes of behaviour. A patient may admit that he cannot see clearly but go on to project his disability by invoking shortcomings in the illumination. He may grumble that the blinds are drawn; that it is night-time; or that the lamps have not been lighted.

Lastly, a patient may admit his blindness but quite casually, without any feeling-tone of despondency or grief. Unless prompted, he does not refer to his affliction, nor does he importune his doctors as to his prognosis and his chances of getting back to work.

Merely to list all these various modes of reaction to cortical blindness, however, is not enough. A patient's attitude may vary from day to day, or even from moment to moment. Inconsistency of response or reaction is characteristic, and it seems to lie outside the patient's awareness. Thus he may one moment deny that he is blind and yet permit nurses to fend for him; lead him around; wash, dress, and feed him.

Other visuopsychic disabilities are likely to be present. Visual memory and visual imagery may both be lacking, and in compensation the patient in his Korsakoff-like state, may confabulate madly.

There is an interesting clinical phenomenon, rarely if ever mentioned in the literature, whereby a patient displays a "confabulatory visual pseudorecognition" of objects before him. Thus when an article is held up for identification, the patient is naturally at a loss, for he can see nothing at all. When, however, it is put within his grasp, he promptly names it. *If a moment later the patient is told to uplift the object before his eyes, he will now stoutly assert that he can see it clearly and identify it.* That he is confabulating is shown, however, as soon as he is asked to describe its appearance and colour. Quite unperplexed, he does not hesitate to proffer preposterous guesses.

We neurologists are in possession of a number of alternative hypotheses to explain these various aspects of anosognosia. One notion maintains that lack of insight is the specific consequence of a right parietal lesion. Opposed to this is the theory of a "denial syndrome" which may stem from brain disease irrespective of site or sidedness. Yet another speculation implicates the nature of the subject's premorbid personality.

I would like to draw attention to yet another way of explaining these cases of defective insight into the consequences of cerebral blindness. This particular theory stresses the pitfalls and artefacts of the "interview situation" and maintains that interpersonal factors are all-important. Jaffé and Slote (1958) explored the physician–patient relationship by means of structured interviews, followed by a content analysis of the patient's responses. Two sets of enquiries were drawn up, one slanted towards minimizing the patient's trouble, and the other directed towards making the most of what defect there was. Contrasting questions were carefully devised, and the patient's replies were closely studied. The authors concluded therefrom that anosognosia represents "a symbolic adaptive mechanism, observed under the conditions of communicative interaction."

If cortical blindness represents the extreme defect after bilateral occipital dysfunction, the stages of restitution are of particular interest to us. It is here that difficulties are likely to occur in the identification of objects, faces, colours, the judgement of distances and rate of movement. Rather than discuss the location within the visual fields of the first glimmerings of returning vision, we will focus our attention more upon the qualities of the phenomena. An ill-defined impression of the surrounding world emerges—what has been termed, not very happily, an "organ sensation." Poppelreuter described six stages of reintegration of visual function. I will not recapitulate these, for I would prefer you to let me quote the account afforded us, not by a neurologist but by an observant ophthalmic surgeon:

> As recovery progresses, an elementary light–dark sensation appears on retinal stimulation, at first in dark adaptation, to disappear in bright illumination. This is the most primitive sensory visual function—a vague formless sentiency with no analysable attributes, a sensation of brightness, subjectively confusing and even vaguely painful, objectively appearing as a diffuse irregular lightening of the visual field, without differentiation or localization and without qualitative or quantitative relation to the position, extensity or intensity of the stimulating light. [Duke-Elder]

The first objective stimuli to be sensed are beams of bright light. Later still, smaller points of illumination may attract attention and be more or less localized. Now, large moving objects may be vaguely detected. Gradually, smaller and less brilliant objects are perceived, and movement no longer becomes essential. Later comes a recognition of shape, a more accurate orientation, and a progressive betterment in visual acuity. White objects are perceived before those which are coloured: Of the latter, the more brilliant and optically significant are observed before the duller and secondary hues. An important step in recovering vision has now been reached, one which may long endure, or even become established. This is the stage of metamorphopsia where the appearance of the environment takes on various illusory features. Aberration may occur in the size or shape of things around. Vertical or horizontal dimensions may seem oblique or tilted; outlines of objects look wavy, blurred, or scintillating. There may be an illusory movement of objects—oscillatory, rotatory, sweeping, or drifting. Or objects may seem alternately to draw near and recede. The patient's localization of surrounding details may be incorrect—blatantly so in the case of optic alloaesthesia so brilliantly described by Hermann and Pötzl. Or chronogenic anomalies may enter, so that objects continue to be sensed long after their removal (visual perseveration) or to reappear unprovoked by any stimulus (palinopsia).

Changes in the semblance of the environment, more tenuous and less tangible, may augment the metamorphopsia. I refer to the sense of unreality, the derealisation, the *jamais vu* phenomenon we know so well, and which may also entail an intense affective colouring, whereby the world may appear sinister, sombre, menacing, or merely horrid and ugly. Throughout this stage, there occurs an upset in the perception of colours, ranging from complete achromatopsia to a total monochrome vision (erythropsia, etc.). More common is a mere muddiness or murkiness which hinders the differentiation of hues.

Nowadays we rarely quote Herbert Parsons on the nature of vision during this period of restoration. Influenced by Henry Head, he sought to trace a dissociation between a late acquired discriminate perception which he called "epicritic" or "photopic" and an older, less vulnerable and more primitive "scotopic" (or "dyscritic") type.

During these conjunctures of recovery, appropriate techniques may reveal other and less obtrusive disorders. Besides simple perimetric defects, more severe limitations may occur in the "effective visual field" of Cibis and Bay. Reduced values for flicker-fusion may be found. Tachistoscopy evokes a number of anomalies, particularly slowness of recognition. These changes, be it noted, are distributed diffusely all over the visual fields and contrast with the focal defects such as scotomas. In other words, symptoms arising from lesions of the higher visual pathways are widespread and range from those which are specific and circumscribed (sector defects) to those which are more general and involve the whole field (Teuber et al.).

Faulty external movements of the eyes themselves constitute a less well-known phenomenon.

During these foregoing stages, the patient may be at a loss to identify some or all of the objects within the range of his vision. He may also fail to recognise the features of bystanders. In this connection, the neurologist commonly speaks of "visual object agnosia" and "prosopagnosia." The temptation to invoke such highest level visuopsychic disorders is all the greater when they arise as independent symptoms due to parieto-occipital disease and without any preceding blindness.

This conception of agnosia as a specific entity of focal nature is one which appeals to neurological didactics, for it is attractive, tidy, and accordant to the idea of neatly demarcated centres representing physical activities and mental attributes. Whether this belief can stand up to the wind of change which now blows through neuropsychology is arguable. To accept a doctrine of agnosia is one thing, seductive perhaps and intellectually cosy, but to condone its correlation with a breakdown of some hypothetical endowment of "gnosis" is quite another thing. And yet the two ideas hang together.

In the past, some of our troubles arose from making a distinction between primary and secondary sensory qualities. A primary sensory quality would presumably entail, or be represented by, a *Sinnesempfindung*, a pure sensation—visual or otherwise—devoid of any qualifying properties. Whether there ever occurs in adult human experience any such pure "sense datum" (Bertrand Russell) or "sense awareness" (Whitehead) is doubtful, or in any event it must be rare. All sensory experiences entail a multiplicity of memories, associations, and embellishments stemming from past experience. Thus all perception is actually a secondary sensory experience: hence Russell Brain's expression "the private perceptual world." To try and equate the subjective predicament of an agnosiac with a being who lives in an environment of primary sensory experiences, or pure sense data, is erroneous and foreign to the facts as we can read them. To invoke the stripping off of some secondary stage of perception, to expose naked, as it were, a primary state of mere stimulus reception, would be a harkback to an unsubstantiated and outmoded hypothesis in philosophy propounded by John Locke.

Even on simple clinical grounds, reasons for scepticism readily come to mind. I will not refer to the classical critics of the mystique of visual agnosia, such as Mauthner, Siemerling, v. Stauffenberg, Poppelreuter, Lange, Pavlov, v. Monakow, Leland Alford, Lashley, Bay, Teuber, Bender, Gereb, among others. I may allude to the mounting reluctance towards attempting a cleavage between higher and lower visuosensory pathways and between perceptual centres as opposed to so-called mnestic or gnostic centres. This attitude has been stressed by numerous Soviet investigators on the basis of a study of conditioned reflexes. As Gereb put it, "The field of perception and the field of association form an anatomical and functional unity."

From my own experiences of parieto-occipital disease, I submit, first of all, that a patient with so-called visual agnosia does not, as a matter of fact, perceive his environment in a normal fashion. The idea that an agnosiac sees objects before him in sharp focus, clear-cut and vivid, as in a painting by Canalletto or Caravaggio, and yet cannot make head or tail of it is, in my submission, at variance with the facts. That the patient discerns the mysterious objects well enough to be able to make an adequate sketch of them is incredible. No agnosiac I have ever studied has claimed that he could see his environment plainly. Indeed speech is scarcely necessary. His whole deportment of peering, groping, visual search, with random eye movements and hesitating answers, bears out eloquently the fact which the agnosiac will usually admit, namely that the surrounding scene is anything but distinct and well defined.

Secondly, I would like to stress that the patient's performance is characteristically variable. Often he utterly fails to identify articles before him; occasionally he succeeds, or he may realize a few of them. Thus he may recognise and name a table knife but not a fork. If the interrogation is continued—or repeated on some later occasion—the situation may be reversed: The patient may now recognise the fork but not the knife. Why one object should be correctly acknowledged but not another is uncertain. Perhaps it depends upon the optical importance of the stimulus object, that is to say, upon such purely physical factors as size, simplicity of shape, brilliancy, colouring, movement, as well as familiarity. Even more, recognition or nonrecognition may be the resultant of the total situation with its intrinsic and extrinsic variables.

In my view, it is a vain pursuit to seek to isolate various subtypes of visual agnosia, e.g., for colours or for faces. But surely, the pinnacle of absurdity is found in an alleged dichotomy between an agnosia for inanimate as opposed to animate objects. As lief might one seek to distinguish an agnosia for knives as against forks, which could equally well be claimed from the case notes of some patients.

Kinetic factors play an important role in perception and must be reckoned with when discussing pathological cases. The act of observing an object is anything but a simple passive perceptual business. On the contrary, identification is the product of a very active process of gazing at an object, of surveying its outlines and surfaces, and finally synthesizing these various visual data. Not inappropriately one often speaks of "visual touch" in this connection, for both the hand and the eye are organs of exploration. Though often forgotten, this analogy of the eyes as optic "tentacles" is an old one, having been eloquently propounded by Diderot in the eighteenth century, and by Sechenov over a hundred years ago. In cases of so-called visual agnosia, this process of integration is gravely disorganized. This can be demonstrated by instrumental recording of the eye movements during visual scrutiny, assimilation, and identification. Naturally, this is technically easier with two-dimensional pictorial equivalents, rather than objects themselves (Yarbuss, Luria, Homskaya). Exemplifying an extreme defect, there is the case reported by Balint and associated with his name. No theory of agnosia can afford to neglect this aspect of disordered motility.

Most writers upon the topic of visual agnosia have glossed over an important clinical phenomenon which is by no means rare, as a matter of fact. The patient who, in typical fashion, does not recognise an object held up before his gaze, surprisingly enough *may also fail to identify the article when it is put into his hands*. Here then is something more than an orthodox visual agnosia. This clinical observation removes the failure of identification from a defect which is purely visual and denotes a far deeper disorder of perception. May I emphasize that cases of this sort are by no means uncommon? Perhaps in the past they have been disregarded, the facts appearing too incongruous and too difficult to explain.*

---

*Teuber has described something similar in alleged cases of visuospatial agnosia, where performance may deteriorate appreciably in the dark. "It is conceivable," wrote Teuber, "that the disorder transcends vision, and is present even if the patient has to orient himself to other than visual cues." Teuber constructed a route-finding exercise where the clues were either tactile or visual. He found that the failures could not be easily ascribed to a visuospatial agnosia, the errors being specific neither for vision nor for somesthesis. They transcended both and therefore failed to adhere to the modality-specific character of a classical agnosia.

Adherents of Gestalt psychology stress a failure to discriminate between figure and background as an important handicap in recognition. This may well play a part. The idea can be put to the test experimentally in the case of two-dimensional sense date in particular. Tonkonoguy, at the Bechterew Institute in Leningrad, prepared photographs of common objects while cluttering up the background with an accumulation of "visual noise." The result would be a picture prepared *en pointillisme*, where figure and background approximate closely in tonal properties, both of them being made up of a system of dots. A graded series of such pictures is then prepared, with the background conforming more and more with the pictorial depiction in the foreground. The patient is confronted with these illustrations and is required to identify the object which is concealed.

Tonkonoguy's test is applicable in the main to meaningful objects. When a picture of a teapot is overlaid and surrounded by visual noise, the associational attributes of the teapot do not arise unless the teapot is perceived. All which comes to sense-awareness is a complex of dots coupled perhaps with certain imaginal associations, as in a Rorschach blot, but devoid of "meaning." The wartime use of camouflage was similarly used to break down a recognizable and identifiable battleship or tank into a sense-datum of patterning which merged into the background. Older neurologists might have said that the visual noise or camouflage converts an object or a picture of an object from a secondary to a primary sense quality. But the point is that meaning depends upon clarity of vision, and this entails a sharp distinction between foreground and background.

In other words, the confusion engendered by a multiplicity of visual stimuli hinders the identification of objects. This may be a factor in some cases of agnosia, though not necessarily in all. The patient cannot cope with too much visual excitation at a time, as can readily be shown at the bedside. Originally stated by Balint, it was more specifically discussed by Wolpert under the term "simultaneous agnosia." Despite the shortcomings of this expression, Wolpert's syndrome highlights the common inability of the patient to realize the essence of a solid object or picture. Isolated items are correctly named, but the patient fails to assemble and synthesize them into a coordinated and meaningful whole. This "bit by bit," or piecemeal, approach constitutes in the visuopsychic sphere an inability to see the wood for the trees. Records of the eye movements confirm this. It is tempting to suggest that perception, when impaired, finds it difficult or impossible to interpret more than one stimulus at a time. Many writers have called attention to this phenomenon, Luria in particular.

My argument therefore is that the so-called agnosiac does not perceive the surrounding world distinctly; or at any rate, not like most normal subjects. Moreover, the shrewd and proper utilization of available clues, often ambiguous or misleading, is a mental operation of an intricate sort. The immediate set or frame of expectation is important in the perception of visual sense-data just as it is in the case of speech. One of the principal adjuvants is the factor of credibility (Ridley). As Marcel Proust wrote, "The evidence of the senses is also an operation of the mind, in which conviction creates the evidence." If then there happens to exist in an agnosiac an intellectual handicap, the performance will be still further hindered, as Bay has stressed so eloquently. The patient not only fails to discern his environment clearly, he furthermore cannot successfully utilize the distorted clues by appropriate adjustment, correction, or interpretation. Such an agnosiac is like a crazy man in a fog or a drunken myope without his spectacles, lacking the capacity to take advantage of the imperfect and distorted visual pointers.

At this juncture I might well be urged to have done with iconoclasm and to proclaim my own views as to the nature of highest level disturbances of vision. According to my *credo* there exists as a consequence of hindmost lesions of the brain a sort of *continuum* of visual defects. The peak of disability obviously comprises cortical blindness, the *Rindblindheit* of German writers. Short of this extremity of defect are the graded qualitative disorders of perception which, I submit, include the difficulties in object recognition usually known as agnosia. In their important monograph of 1961, Hoff, Gloning, and Gloning have stated that there are no object agnosic disorders without a primary visual disorder with a change of function *(Funktionswandel)* caused by it. They went on to state, however, that the agnosic disorder far exceeds the primary visual disorder and cannot be explained by this alone. It is over this latter statement where I believe a legitimate doubt may be said to exist.

Also within this broad spectrum of disordered perception lie the subtotal occipital defects which may arise either per se or as restitution phenomena after a preliminary amblyopia. Here belong the cases of pinhole or tubular vision due to extreme constriction of the visual fields. Again I do not believe that in these attenuated circumstances qualitatively normal vision exists. Recognition of objects and of pictures may be possible, but the performance is slow and depends upon exaggerated sweeping and exploring movements of the eyes (Wilbrand's manoeuvre). In my opinion, no case of tubular vision can occur without other visuopsychic defects, such as a loss of topographical conception or memory, or of colour appreciation.

My plea therefore is for more studies in detail of the patients who show hesitation or slowness in identifying their environment. We must record faithfully each patient's performance, his answers, and his comportment during the interview. Instead of interpreting the patient's behaviour, we should simply report it accurately, without shrinking from taking note of data that may appear anomalous or nonconforming.

I believe that henceforth we shall be compelled to relegate the visual agnosias within a scale of defect, varying in intensity according to numerous factors including *inter alia* site of lesion, size of lesion, abruptness of onset, together with diverse subtle situational variables. Lastly I hazard the plea, with some trepidation in this august city, for the abandonment of the term "agnosia" suggested in 1891 by Freud. Though at that time it might have been appropriate, subsequent writers have debased the currency. To speak of "finger agnosia," "pain agnosia," "agnosia for danger," "spatial agnosia," and so on and so forth is to outrage both thinking and language. What should we put in its place, so as to indicate that condition which we all have in mind and which is now loosely spoken of as "agnosia"? I prefer some noncommittal term like "disorder of perception" or "perceptual defect"; or even—turning back the pages of neurological history over 100 years—"imperception," as Hughlings Jackson suggested.

Developmental Dyslexia: A Brief Overview

The literature on the subject of developmental dyslexia has become grossly overloaded. In 1969 it was estimated that more than 20,000 papers had been published dealing with this topic. In the 15 years that have elapsed, this figure may well have increased fivefold.

The only excuse I can offer for adding to this literary extravagance is an experience which is perhaps unusual. The first dyslectic patient I encountered was in 1925, when I demonstrated this child before the Neurological Society in London. Two years later I delivered my first paper upon the subject, with obvious lack of interest on the part of my audience. Over the last 20 years I have had the opportunity of examining and recording in the greatest detail no fewer than 3,500 cases.

Rather than embark upon a critical overview of this well-worn subject, it might be wiser if I were to select a few aspects that are still obscure or else controversial, and which are ripe for discussion.

1. Logically, one should first consider the *history of developmental dyslexia*. I have often been asked why it is only lately that dyslexia has attracted attention. Actually it has had a place in the *corpus* of medicine for almost a century and probably much longer. I say that because I have come across a remark made by Thomas Willis in 1672 in his *De Anima Brutorum* which almost certainly refers to young persons with an inborn delay in learning to read and write.

2. The question of *nomenclature*. The word "dyslexia" was employed as far back as 1887, but it was in the context of an *acquired* defect of reading in adults. "Congenital word-blindness" was the earliest of the proposed terms. By 1909, however, many alternatives had been suggested, such as legasthenia, bradylexia, typholexia, word amblyopia, amnesia visualis verbalis, script blindness, and analphabetia partialis.

Recently, and especially in the United States, a vague and noncommittal term, "learning disability" (even the acronym LD) has become widely used. This I deplore as not being sufficiently specific.

Professor Cruickshank of New York has shrewdly pointed out the terminological muddle that exists in America. In his own words: "If the child diagnosed as dyslexic in Philadelphia moved to Bucks County, 10 miles north, he would be called a child with a language disorder. In Montgomery County, Maryland, a few miles south, he would be called a child with a perceptual disturbance. In California he would be called either a child with educational handicaps or a neurologically handicapped child. In Florida and New York State he would be called a brain-injured child. In Colorado the child would be classified as having minimal brain dysfunction."

Just when the term "dyslexia" became used in its present context is uncertain. S. T. Orton was certainly using it occasionally in 1925, though he preferred his own favoured designation "strephosymbolia."

In Great Britain, for many years, educational authorities at a governmental level resisted the term dyslexia and put forward as an alternative "congenital reading retardation." But this expression is unacceptable, for developmental dyslexia embraces a dimension of language which transcends mere difficulty in reading, something which is only the tip of a veritable iceberg. As a matter of etymology, "dyslexia" is a very appropriate word, for its literal translation from the Greek is "difficulty in the use of words," which is exactly what developmental dyslexia represents.

3. *How prevalent is developmental dyslexia?* Two chief difficulties arise here. First, most cases probably go unrecognised. Second, there are two very distinct types of dyslexia, and these are only too often confused. This criticism particularly applies to some of the oft-quoted geographical surveys of backward readers.

Thus the *Bullock Report* of 1975 quoted a full-scale profile of children in Great Britain. It was found that of the 12-year-olds 22.6% were below average in their standard of reading, and of the 14-year-old group the figure was 20.1%. These estimates are not scientific, however, being embrangled by the fact that their community of poor readers was probably a heterogeneous one.

Let us look at the census figures for the United States. Out of a population of 205 million, 1.5 million could not read at all. Eight million schoolchildren needed additional academic help. Five million job-seekers were functionally illiterate, and 20 million Americans over 16 years of age were unable to complete the standard application form for a driver's licence.

Developmental dyslexia corresponds with what might be called *primary* or *specific* dyslexia, affecting children of any intellectual level, boys more often than girls, and occurring in families. No pathological basis is yet known. *Secondary dyslexics* are those with delayed literacy, most of whom have suffered perinatal trauma leading to minimal brain dysfunction. Differential diagnosis is a medical problem and often an extremely difficult one, requiring all the special facilities of a neurological clinic to make certain of the diagnosis. No wonder then that confusion occurs, for this kind of teamwork is exceptional.

Although in many ways alike, these two types need to be sharply differentiated, for the prognosis is different, and sociofamilial implications are important.

My guess is that in Great Britain the prevalence of true cases of specific developmental dyslexia is at least 1% of all schoolchildren. Many would regard this figure as an underestimate. Because of the genetic properties of developmental dyslexia, this figure of 1% is likely to increase over the years rather than diminish.

4. *Are there subtypes of specific developmental dyslexia?* Many affirm that there are, and that it is possible to isolate what they call "neural models," distinguishing a type where there is a visile or visuoperceptual problem from an audioperceptual

type. Boder would add a third or mixed group, incidentally speaking of a dyseidetic group. Zangwill visualized three subtypes on the basis of cerebral dominance. Bakker divided dyslexics into R-types and L-types, claiming that in the former the right half of the brain is functionally overdeveloped, whereas in the latter the reverse is true.

To medical men like myself such efforts are not impressive and seem premature and speculative. A doctor prefers to speak of "a dyslectic child" rather than "a case of dyslexia," for he realises that no two instances can possibly be identical, any more than any two individuals are exactly the same, either in sickness or in health. Therefore, to make a rigid parcellation within the clinical picture of developmental dyslexia is going too far. The syndrome is not a sharply demarcated, recurring, clinical isolate. Such a belief is an affront to neurological thinking and, indeed, out of harmony with the discipline of medicine.

5. *The sex incidence in developmental dyslexia.* All who have written on the subject agree that dyslectic boys outnumber girls. Most statistics show that the ratio is roughly four boys to one girl. In 1968, in a personal series of 616 children with dyslexia, 79% were boys, that is, 1 girl to 3.8 boys. Over the following years, however, the proportion of dyslectic girls rose, and by 1983 the ratio was more like 1 girl to 2.5 boys. My sample, though a large one, was not wholly representative in that all the parents who consulted me about their children belonged to the upper three social classes. There seemed to be an increasing tendency to devote more care and concern to the education of their daughters, compared with the practice 20 to 30 years earlier.

One unexpected factor must not be overlooked when contemplating these figures. In paediatric hospitals there is a greater number of boys than girls in the incidence of a medley of physical maladies, as though in some cryptic fashion boys were more vulnerable subjects than their sisters.

6. *Are there any preschool anomalies that characterize candidates for developmental dyslexia?* No abnormalities are to be expected in the attainment of the developmental milestones in infants who later prove to be specific dyslexics. Parents and grandparents have the impression of a perfectly normal infant. When at his first school the teacher finds that he is lagging behind his peers in learning his letters, the news comes as a surprise to all.

Let me qualify these remarks. Some, like T. R. Miles, allege that the predyslexic often skips the stage of crawling, learning to stand and walk unaided at the usual ages, but after a period of bottom-shuffling. This, however, is not a wholly reliable index. The percentage of infants who never crawl is said to be seven; but no follow-up has been made to ascertain how many of these become dyslexic. A retrospective study of my random sample of 125 cases of developmental dyslexia revealed that 21 had never crawled (16.8%). Clearly, this is a point that might repay properly controlled investigation.

The dyslectic child is sometimes said to have been a *late talker* and that for a time his speech was indistinct. Some had required a short period of therapy. In my sample of 125 dyslectic children, 41 (32.8%) had been late in the acquisition of clear, articulate utterance, a figure which must be higher than in a nondyslectic population. This is not surprising for, as I continually emphasize, dyslexia is a disorder of "the use of words" in the broadest sense of the term.

Learning to tell the time is also a late accomplishment in many dyslexics. Something artificial attends this observation, however. Children have to be taught this skill; it is not a natural one. Perhaps they are late in learning a clock simply because parents and others have been dilatory in showing them how. This is unlikely to be the whole explanation. Some dyslexics go through a phase of being hazy about spatial relationships and confuse front/back, up/down, below/above, and, characteristically, right/left. One dyslexic shrewdly asked why the long hand of a clock showed the minutes and the short hand the hours, when hours were so much longer in time than minutes. The introduction of digital watches and clocks has still further complicated the issue.

Over and above the foregoing, some workers, notably de Hirsch and Jansky, have considered they could isolate a constellation of minor manifestations that occur in those children around the age of five and who subsequently prove to be dyslexic. They drew up what they called a "predictive index." During the 22 years that have elapsed since their original papers, surprisingly few communications have appeared in the literature supporting this notion. Personally I am sceptical of any such attempts to forecast within a family setting those siblings who will turn out to be dyslexic and those who will not.

7. *The question of "soft neurological signs."* It was Schilder who invented this term, by which he meant anomalies that escape routine examination of the nervous system but which come to light only after what he called an "extended" neurological examination. Among the features claimed by various authors at various times as typical of a dyslexic are clumsiness, incoordination, inability to catch a ball or to hop or skip; right–left confusion; hyperactivity; failure to imitate a tapped-out rhythm, to draw (as in the Goodenough test), and to reproduce a geometrical shape from memory after the model has been briefly displayed and then withdrawn (Benton's test); vague ideas of time as well as of space; poor figure/background discrimination; motor impersistence; faulty colour-naming; the presence of postural reflexes; and motor synkinesia.

Without hesitation I would assert that the majority of these phenomena occupy no place in the diagnosis of developmental dyslexia. When some or all of them are found in a child who is late in learning to read and write, the case, in all likelihood, is one of secondary dyslexia, the sequela of minimal brain damage. Here again, we witness the chaos which results from failure to separate specific developmental dyslexia from the dyslexias resulting from established cerebral disorders. One or two points require elaboration.

Clumsiness is the term parents sometimes use when they wish to indicate a certain awkwardness or *gaucherie* in their child. In the neurological sense of the word, clumsiness is something quite different and quite unmistakable. Several possible factors underlie this symptom—pyramidal, extrapyramidal, sensory, cerebellar, or apractic. I have found that most dyslectic children are anything but clumsy, even if sometimes bungling and ungainly. On the contrary, dyslectic boys usually show enjoyment and skill in things mechanical, constructional, or electrical. They often excel at games. Indeed I know two Olympic gold-medallists who are dyslexic. Many dyslectic girls are dainty dancers and are deft at needlework and art.

Overactivity and restlessness are not symptoms of developmental dyslexia. The hyperkinetic child and the dyslectic child are poles apart. The most I will admit is that short-term memory and difficulty in concentration may provoke inattention during those particular lessons which dyslexics may find dull and difficult.

Colour-naming is, of course, something that is learned and not spontaneously achieved. My routine testing always includes an item where colours are named, and I can confidently assert that I have not encountered any difficulties except in a few boys who, on more searching procedures, proved to have an unsuspected colour blindness.

Postural reflexes and synkinesis are a different matter. They are present in all young children and usually disappear by the age of six or seven. In some children with developmental dyslexia aged seven or even eight, they may still be demonstrable, which means nothing more than a delay in maturation. This is not surprising in a child with developmental dyslexia, a condition which may well be the expression of a cerebral immaturity.

Infirm Cerebral Dominance

The possibility of interhemispheric rivalry and noncooperation was first mooted by Orton in 1925. His observations were arresting, though his conclusions were not accepted in their entirety. After Orton's death, this aspect of dyslexia was relatively neglected in favour of other interesting considerations. However, over the past 10 to 15 years there has been a revival of interest, possibly to an inordinate degree. Four factors have contributed to the upsurge in attention to this matter of right–left cerebral equipotentiality: (1) an increasing preoccupation with the possible functional role of the minor parietal lobe; (2) the realisation that even in right-handers the right cerebral hemisphere is not entirely devoid of language function; (3) a growing search for anatomical asymmetries in the convolutions of the brain; and (4) the techniques of dichotic listening.

There seems to be little doubt but that within the population of developmental dyslexics the proportion of so-called sinistrals is somewhat greater than in nondyslexics. Furthermore, the incidence of crossed laterality is a little higher among dyslexics. Even more impressive is the observation that dyslectic children in their early attempts at writing show a definite perplexity as to right–left orientation of letters. This is revealed when they so often rotate letters, confuse *b* and *d*, reverse short words (dog/god, saw/was), and perpetrate internal reversals (film/flim, girp/grip). Frank mirror-writing occasionally occurs in the case of dyslectic sinistrals.

These matters cannot, however, be of crucial importance, for there are still many children with developmental dyslexia who are right-handed and not crossed laterals. Furthermore, crossed laterality is often met with in non-dyslectic subjects.

One of the fundamental problems is not yet fully realised, even by those who have devoted thought to the vexed question of manual preference. How does one decide whether a person is right- or left-handed? The tests that have been devised are multifold but of unequal merit. The manner of writing, the preferred hand in the use of tools, the choice of hands in wielding a cricket or baseball bat, a golf club, a hockey stick, a spade or shovel—these may be learned activities ordained by instructors rather than being natural to the individual. Some other activities are automatic, such as the mode of folding arms, interlacing the fingers, clapping hands, clasping hands behind the back. Then there are different ways of performing bimanual tasks, such as threading a needle, scrubbing the nails, and opening a bottle of champagne. Social and religious taboos must also be considered. In India the right hand is always used for feeding, the left being reserved for anal toilet; in China chopsticks are manipulated with the right hand, even by a natural left-hander.

It would be simple if all these various tests for handedness correlated in a tidy fashion, but unfortunately they do not. The same discrepancies occur in tests for footedness, eyedness, and aural performance. Then, too, there is the important matter of the favoured direction of lateral gaze, something that almost always proceeds from left to right (except perhaps with Arabs).

In other words, there is no one single reliable test for handedness. It is therefore impossible to make a sharp cleavage between right- and left-handers. Doubtless in time one will be able to assign marks to each test and then to describe a person as being, say, 64% right-handed and 36% left-handed, or vice versa. And when ocular, pedal, and aural preferences are included, one will have to distinguish *degrees* of cerebral dominance in a manner which today is impossible.

Perplexity grows the deeper one probes. Masland, indeed, has written upon "the advantages of being dyslexic," implying that the minor hemisphere is not quite so subordinate as it is in nondyslexics.

In my opinion, this aspect of the dyslexia story is still *sub judice*.

Profile of Imperfect Literacy in the Adult Dyslexic

When we examine the question of imperfect literacy we are on firmer terrain than when isolating soft neurological signs. Developmental dyslexia presents a muster of literary shortcomings still discernible long after school-leaving age. This assortment of defects so aptly subsumed by the word "dyslexia," or difficulty in the use of words, forms a profile of imperfect literacy.

Reluctance to read is outstanding even when the dyslexic has advanced to the stage of being able to read for all practical purposes, except the most abstruse material. He prefers to be doing things rather than sitting and reading. If he has an intriguing hobby such as gardening or motorcycling, he may subscribe to an appropriate magazine, but it is unlikely that he will do much more than skim the headlines and study the illustrations. The same applies to newspapers, where the football results are perhaps the sole items to attract his notice. Even those established executives whose school days were plagued by a dyslexia will try to avoid studying printed reports, memoranda, briefs, parliamentary white papers, and the like. They will probably contrive for a junior colleague or personal assistant, either to read the paperwork aloud to them or perhaps to peruse the document in private and then extract the nub or salient point of the subject matter.

The adult dyslexic does not browse in libraries or secondhand bookshops. Nor is he ever a bibliophile or book collector, even for the mere sake of their bindings or their rarity.

Not only is he a reluctant reader, he is, moreover, a slow reader. This is a feature insufficiently stressed by most writers on dyslexia. Despite the deliberation with which he pores through a printed page, he tends to be inaccurate. Long words he may misread; more often still, he is tripped up by the small "filler" words. He may read *this* for *that, but* for *and*. A still more common habit is completely to overlook a short word, even such an all-important adverb as "not," with utter disaster to the comprehension of the text. Should he be reading aloud, the mistakes may increase in number and become obvious to others. One interesting and unexpected error is for him to read the word in silence and with understanding, and then to come out with a synonym when reading it aloud. Thus if the word is *sombre* he may say *gloomy*, or *ale* for *beer*. This is what may be called "narremic substitution" and it corresponds with the "deep dyslexia" of Newcombe and Marshall that is found in some patients with aphasia.

He may recall vividly the embarrassing occasions when during his scholastic examinations he misread a question with disastrous consequences.

His written work is revealing. Again he is disinclined to put pen to paper, for he is aware that he has difficulty in expressing his ideas in writing with lucidity, piquancy, and in a logical order. And yet he has no trouble in expressing himself by word of mouth. Indeed he may be a fluent public speaker, eloquent and inspiring. He shows no hesitancy in dictating to his secretary or into a tape recorder.

The first draft of what he writes is always a slow and painful business. Not only is it conspicuously brief, it is full of errors including those of grammar, punctuation, and style. The word bank at his disposal is meagre. He is cliché-bound and repeats himself in respect of both individual words and phrases. Spelling mistakes are copious, some of which he has detected and erased, others remaining unrealised. There are inconsistencies too in the spelling, for even on the same page a word might be written correctly in one place and incorrectly in another. A longstanding difficulty in sequencing has probably not been fully surmounted. Hence it might prove a slow and tedious job to consult a dictionary or even to turn up a name and number in a telephone directory.

As a rule, the handwriting too is untidy and immature in character, the individual letters being ill-formed. Not infrequently the childish practice of "manuscript" writing takes the place of a flowing script. The overall picture, or "form level" as graphologists say, is easily identified as the work of a dyslexic.

Some writers of prose and verse find an almost sensual pleasure in words for their own sake—their euphony, their singularity, their appearance. Such authors select and assemble words like a jeweller singling out this precious gem and rejecting that one, arranging them so as to form an exquisite piece of *bijouterie*, or like a Japanese immersed in a flower arrangement. Dylan Thomas, Ruskin, H. G. Wells, and Walter Pater shared this attribute. No such connoisseur in words could have been dyslexic, despite what has been alleged about Théophile Gautier.

Favourable and Unfavourable Prognostic Indications

When the diagnosis of developmental dyslexia is first made, the parents naturally enquire as to the outlook. Is their particular child a mild or a severe case? What sort of scholastic progress is to be expected? And what of the remote future? Much variability exists from one case to another, but in my experience there are five favourable factors which, when present in combination, augur well for the child. These are (1) good intelligence; (2) early recognition; (3) an understanding and caring attitude on the part of parents and teachers; (4) availability of individual coaching by specialist teachers; and (5) ambition and sheer determination on the part of the dyslectic child. Of that prognostic pentagon the last is probably the most important.

On the other hand, there are certain circumstances which act in an unpropitious manner. (1) An intellectual level which is either too low or exceptionally high. In other words a dyslexic who is a dullard has an upward task before him. So for that matter has a gifted child who happens to be dyslexic. (2) Bilingualism and poly-glottism in the household. (3) Too frequent changes of school. (4) Excessive absenteeism, especially when this is the result of chronic ill health. (5) Dyslexia in both parents. This last-named is something I have never seen mentioned in the literature, but it is, I am convinced, a very real problem. Such children make slower headway with reading and writing throughout the whole of their school careers. It is by no means an uncommon occurrence, for dyslectic adolescents of both sexes tend to establish contact with each other and often marry.

Definition

Time does not permit me to deal with the very many aspects of developmental dyslexia. I will, instead, finish by giving the lie to that oft-repeated assertion that there is no definition of this condition. Indeed, there are many, but most, if not all, have come in for criticism. May I, therefore, put in my own which I hope is foolproof and generally acceptable?

> A learning disability which initially shows itself by difficulty in learning to read, and later by erratic spelling and by lack of facility in manipulating written as opposed to spoken words. The condition is cognitive in essence, and usually genetically determined. It is not due to intellectual inadequacy or to lack of sociocultural opportunity, or to faults in the technique of teaching, or to emotional factors, or to any known structural brain defect. It probably represents a specific maturational defect which tends to lessen as the child grows older and is capable of considerable improvement, especially when appropriate remedial help is afforded at the earliest op-portunity.—Critchley and Critchley, 1978

Developmental Dyslexia Complicated by Multilingualism

I am well aware how presumptuous it is on my part to venture to discuss the topic of polyglottism here in Switzerland of all places, "the most romantic region in the world," as Lord Byron wrote. For many reasons, I believe it logical to discuss the complicated problems of polyglottism and the merits and demerits of a bilingual accomplishment before proceeding to consider how bilingualism affects dyslexia and vice versa. I will therefore deal with the bilingual dyslexic in the latter part of this presentation.

My own claims for multilingual status are slender, but I have long realized that the subject of polyglottism, even bilingualism, is far more intricate than might appear at first sight. Although my experience is largely theoretical, I can certainly claim considerable personal knowledge of adult polyglots who, through disease, have sustained severe difficulties in communication, and, what is more pertinent today, of dyslectic children who are being educated in an environment where more symbol systems than one have to be acquired.

The advantages of being able to talk and to read and write in one or more foreign languages are obvious. Such an accomplishment considerably extends the cultural and social ambience of the fortunate polyglot. The benefits are often reciprocal in that a knowledge of French and certainly of Latin and Greek may go far to enhance the vocabulary and ennoble the syntax of one's own idiolect.

Yet it has been widely believed, perhaps less so nowadays than in the past, that bilingualism carries with it certain disadvantages. The philologist, Schuchardt, asserted in 1885 that if a bilingual has two strings to his bow, both are rather slack. The ancient Roman used to boast of his three souls, derived from his ability to speak three different languages, but, after all, they were three very indifferent souls. Jesperson, another linguist, believed that the advantage of familiarity with two languages may be, and usually is, purchased too dear. Later writers have demurred, some indeed having adopted a diametrically opposite opinion.

Perhaps we have been confused by a lack of precision in our terminology. Bilingualism is by no means the same as "equilingualism," an entity which must be conceded as rare. Words carry with them so many overtones and mental associations that they can rarely, if ever, be completely shared. Some prefer to speak of "pseudobilingualism" where the first tongue is supplemented by a second language which, however rich, never matches the so-called mother tongue, or, to

---

Lecture delivered in Geneva, October, 1982.

be more accurate, the language the speaker employs most commonly. In other words, there are degrees of bilingualism ranging from zero to a notional 100% competence in both. The latter, I suggest, is scarcely ever attained, and probably few if any multilinguals move with equal ease along the corridors of two or more linguistic systems. The philosopher's *homo utrimque linguae* may well turn out to be a *homo fabulosus*, a mere mythological creature. Not only is there the matter of matching two or more vocabularies, the problem always remains of sharing the emotional attachments of each language, as well as the overtones and linguistic associations mentioned earlier. What about such considerations as the use of slang, of witticisms, innuendoes, and verse? To quote an anonymous literary critic (1955): "Poetry is so rooted in the local usage of a language, that all attempts to transplant it are futile... we can only appreciate the poetry of a dead language by analogy; and even in the case of a living language, unless we are genuinely bilingual (a rare condition), we have about the same relation to the poetry of that language as we have to a lark's song."

Language is a firmly built-in aspect of one's mode of thinking and behaviour. To switch successively from one tongue to another, the speaker must alter his total personality like the Player in Hamlet. A range of gestural and paralinguistic mannerisms must be shed and others adopted. Not an easy matter.

Dictionary equivalents are by no means absolute. A Russian referring to the colour "red" uses the term "*krasniy*," which also carries with it the implication of beauty. Again, the Russian for "friend" is "*drug*," but the precise social circumstances whereby a Russian refers to another person as "*drug*" are not at all the same as those under which we call someone a friend. In the same way, the French "*ami*" and the German "*Freund*" are not wholly equivalent.

Many many other examples could be given from other languages, including—be it noted—American versus Standard Received English.

The circumstances which underlie bilingualism may differ considerably. There are some who are reluctantly compelled to learn a second language, whereas some others willingly choose to do so. When change of habitat is a factor, one must distinguish between the emigré and the refugee. Of the 203 million in the United States, 20 million are said to be endowed with a mother tongue other than English.

A multilingual state of affairs may be either natural or mandatory. Thus one special circumstance exists in those geographical regions where more than one socio-political-racio-cultural environment is operative, e.g., Switzerland, Luxembourg, Belgium, the Basque provinces, parts of Wales, and vast areas of India and Africa. The situation may often be fostered by extreme nationalistic motives as in the promotion of Afrikaans in the Republic of South Africa and of the vernacular in the emergent Zimbabwe. Despite strong special pleading from local educationalists, the problem is usually one of pseudobilingualism where chauvinistic considerations outweigh those that are logical and linguistic, with resulting harm to both symbol systems. The need for a pervading *lingua franca*, usually English, holds a special place in the Babel-like plight in India with its 225 languages and in Africa with almost as many.

Quite different is the situation often encountered in Great Britain where one parent, or both, is not English. The parents might deliberately decide that it would be in their child's best interests—educationally and culturally—to be raised as a bilingual. Their decision is made for motives that are altruistic and discerning. If the experiment is successful, the benefits are obvious. How to bring about a wholly bilingual upbringing is another matter.

Such well-meaning, synthetic bilingualism is not devoid of hazard, however. To attain real proficiency in more languages than one demands a superior verbal intelligence, as well as freedom from any trace of dyslexia.

Turning for a moment to clinical medicine, I can recall many instances of aphasia in polyglots. The conventional teaching is that in such cases the mother tongue suffers less than languages that had been acquired later in life, even though many years may have elapsed since the first language had been employed. Experience, however, shows that there are more exceptions than adherents to this rule. Much depends upon the most recent place of residence of the patient; the language of those around him; and various subtle emotional factors which may have become attached to the linguistic background. When discussing the fragmentary linguistic skills of a multilingual aphasic, one has to take into account such factors as *what* the patient is struggling to say; *in what circumstances*, immediate and remote; and *in conversation with whom*.

May I briefly quote a famous case reported by Professor Minkowski of Zürich? The patient had been born and brought up in that city, his first "little language" having been *Schweizerdeutsch*. At school his lessons were conducted in High German, which was the tongue spoken in his home and by his playmates and by almost everyone around him. As second and third languages he was taught French and some Italian. After attaining his degree at the University of Zürich, he was appointed a lecturer in physics. At the exceptionally early age of 30 he was elected to a professorial chair at Neuchâtel, where it became necessary for him to speak nothing but French in the lecture theatre, the laboratory, and his home. Fourteen years went by, and then he became aphasic as the result of a stroke. Slowly and painfully he regained his French, so much so that after 3 years he was sufficiently fluent to resume his teaching duties. Literary German followed, and then Italian. He never regained his Swiss–German mother tongue, even though he eventually left Neuchâtel and retired to Zürich, his home town. As Minkowski explained, French was the language which corresponded most with this man's affections and represented a deep-rooted symbol of social and professional success.

Let me leave the protean and fascinating subject of polyglot aphasia to consider for a moment a state of affairs which in many ways represents the opposite of speech impairment. I refer to the psychoanalytic interview. A certain Dr. Krapf, by birth a Viennese, was a polyglot practitioner who migrated to Buenos Aires. His clientèle was of many nationalities, and he often noticed that the analytic interview might commence in the local Spanish, but later, when certain significant or embarrassing circumstances from the patient's earlier life came to light, he might switch so as to proceed with the interview in German, English, or some other mutually comprehended tongue. Later, when the emotional pressure had eased, he would revert to his native Spanish.

Dyslectic Bilinguals and Polyglots

Almost all of those who have written upon the subject of bilingualism have concentrated upon the spoken form of the languages concerned. Relatively scant attention has been given to the important topic of proficiency in reading, writing, and spelling in the bilingual. These, however, are precisely the skills which are at risk when the polyglot child turns out to be dyslexic.

It seems simple for any child to pick up the sound and significance of two languages he hears spoken around him by other members of the family, servants, and friends. But in reality, bilingualism is something more profound: It is a matter of biliteracy. Common sense suggests that the task of mastering twice as many terms as a monoglot imposes an extra burden upon any child. Still more so if he is dyslexic. The young bilingual, moreover, must avoid confusing the terms and must understand when it is appropriate to say *cheval*, as opposed to *Pferd* or *horse*. Confusion is less likely to occur if the mother consistently addresses the child in one language and the father in another. These "universes of discourse," as they have been called, should, according to some educationalists, be always kept distinct.

In my experience, bilingual or multilingual dyslexics do not appear to be handicapped in this preschool stage. They are not necessarily late in learning to talk. Whether so-called reading-readiness is delayed is uncertain and may well be the case. However, it is not easy to prove or disprove this contention. Trouble certainly begins when the rudiments of reading and writing appear on the scene. If the parents demand, or desire, that their child aim at mastering two symbol systems, despite his dyslexia, many questions will arise. In the first place—and this applies to all bilinguals—at what age should literacy be started in the two languages? There is no unanimity. Most authorities are in favour of starting as early as possible, the argument being that all children, monoglot or polyglot, dyslexic or eulexic, pick up their mother tongue with a mysterious facility which is never experienced at a later age. In other words, the mother tongue of a bilingual is potentially a binary or duplex phenomenon, a forked tongue in fact.

Others disagree and advocate that book learning in the second language should be deferred until the age of 10 or even 12.

From the standpoint of a dyslexic growing up in a multilingual environment, trouble becomes obvious after the first few months at school, and it will continue throughout the whole period of schooling and subsequently. Moreover, the dyslexia will present itself and affect all languages in the curriculum, though not necessarily to an equal degree.

Even in the case of monoglots, few teachers would deny that if they are dyslexic they fare badly when they have to study foreign languages for the purpose of formal examinations. Not only do they fail to keep pace with their peers in the written aspect of a second or third language, but their attempts to do so hinder their acquisition of literacy in their mother tongue. The time and stress expended in grappling with a second language could be more wisely dedicated to the difficult task of attaining competency in their natural medium of communication. In my experience, very few dyslexics in Great Britain succeed in passing examinations in French or Latin. Indeed, my practice is to recommend strongly that these languages be dropped. Of course, I am speaking of English dyslexics. Teachers do not always accept my advice, or, to be more precise, accept it to begin with. As the years slip by, the attitude of the school authorities may alter, but valuable time has been squandered.

Although there is general awareness that developmental dyslexics find foreign languages inordinately difficult, there is relatively little on this topic in the extensive literature upon learning disorders. In 1959 M. Yves Chesni studied 1,809 school-children by way of a questionnaire sent to 75 teachers in and around Geneva. Of these, 93 (5.14%) were regarded as being dyslexic. A closer study was carried out upon 86 of these children, and 6 were rejected because of their relatively low intelligence. The remaining 80 represented 4.42%. Of these 80, 16 were Franco-German bilinguals, that is, 22.5%. The author did not state how many of the nondyslexics were bilingual.

Professor T. R. Miles of the University of Bangor has told me that no figures are available on the incidence of dyslexia among Anglo-Welsh bilinguals. His wife's impression is that when a dyslexic's first language is English he makes disappointing progress with Welsh, which seems actually to be an obstructive element in the curriculum. Dyslectic children whose mother tongue is Welsh respond well to individual instruction; they also fare better in reading English, but their spelling is faulty. It appears important that, in general, English is the principal medium of their environment.

Kline and Lee (1976) studied a series of Chinese children in Vancouver who had difficulty reading English as well as their mother tongue. The rate of improvement in both English and Chinese was so rapid as to raise doubts in my mind whether the original difficulties were really dyslexic.

The position in Ireland is easier to understand. Following the establishment of the Republic, Irish became a compulsory language in all state schools as well as the national universities. According to Finnegan, the general progress of 25% of the children was deemed "unsatisfactory." Furthermore, 25% had difficulties with English, 48% with arithmetic, and 50% with Irish. The fact that all elementary school children in the Republic of Ireland learn a second language was regarded as a possible source of learning difficulties. Since 1970, Irish is no longer obligatory in schools there.

Summary

It is obvious from what has been said that certain conclusions appear warranted on the topic of dyslexia complicating and complicated by multilingualism.

1. Purely from the standpoint of dyslexia, multilingualism is unfortunate and should not lightly be encouraged.

2. When two or more languages are taught to a dyslexic purely as articulate exercises, no great harm is likely to result.

3. Despite the demerits of bilingualism in the education of a dyslectic child, there may be various circumstances which ordain that the exercise is justified.

4. In the context of compulsory bilingualism where the learning of an indigenous language is imposed upon a community for purely political or ethnic reasons, a great and intolerable burden is imposed upon a dyslexic.

5. The decision whether a young child should be brought up as a bilingual is the responsibility of the parents. They should be made aware of the possible disadvantages, however. It is unfortunate that this resolution has to be taken very early in life, that is, before it is realised that the child may be dyslexic.

6. As soon as the diagnosis of dyslexia is established, the parents and the teachers should be made aware that the simultaneous acquisition of two languages will present peculiar difficulties. The parents may then decide that in the circumstances it would be in the child's interests to sacrifice one language. In this way, mastery of the other tongue would be facilitated.

7. If bilingualism is insisted upon, the problem will arise, if biliteracy is to be achieved, of finding *two* specialist teachers, experienced in the techniques for helping dyslexics, who will provide coaching in reading, writing, and spelling, and the full use in fact of the two languages in question. To find the ideal would indeed be difficult in a country such as Great Britain.

8. Moreover, if the dyslexic is to continue his role as a bilingual, the parents and their advisers will have to consider seriously the advantages of a bilingual over a monoglot school. In both the private and the public sectors, bilingual schools are few in number, sparsely distributed, and usually expensive. Sometimes their general academic standards comprising verbal and "content subjects" are excessively high. All these considerations certainly apply strongly to the schools in Great Britain.

9. The parents of a bilingual dyslexic living in England will be more likely to find the ideal school in Switzerland than at home.

10. The term "bilingual school" is not always clear, and the system of instruction may differ from one institution to another. This is exemplified in the manner in which the various "content subjects" are taught. Thus in Anglo-French bilingual schools, mathematics may be taught in French in one of them and in English in another.

11. Here in Switzerland you have unparalleled opportunities for helping dyslexics in a bilingual context. What is more, you have stupendous opportunities for research into the obscurities which still surround the conundrum of the multilingual dyslexic.

Dr. Samuel Johnson's Stroke and Consequent "Impediment in Utterance"

Descriptions of aphasia were uncommon before the start of the nineteenth century, and personal accounts written retrospectively were even rarer. Dr. Samuel Johnson's own record of his stroke with subsequent disturbance of speech is therefore important. It seems odd that the copious literature on Johnson, even those studies dealing with his medical record, should so lightly pass over this particular event.

The clinical story can be assembled from various sources. Boswell is obviously a valuable witness, and Hawkins supplied additional material, though not always accurate. Mrs. Thrale's correspondence is also helpful. Most important of all are the letters Dr. Johnson himself wrote throughout his illness, something that is quite unusual in the annals of aphasiology.

The facts are as follows. Dr. Johnson, in poor health for some years, had been particularly cantankerous during the spring of 1783, while living at Bolt Court, Fleet Street. Restlessness and spasms in the chest were interfering with his sleep, and he was experiencing sensations which he likened to "flatulence or intumescence," finding them difficult to describe more accurately. He was considerably overweight and had long been a slave to voracious and intemperate overeating; he was breathless, bronchitic, and gouty. Some years before, he had eschewed alcoholic beverages altogether, but he had not controlled his gluttony. Always obsessed with his health, he kept in close touch with many medical men socially and professionally. There were apothecaries, too, within his immediate circle, and one had actually lived in Bolt Court as a lodger.

On 16 June 1783 he was actually a trifle better than usual. Feeling "light and easy" he began to plan "schemes of life." He spent a fairly busy day and during the afternoon had sat for his portrait at the studio of Miss Frances Reynolds. This particular portrait was never to his liking, and he dubbed it a "grimly ghost." (Incidentally, it has been unkindly said about Frances Reynolds that her work made everybody laugh and her brother Joshua cry.) After his sitting Johnson went home and retired at the customary hour. In the middle of the night (at 3 a.m. he believed)

Reprinted from Critchley, M. (1962): *Medical History*, vol. 6, and Critchley, M. (1964): *The Black Hole*. Pitman Medical, London. A revised version appears in the *1986 Medical and Health Annual*, published by Encyclopaedia Britannica, Inc., Chicago © 1985.

he awoke and immediately realised that he had sustained a stroke. The subjective sensations that befell him we can only surmise. Later, Johnson spoke of a confusion and indistinctness in the head lasting half a minute. Maybe he noticed some discomfort in a limb. Perhaps he tried to speak aloud in the solitude of his room only to find that words eluded him. We do not know. There is no question, however, but that he proceeded to carry out a mental test of an unusual type: he composed a prayer in Latin verse. According to R. W. Chapman, the text was the following:

Summe Pater, quodunque tuum de corpore Numen
Hoc statuat, precibus Christus adesse velit;
Ingenio parcas, nec sit mihi culpa rogasse,
Qua solum potero parte, placere tibi.

[Almighty Father, whatever the Divine Will ordains concerning this body of mine, may Christ be willing to aid me with his prayers. And let it not be blameworthy on my part to implore that Thou spare my reason, by which faculty alone I shall be able to do Thy pleasure.]

Hawkins, on the other hand, said that Johnson attempted to repeat the Lord's Prayer first in English, then in Latin, and after that in Greek, succeeding in only the last attempt.

Mrs. Thrale, in her *Anecdotes*, reported the incident thus:

Fear was a sensation to which Mr. Johnson was an utter stranger, excepting when some sudden apprehension seized him that he was going to die; and even then he kept all his wits about him, to express the most humble and pathetic petitions to the Almighty; and when the first paralytic stroke took his speech from him he instantly set about composing a prayer in Latin, at once to deprecate God's mercy, to satisfy himself that his mental powers remained unimpaired, and to keep them in exercise that they might not perish by permitted stagnation. This was after we parted; and he wrote to me an account of it, and I intend to publish that letter and many more.

According to Fanny Burney, Dr. Johnson first composed this Latin prayer "internally"; but when he tried to say it aloud, he found his voice was gone.

The evidence suggests that Dr. Johnson's prayer did not entail the recital of some well-remembered lines, but was a spontaneous *ad hoc* composition. The task was performed to his qualified satisfaction, and his awareness of any possible shortcomings was to him a true indication that his intellect was not gravely disturbed.

Immediately afterwards, Johnson carried out another interesting act. Hoping to loosen his tongue, as it were, he deliberately broke his habit of abstinence and drank some brandy (according to Hibbert, two glasses of wine). Whether it had any effect on his speech is not known, but he immediately fell asleep again.

Next morning when he awoke, or on being aroused perhaps, his speech was still impaired. His black servant Frank* came into the bedroom talking and was aston-

---

*Francis Barber was a Jamaican slave who was freed and brought to England by Dr. Bathurst. Later he entered Dr. Johnson's employ, remaining a faithful companion until Johnson's death. According to Hibbert, he died in penury in 1801, having sold all the gifts Johnson had bequeathed him including a watch with a tortoise-shell case, which Johnson had originally bought for 17 guineas.

ished to find his master speechless, or maybe just incoherent, for he put into his hand a note asking Mr. Samuel Allen, his next door neighbour, to be summoned, as well as Dr. Heberden, his physician and friend.

Throughout that day Johnson wrote other letters, though with some difficulty. Heberden came and prescribed a mixture containing aromatic carbonate and aloes, and ordered blisters to his head and throat. Dr. Johnson's disability diminished in severity during the next few days so that by the end of the week little or no impairment in language remained. At no time was there any paralysis. He was a difficult patient, at first taking his medicine very reluctantly. He argued with his apothecary over the salve which, he insisted, should have been prepared according to the Edinburgh dispensatory.

Let Dr. Johnson's letters tell their own tale. The original note thrust into the hands of his servant is not available. But during the first 24 hours of his illness he had written the following letters (which I have been permitted to study and reproduce through the great kindness of Mr. and Mrs. Donald Hyde).

Letter 1: first day of illness (847 Chapman Collection); to Edmund Allen:

> Dear Sir, It hath pleased almighty God this morning to deprive me of the powers of speech; and, as I do not know but that it may be his farther good pleasure to deprive me soon of my senses, I request you will, on the receipt of this note, come to me, and act for me, as the exigencies of my case may require. I am, sincerely yours, S. Johnson. June, 17, 1783.

The present whereabouts of this letter is not known. The following letter is reproduced through the courtesy of the New York Public Library (Berg Collection).

Letter 2: first day of illness (848 Chapman Collection); to the Rev. Dr. Taylor*:

> Dear Sir, It has pleased God by a paralytick stroke in the night to deprive me of speech.
>
> I am very desirous of Dr. Heberden's assistance as I think my case is not past remedy. Let me see you as soon as it is possible. Bring Dr. Heberden with you if you can, but come yourself, in all events. I am glad you are so well, when (when) I am so dreadfully attacked.
>
> I think that by a speedy application of stimulants much may be done. I question if a vomit vigorous and rough would not rouse the organs of speech to action.
>
> As it is too early to send I will try to recollect what I can that can be suspected to have brought on this dreadful distress.
>
> I have been accustomed to bleed frequently for an asthmatick complaint, but have forborn for some time to Dr. Pepys's persuasion, who perceived my legs beginning to swell. I sometimes alleviate a painful, or more

---

*John Taylor had been at school with Samuel Johnson in Lichfield. He entered the church and resided principally in Ashbourne, Derbyshire. When appointed prebendary of Westminster, he was often in London residing in the Cloisters, Little Dean's Yard. Johnson often wrote Taylor's sermons for him at two guineas a time.

properly an oppressive constriction of my chest, by opiates, and have lately taken opium frequently but the last, or two last times in smaller quantities. My largest dose is three grains, and last night I took but two.

You will suggest these things, and they are all that I can call to mind, to Dr. Heberden. I am etc., Sam: Johnson June 17. 1783.

Dr. Brocklesby will be with me to meet Dr. Heberden, and I shall have previously made master of the case as well as I can.

Letter 3: second day of illness (849 Chapman Collection); to Mr. Thomas Davies*:

Dear Sir, I have had, indeed, a very heavy blow; but God, who yet spares my life, I humbly hope will spare my understanding, and restore my speech. As I am not at all helpless, I want no particular assistance, but am strongly affected by Mrs. Davies's tenderness; and when I think she can do me good, shall be very glad to call upon her. I had ordered friends to be shut out; but one or two have found their way in; and if you come you shall be admitted: for I know not whom I can see that will bring more amusement on his tongue, or more kindness in his heart.

I am, etc. Sam. Johnson. June 18. 1783.

Letter 4: third day of illness (850 Chapman Collection); from the Hyde Collection; to Mrs. Thrale, in Bath†:

Dear Madam, I am sitting down in no chearful solitude to write a narrative which would once have affected you with tenderness and sorrow, but which you will perhaps pass over with the careless glance of frigid indifference. For this diminution of regard, however, I know not whether I ought to blame you, who may have reasons which I cannot know, and I do not blame myself who have for a great part of human life done you what good I could, and have never done you evil.

I have been disordered in the usual way and had been relieved by the usual methods, by opium and catharticks, but had rather lessened my dose of opium.

On Monday the 16th I sat for my picture, and walked a considerable way with little inconvenience. In the afternoon and evening I felt myself light and easy, and began to plan schemes of life. Thus I went to bed, and in a short time waked and sat up as has long been my custom, when I felt a confusion and indistinctness in my head which lasted, I suppose about half a minute: I was alarmed and prayed God that however he might afflict my body he would spare my understanding. This prayer, that I might try

---

*Thomas Davies (1712–1785), of 8 Russell St., Covent Garden, was a bookseller, actor, and author. His wife, Susanna, a former actress, was a great beauty. Davies was a friendly, hospitable, and entertaining man, if somewhat pompous. He was a clever mimic and could imitate Johnson's voice and mannerisms.

†Her husband was to die in April 1784 when Mrs. Thrale was left a rich widow. Her attitude towards Dr. Johnson had for some time already been cooling. She eventually disposed of her comfortable house in Streatham. Johnson knew nothing of her growing attachment to Gabriel Piozzi, her daughter's Italian music teacher.

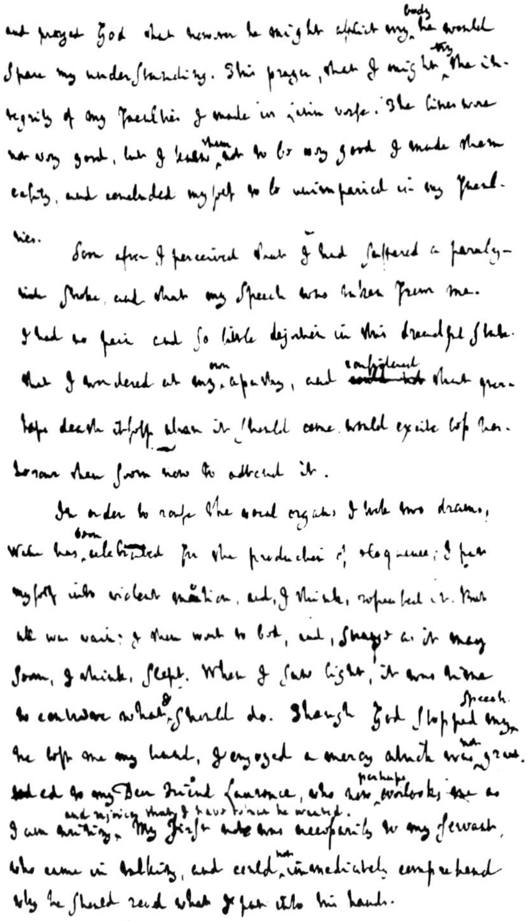

[Figure: handwritten letter — facsimile]

FIG. 1. Second page of Dr. Johnson's letter to Mrs. Thrale, written on the third day of his illness, 19 June 1783. (850 Chapman Collection.)

the integrity of my faculties I made in Latin verse. The lines were not very good, but I knew them not to be very good. I made them easily, and concluded myself to be unimpaired in my faculties. (See Fig. 1.)

Soon after I perceived that I had suffered a paralytick stroke, and that my Speech was taken from me. I had no pain and so little dejection in this dreadful state that I wondered at my own apathy, and considered that perhaps death itself when it should come, would excite less horrour than seems now to attend it.

In order to rouse the vocal organs I took two drams. Wine has been celebrated for the production of eloquence*; I put myself into violent motion, and, I think, repeated it. But all was vain; I then went to bed, and strange as it may seem, I think, slept. When I saw light, it was time

---

*Dr. Johnson was probably conversant with the words of Aristotle: "Why do those who hesitate in their speech become. . . . better under the influence of drunkenness?"

to contrive what I should do. Though God stopped my speech he left my hand, I enjoyed a mercy which was not granted to my Dear friend Laurence,* who now perhaps overlooks me as I am writing and rejoices that I have what he wanted. My first note was necessarily to my servant, who came in talking, and could not immediately comprehend why he should read what I put into his hand.

I then wrote a card to Mr. Allen, that I might have a discreet friend at hand to act as occasion should require. In penning this note I had some difficulty, my hand, I know not how or why, made wrong letters. I then wrote to Dr. Taylor to come to me, and bring Dr. Heberden, and I sent to Dr. Brocklesby, who is my neighbour. My Physicians are very friendly and very disinterested, but give me great hopes, but you may imagine my situation. I have so far recovered my vocal powers, as to repeat the Lord's Prayer with no very imperfect articulation. My memory, I hope, yet remains as it was. But such an attack produces solicitude for the safety of every faculty.

How this will be received by you I know not, I hope you will sympathise with me, but perhaps

> My mistress, mild and good
> Cries, Is he dumb? 'tis time he shou'd†

But can this be possible, I hope it cannot, I hope that what, when I could speak, I spoke of you, and to you, will be in a sober and serious hour remembered by you, and surely it cannot be remembered but with some degree of kindness, I have loved you with virtuous affection, I have honoured you with sincere Esteem. Let not all our endearment be forgotten, but let me have in this great distress your pity and your prayers. You see that I yet turn to You with my complaints as a settled and unalienable friend, do not, do not drive me from You, for I have not deserved the neglect or hatred.

To the Girls, who do not write often, for Susy has written only once, and Miss Thrale owes me a letter, I earnestly recommend as their Guardian and Friend, that They remember their Creator in the days of their Youth.

I suppose you may wish to know how my disease is treated by the Physicians. They put a blister upon my back, and two from my ear to my throat, one on a side. The blister on my back has done little, and those on my throat have not risen. I bullied and bounced (it sticks to our last sand) and compelled the apothecary to make his salve according to the Edinburgh dispensatory, that it might adhere better. I have two on now of my own prescription. They likewise give me salt of hartshorn, which I take with no great confidence, but satisfied that what can be done is done for me.

Oh God, give me comfort and confidence in Thee, forgive my sins, and if it be thy good pleasure, relieve my distress for Jesus Christs sake, Amen.

---

*Dr. Thomas Lawrence (1711–1783), sometime President of the Royal College of Physicians, had been Johnson's medical adviser. He had died about 2 weeks before, paralysed and presumably aphasic.
†A quotation from Swift.

I am almost ashamed of this querulous letter, but now it is written let it go.

I am, Madam, your most humble servant,

Sam: Johnson Bold*[sic]*Court, Fleet Street, June 19 1783.

Letter 5: fourth day of illness (851 Chapman Collection); to Mrs. Thrale in Bath:

Dearest Lady, I think to send you for some time a regular diary. You will forgive the gross images which disease must necessarily present. Dr. Laurence *[sic]* said that medical treatises should be always in Latin.

The two vesicatories which I procured with so much trouble did not perform well, for, being applied to the lower part of the fauces always in motion their adhesion was continually broken. The back, I hear, is very properly played *[sic]*.

I have now healing application to the cheeks and have my head covered with one formidable diffusion of Cantharides, from which Dr. Heberden assures me that experience promises great effects. He told me likewise that my utterance has been improved since yesterday, of which however I was less certain. Though doubtless they who see me at interval can best judge.

I never had any distortion of the countenance, but what Dr. Brocklesby called a little prolapsus which went away the second day.

I was this day directed to eat Flesh, and I dined very copiously upon roasted lamb and boiled pease. I then went to sleep in a chair, and when I waked I found Dr. Broaclesby *[sic]* sitting by me, and fell to talking to him in such a manner as (as) made me glad, and, I hope, made me thankful. The Dr. fell to repeating Juvenal's tenth satire,* but I let him see that the province was mine.

I am to take wine to night, and hope it may do me good.

I am, Madam, your humble Servant

Sam: Johnson. London June 20 1783.

Letter 6: fourth day of illness (852 Chapman Collection) from the Hyde Collection:

Sir, you know I suppose that a sudden illness makes it impracticable for me to wait on Mr. Barry,† and the time is short. If it be your opinion that the end can be obtained by writing. I am very willing to write, and, perhaps it may do as well; it is, at least, all that can be expected at present from,

Sir, your most humble servant, Sam: Johnson Friday, June 20th. 1783 if you would have me write, come to me: I order your admission.

Orandum est, ut mens sana in sano corpore, X 356. (Pray that a healthy mind be in a healthy body.)

†This is presumably Spranger Barry (1719–1777) the "silver-toned" actor, who, along with David Garrick, had appeared in Johnson's play *Mahmet & Irene*.

Letter 7: fifth day of illness (853 Chapman Collection); to Mrs. Thrale in Bath:

Dear Madam, I continue my Journal. When I went to bed last night I found the new covering of my (my) head uneasy, not painful, rather too warm. I had however a comfortable and placid night. My Physicians this morning thought my amendment not inconsiderable, and my friends who visited me said that my look was spritely and cheerful. Nobody has shown more affection than Paradise.* Langton† and he were with me a long time yesterday. I was almost tired. When my friends were gone, I took another liberal dinner such as my Physicians recommended and slept after it, but without such evident advantage as was the effect of yesterday's *siesta*. Perhaps the sleep was not quite so sound for I am harrassed *[sic]* by a very disagreeable question of the Cantharides which I am endeavouring to control by copious dilution.

My disorders are in other respects less than usual, my disease whatever it was seems collected into this one dreadful effect; My Breath is free, the constrictions of the chest are suspended, and my nights pass without oppression.

Today I received a letter of consolation and encouragement from an unknown hand without a name. Kindly and piously, though not enthusiastically written. I had just now from Mr. Pepys,‡ a message enquiring in your name after my health, of this I can give no account.

I am, Madam, Your most humble servant,
Sam: Johnson, London June 21, 1783.

Letter 8: seventh day of illness (845 Chapman Collection); to Mrs. Thrale in Bath:

Dear dear Madam, I thank you for your kind letter, and will continue my diary. On the night of 21st. I had very little rest, being kept awake by an effect of the cantharides not indeed formidable, but very irksome and painful. On the 22 the Physicians released me from the salts of . The Cantharides continued their persecution, but I was set from it at night. I had however not much sleep but I hope for more to night. The vesications on my back and face are healing, and only that on my head continues to operate.

---

*Dr. John Paradise, F.R.S. (1743–1795) had large estates in Virginia and was married to a very beautiful lady. He was described as "a very cultivated man, a great scholar, a poet, a critic, and very soft mannered and obliging." He was a member of the Essex Head Club.

†Bennet Langton (1737–1801), when quite a young man, was so impressed with *The Rambler* he left Leicestershire for 3 months in order to meet Johnson. A tall (6 feet 6 inches), thin gangling adolescent, he was likened to a stork on one leg. He was a very intense individual whose speech would pour out in incoherent torrents when excited. He was of very distinguished ancestry; he joined the militia on leaving Oxford.

‡This is possibly Sir William Walter Pepys Bt. (1740–1825), master in Chancery, but more likely his brother, Sir Lucas Pepys Bt. (1742–1830) who was a physician and a friend of Mrs. Thrale. Johnson disliked his brother, William Walter.

My friends tell me that my power of utterance improves daily, and Dr. Heberden declares that he hopes to find me almost well tomorrow.

Palsies are more common than I thought, I have been visited by four friends who have each had a stroke, and one of them, two.

You offer, dear Madam, of coming to me is charmingly kind, but I will lay up for future use, and then let it be considered as obsolete. A time of dereliction may come when I have hardly any other friend, but in the present exigency, I cannot name one who has been deficient in activity or attention. What man can do for man, has been done for me.

Write to me very often, I am Madam, Your most humble servant. Sam: Johnson. June 23. 1783 London.

Letter 9: eighth day of illness (855 Chapman Collection); from the Prime Minister's Collection; to Mrs. Thrale:

Dear Madam, The journal now like other journals grows every day, as it is not diversified either by operation or events. Less and less is done, and, I thank God, less and less is suffered every day. The physicians seem to think that little more needs to be done. I find that they consulted today about sending me to Bath, and thought it needless. Dr. Heberden takes leave tomorrow.

This day I watered the garden and did not find the watering jobs more heavy than they have hitherto been, and my breath is more free.

Poor dear... has just been here with a present. If it ever falls in your way to do him good, let him have your favour.

Both Queeny's* letter and yours gave me today great pleasure. Think as well and as kindly of me as you can but do not flatter me. Good reciprocations of esteem are the great comforts of life, hyperbolical praise only corrupt the tongue of one and the ear of another.

I am, dear Madam, Your most humble servant. Sam: Johnson London, June 24, 1783. Your letter has no date.

Letter 10: ninth day of illness (856 Chapman Collection); from the Hyde Collection; to Lucy Porter† (Lichfield):

Dear Madam, Since the papers have given an account of my illness, it is proper that I should give my friends some account of it myself.

Very early on the morning of the 16th of this month, I perceived my speech taken from me. When it was light I sat down, and wrote directions as appeared proper. Dr. Heberden and Dr. Brocklesby were called. Blisters were applied, and medicines given; before night I began to speak with some freedom, which has been increasing ever since, so that I now have very [little] impediment in my utterance. Dr. Heberden took his leave this morning.

---

*Queeny: Hester Marie (1764–1859) eldest daughter of Mr. and Mrs. Thrale; afterwards Viscountess Keith.
†Lucy Porter (1715–1786), Dr. Johnson's stepdaughter.

Since I received this stroke I have in other respects been better than I was before, and hope yet to have a comfortable summer. Let me have your prayers.

If writing is not troublesome let me know whether you are pretty well, and how you have passed the Winter and the Spring.

Make my compliments to all my Friends.

I am, dear Madam, Your most humble servant,

Sam: Johnson. London. June 25. 1783.

Letter 11: 13th day of illness (858 Chapman Collection); New York Public Library, Berg Collection; Torn; postmark 30.VI; date added by Mrs. Piozzi,* 29 June 1783; to Mrs. Thrale in Bath:

I climbed up stairs to the garret, and then up a ladder to the leads, and talked to the artist rather too long, for my voice though clear and distinct for a little while soon tires and falters. The organs of speech are yet very feeble, but will I hope be by the mercy of God finally restored, at present like any other weak limb, they can endure but little labour at once. Would you not have been very [sorry] for me when I could scarcely speak?

Letter 12: 17th day of illness (861 Chapman Collection); to James Boswell (Edinburgh):

Dear Sir, Your anxiety about my health is very friendly, and very agreeable with your general kindness. I have, indeed, had a very frightful blow. On the 17th of last month, about three in the morning, as near as I can guess, I perceived myself almost totally deprived of speech. My organs were so obstructed that I could say *no*, but could scarcely say *yes*. I wrote the necessary directions for it pleased God to spare my hand, and I sent for Dr. Heberden and Dr. Brocklesby. Between the time in which I sent for the doctors I had, I believe, in spite of my surprise and solicitude, a little sleep, and Nature began to renew its operations. They came, and gave the directions which the disease required, and from that time I have been continually improving in articulation. I can now speak, but the nerves are weak, and I cannot consider discourse long; but strength, I hope will return. The Physicians consider me as cured. . . .

July 3. 1783.

Letter 13: 19th day of illness (862 Chapman Collection); from the Hyde Collection; to Lucy Porter (Lichfield):

Dear Madam. . . My disease affected my speech, and still continues in some degree to obstruct my utterment, but voice being distinct enough for a while, but the organs being yet weak are quickly weary. But in other respects I am, I think, rather better than I have lately been, and can let you know my state without the help of any other hand.

---

*Mrs. Thrale married Gabriele Piozzi on 25 July 1784.

In the opinion of my friends, and in my own I am gradually mending. The Physicians consider me as cured, and I had been four days ago to wash the Cantharides from my head. Last Tuesday I dined at the Club. . . .
    July 5. 1783.

Letter 14: 22nd day of illness (865 Chapman Collection); to John Ryland* (Cranbrook):

Dear Sir. . . My recovery, I think, advances, but its progress is (is) not quick. My voice has its usual tone, and a stranger in the beginning of our conversation does not perceive any depravation or obstruction. But the organs of articulation are weak, and quickly tire. I question if I could read, without pausing, a single page of a small book.
    July 8. 1783.

Letter 15: 29th day of illness (867 Chapman Collection); to William Strahan Esq., M.P.† (London):

Sir. . . My breath is more free, and my nights are less disturbed. But my utterance is still impeded, and my voice soon grows weary with long sentences.
    July 18. 1783.

Letter 16: 36th day of illness (869 Chapman Collection); to Mrs. Thrale in Bath:

I am very well except my voice soon falters. . . .
    July 23. 1783.

Letter 17: 37th day of illness (871 Chapman Collection); to the Rev. Dr. John Taylor (Ashbourne):

. . . My voice in the exchange of salutations, or on other little occasions is as it was, but in a continuance of conversation it soon tires. I hope it grows stronger but it does not make very quick advance. . . .
    July 24. 1783.

Letter 18: 37th day of illness (871.2 Chapman Collection); from the Hyde Collection; to Wm. Bowles‡ (Heale):

---

*John Ryland (1717?–1798) was a friend of Johnson and fellow member of the Kings Head Club in Ivy Lane. He was a West Indian merchant of Tower Hill, though originally a lawyer. A dissenter, he was known as a Whig of the old school. Johnson, a staunch Tory, dubbed him "a republican and a roundhead."

†William Strahan (1715–1785) was a Scot and Johnson's printer and unofficial banker. His premises were in New St., off Fleet St., and in order to be close by while compiling his dictionary, Johnson took a house in Gough Square, with Gunpowder Alley in between. Strahan entered Parliament and tried to persuade Johnson to do the same, but nothing came of it. Years later Johnson arranged for Strahan's son George to secure a place at the Henry Bright College, Abingdon, Berks.

‡William Bowles (1755–1826), of Heale Court, Upper Woodford, near Salisbury, was "a man of exemplary religious order in his family."

Dear Sir, You will easily believe that the first seizure was alarming. I recollected three that had lost the voice, of whom two continued speechless for life, but I believe, no means were used for their recovery. When the Physicians came they seemed not to consider the attack as very formidable, I feel now no effect from it but in my voice, which I cannot sustain for more than a little time.
July 24. 1783.

Letter 19: 57th day of illness (875 Chapman Collection); to Mrs. Thrale (Weymouth):

I am now broken with disease, without the alleviation of friendship, or domestick society. I have no middle state between clamour and silence, between genial conversation and self-tormenting solicitude. . . .
August 13. 1783.

. . . .

The evidence as to Dr. Johnson's illness points clearly to a cerebrovascular accident followed by a disorder of speech, by no means severe, and comparatively brief. That the problem was not one of pure dysarthria but a dysphasic one is shown by defects in his written compositions. Nevertheless, the speech disorder included a strong element of dysarthria which continued even after the availability of words had returned. Such, at any rate, was Johnson's belief. The opinion of his doctors and of those around him might have been different. His aphasia seems, therefore, to have belonged to that category often referred to as aphemia, or Broca's aphasia. Such a diagnosis might even now be supported by those neurologists who are uncritical of systems of classification of the aphasias. It is interesting that, like so many aphasiacs, Johnson experienced a temporary difficulty with the particles *yes* and *no*, and found that the negative term came more readily to his lips than the affirmative. Might this be an outcome of the patient's previous personality?

Study of the original manuscript letters that Johnson wrote over the ensuing month reveals a number of departures from his usual literary style. For one thing, the penmanship was more untidy than was customary. Johnson made no mention of any weakness of the hand with which he held the pen, and the fault must have been at a higher level. In addition, many examples of verbal misuse, omissions, and iterations can be seen. Some mistakes were detected by Johnson and corrected, but not all. These features are shown, for example, in letter 4, where we find (see Fig. 2):

Line 8: two illegible words erased, and "human life" inserted
Line 10: "had" changed to "have" and "been" inserted
Line 18: illegible word erased, and "my head" inserted
Line 20: "body" inserted
Line 21: "try" inserted
Line 23: "them" inserted
Line 29: "own" inserted, "could not" erased, and "considered" inserted
Line 33: "been" inserted
Line 34: "a" changed to "o" in "motion"

FIG. 2. Enlargements displaying the writer's emendations. (1) "...however he might afflict my [body] he would spare my understanding. This prayer, that I might [try] the integrity of my faculties...." (2) "...I wondered at my own apathy and [considered] that perhaps death..."(3)"...Wine has [been] celebrated..." (4) "...Though God stopped my [speech]..."

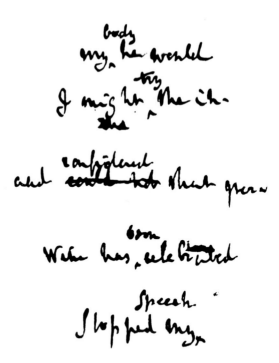

Line 37: "I" inserted; "speech" inserted
Line 38: "not" inserted
Line 39: illegible erasure; "perhaps" inserted
Line 41: "not" inserted
Line 50: "recovered" misspelt but corrected
Line 58: "you" erased, "That" inserted
Line 67: erasure of "on each way" and "from my ear" inserted
Line 72: "now" inserted

The content of the foregoing correspondence is also worthy of comment. In all the letters Johnson wrote just after his stroke we find a preoccupation with his symptoms. Those letters in particular addressed to Mrs. Thrale constitute a series of medical bulletins that must have proved wearisome to the recipient. The style of much of the writing is unusual; and in his efforts to express himself, he is often less than successful. Many sentences show a departure from the trenchant, vigorous—if pedantic—prose we associate with Samuel Johnson. His wording is simpler the more concrete the subject matter he is committing to paper. When wrestling with ideas of an abstract nature his phraseology becomes less cogent and less crisp. These imperfections are obvious in letter 4 written on the third day of his illness.

In the later stages, his aphasia is betrayed by an asthenolalia or ready fatiguability involving the volume of his voice.

Dr. Johnson was fortunate in escaping any paralysis of his limbs. Nothing more was evident than a temporary facial asymmetry, or prolapsus as Dr. Brocklesby called it. We do not know whether it was the right or the left side which was at

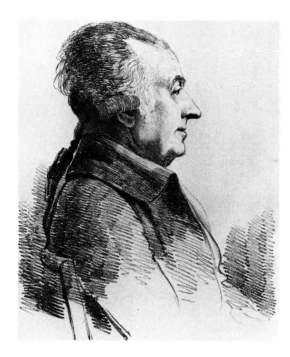

FIG. 3. Dr. Richard Brocklesby (1722–1797). (Courtesy of the Royal College of Physicians.)

fault. A week later Johnson was apparently himself again, for on 24 June Mrs. Thrale was writing in her diary that she had received a letter from him "in his usual style."

By November of that same year, that is, 5 months later, Johnson was exclaiming to Sir John Hawkins: "What a man am I! Who have got the better of three diseases, the palsy, the gout and the asthma, and can now enjoy the conversation of my friends, without the interruption of weakness or pain!"

Scrutiny of the medical evidence unfortunately does not indicate which cerebral hemisphere was the one involved by the presumed vascular accident. Only by assembling indirect evidence or clues can we suspect that it was the left side of the brain that was probably affected.

At this point some data as to the identity of Dr. Johnson's medical advisers might be interpolated.

Dr. Richard Brocklesby (1722–1797) was born in Minehead, Somerset, of Quaker parents, but at an early age went to live in Ireland (Fig. 3). He studied at the Edinburgh School of Medicine, qualified at Leyden, and practised in Norfolk Street, Strand. He was a friend of Edmund Burke and also the medical attendant of Samuel Wilkes, Burke's political antagonist. Brocklesby was a close friend of Johnson to whom he offered a home and an annual stipend of £100.

Dr. William Heberden (1710–1801) was one of the greatest of the eighteenth century physicians (Fig. 4). At the time of Johnson's illness he was practising at Cecil Street, Strand, though later he moved to what had been Nell Gwyn's house in Pall Mall. Johnson spoke of Heberden as "the *ultimus Romanorum*; the last of

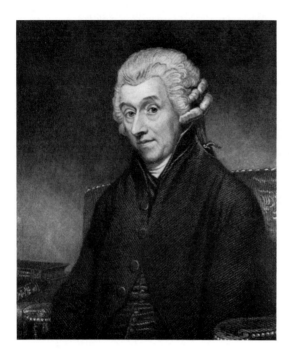

FIG. 4. Dr. William Heberden (1710–1801). (Courtesy of
the Royal College of Physicians.)

our learned physicians," though in another mood he also referred to him as the
"timidorum timidissimus." Heberden's private case books, now in the library of
the Royal College of Physicians, unfortunately contain no certain note as to the
problem of his distinguished patient. True, Dr. Squibb, writing in 1849, believed
he discovered a reference to Johnson's case in Heberden's *Index Historia Morborum.*
Although this statement was accepted at face value by Chaplin, I am by no means
convinced. The date is wrong and the information too meagre. I can but conclude
that Heberden made no specific mention of this important case. Quite recently, L.
McHenry stated (*J. R. Soc. Med.*, 78:485, 1985) that he has identified the probable
reference to Johnson in Heberden's *Index.*

Heberden was also one of London's most fashionable practitioners, and there
was a jingle popular at the end of the eighteenth century:

> You should send, if ought should ail ye
> For Willis, Heberden or Baillie.
> All exceeding skilful men
> Baillie, Willis, Heberden;
> Uncertain which most sure to kill is
> Baillie, Heberden or Willis.

Neither Heberden nor Brocklesby would accept fees from Johnson, who later
bequeathed to them and to each of his other doctors copies of his writings. Dr.
Johnson had an exceptionally wide acquaintance with surgeons, physicians, and

apothecaries in London, and J. P. Warbasse (1907) was able to enumerate no fewer than 59 medical men among his friends.*

Concerning doctors, Dr. Johnson is reported to have said:

> A Physician in a great city seems to be the plaything of fortune; his degree of reputation is, for the most part, casual: they that employ him know not his excellence; they that reject him know not his deficience.

Neurologists with the Johnson case report before them may well ponder why the aphasia was so mild and so short-lived. Various possible explanations occur to one. In the first place, the pathological lesion within the brain might have been small and ischaemic rather than embolic or haemorrhagic in nature. It might conceivably have been either in the category of Pierre Marie's lacunar disintegration or what Denny-Brown would have called a "haemodynamic crisis." In addition to these rather obvious suggestions it is tempting to invoke a more endogenous factor and to argue that the very magnitude of Johnson's literary capacity might have assisted the process of restoration of function. Johnson was not only a master of language but a polyglot, a lexicographer, and a man of prodigious verbal memory who could read and assimilate a printed text with astonishing speed. True, his literary style was ponderous and mannered. As Hazlitt complained, "There is no discrimination, no selection, no variety in it. He uses none but 'tall, opaque words,' taken from the 'first row of the rubric'—words with the greatest number of syllables, or Latin phrases with merely English terminations." Macaulay spoke of "Johnsonese." His letters were different, being elegant and attractive. But his linguistic talents were undoubtedly best shown in his conversation, where his phraseology and his wit were dazzling and of a class rarely equalled.

R. T. Davies (quoted by Hibbert) was less critical about Dr. Johnson's prose. "A conspicuous ingredient of Johnson's ample style," he wrote, "is his polysyllabism. He used big words deliberately and typically, and it is something to which his style shows itself to be the man. One may sometimes suspect that he was partly laughing at himself as he played this role of the orotund man of learning or magnificent moralist. In the final *Rambler* essay, however, he justified his use of big words by explaining that he had "familiarized the terms of philosophy" where "common" words would be "less pleasing to the ear or less distinct in their magnification."

Such a stylistic background may partly account for the nature of Johnson's dysgraphia and explain why the literary level continued so high. We recall his note to Mr. Davies written on the second day of his illness: "If you come you shall be admitted: for I know not whom I can see that will bring more amusement on his tongue, or more kindness in his heart"—lines which no ordinary man could compose and few aphasiacs emulate. Witness too the phrase in letter 9: "Good reciprocations of esteem are the great comforts of life, hyperbolical praise only corrupt the tongue of the one and the ear of the other." Johnson's experience as a dictionary

---

*In 1782, the year before Johnson's stroke, there were 149 physicians in London, 274 surgeons, and 351 apothecaries. The population of London was at that time 650,845. In other words, one person in every 840 had some form of medical qualification.

compiler no doubt accounts for the vocabulary of his letters, so unusually rich for one afflicted with an aphasia. Some quite unexpected terms appear in the text and are therefore arresting and yet wholly appropriate ("exigencies," "integrity," "discreet," "endearment," "unalienable," "salve," "querulous," "dereliction"). These words that one does not expect to find in the letters of the average aphasiac; however, Johnson was by no means an average man, but one who was very much *hors de série*. One or two of the terms which appear in the Johnson letters strike the modern reader as so unusual as to raise the question of whether they might be metonymous, paragraphic errors. For example, one may take the words appearing in letters 4 and 7: "disinterested" (for "interested" or "caring"); "solicitude" ("anxiety"); and "obsolete" (in the sense of "rejected"). Some light can be thrown upon this point by referring to Johnson's own dictionary where his personal views as to the meanings, definitions, synonyms, or verbal equivalents for these unexpected terms can be found, and where they are seen to be not quite appropriate. Certain fragments of his letters contain genuine paragraphic errors as shown from a study of the original text. Even as late as 24 July, i.e., 37 days after the stroke, a note to William Bowles (letter 18) contains a word that Chapman read as "poriting," which might be a neologism if it is not a simple misreading of "posting."

Johnson's aphasia is also betrayed here and there in his letters by the phenomenon of "contamination" whereby a word, evoked in one context, shortly afterwards crops up in another. This is, however, rare in the Johnson letters, and one indeed can but remain astonished at the amazing vocabulary which he continued to employ. If we adopt a statistical analysis of his writings and estimate the type/token ratio of his letters, we find no great difference in those written *before* and those written *after* his stroke. This is illustrated in Table 1.

Another statistical study—a differential punctuation count—of Johnson's writings before and after his stroke is worthwhile. Chapman said that Johnson was ordinarily

TABLE 1. *Type–token ratio before and after Johnson's stroke*

	Letter	Date	Total no. of words, i.e., "tokens"	No. of different words, i.e., "types"	Type–token ratio
Before the stroke	373	20.1.75	169	90	0.53
	844	4.6.83	123	80	0.65
	845	5.6.83	266	170	0.64
	846	13.6.83	298	185	0.62
After the stroke	847	17.6.83	69	49	0.71
(16/17.6.83)	848	17.6.83	253	137	0.54
	849	18.6.83	117	82	0.70
	850	19.6.83	887	352	0.39
	851	20.6.83	255	175	0.68
	852	20.6.83	80	56	0.70
	853	21.6.83	232	159	0.68
	854	23.6.83	232	141	0.60

TABLE 2. *Punctuation count before and after Johnson's stroke*

Punctuation mark	Before Actual	%	After (Chapman enumeration) 847	848	849	850	851	852	853	%
Comma (,)	72	55	8	12	10	85	18	13	15	59
Full stop (.)	43	33	3	13	6	40	13	4	13	34
Semicolon (;)	12	9	1		4	3				3
Colon (:)	3	2		1	1	1	1	3	1	3
Dash (—)										
Question mark (?)										
Exclamation mark (!)						1				
Total	130		12	26	21	130	32	20	29	

rather erratic in his use of punctuation marks. He used them freely with a partiality for semicolons. Table 2 compares the punctuation counts of his letters written before and shortly after the stroke. The difference, though not great, shows itself in an apparent reduction in the use of semicolons.

Another possible explanation of the mild and transient nature of Dr. Johnson's aphasia comes up for discussion. Could it be that he was left-handed and that no real unilateral cerebral dominance existed? We know that left-handers with lesions of either hemisphere, if followed by an aphasia, do well, the language disorder usually being benign in character. From a study of Johnson's upbringing it is not possible to determine with confidence whether he was naturally right-handed or left-handed. His own diary informs us that when he was quite young, an "issue," or seton, was cut in his left arm and deliberately kept open and not allowed to heal until he was 6 years of age. The purpose of this surgical measure is not known. Probably it was a device whereby his defective eyesight might be cured, according to a popular superstition. Conceivably it might have been intended to overcome an incipient left manual preference. The commonsense view is that whatever the object of the seton it was deliberately inserted into the nonpreferred limb, leaving the masterhand free and unimpeded.

Certainly the doctor used the right hand for writing, but this must not be taken as proof of inherent right-handedness: The orthodox way to hold a pen might have been imposed upon him. Contemporary portraits show that Johnson usually used the right hand for holding a book as well as a walking stick. Only one picture might appear to argue in favour of a left-sided preference. In the illustration in which Johnson is entertaining two pretty Methodist ladies at the Mitre Tavern, his teacup is on the table in front of him and just to the left-hand side. As this picture was painted many years after Johnson's death by Dante Gabriel Rossetti, it has no clue in this present context.

Some would argue that the problem of Dr. Johnson's handedness is solved in his last portrait—that by James Roberts (Fig. 5). Here the doctor sits with his hands clasped before him in a natural attitude of repose. The little finger of the right hand lies lowermost (Fig. 6). This purely automatic posture argues to some au-

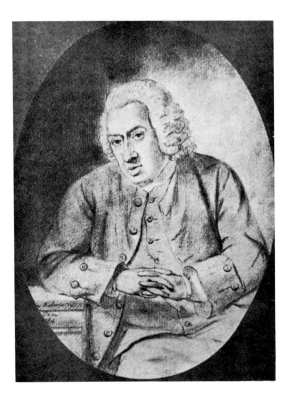

FIG. 5. Last portrait of Dr. Johnson (by James Roberts).

FIG. 6. Enlargement of the clasped hands in Dr. Johnson's portrait.

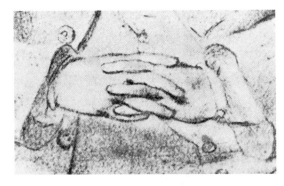

thorities in favour of right-handedness. Unfortunately, this procedure does not stand up well to statistical analysis. In 1978 Critchley and Critchley published the results of a comparison between preferred hand for writing and manner of interlacing the fingers. Their series comprised 676 children with developmental dyslexia (493 boys, 183 girls), chosen randomly. Of those who preferred to hold a pen with the right hand, 39% showed a left-handed type of handclasp; among those writing with the left hand, 38% interlaced their fingers in a right-handed way. It was found, then, that out of five persons conformity between preferred hand for writing and mode of interlacing fingers was seen in three and nonconformity in two.

Therefore, although we cannot prove that Johnson was right-handed, we are able to assert that no evidence exists that he was left-handed.*

Although Johnson suffered no change in intellectual powers after the stroke, he developed a marked depression which followed a brief period of apathy. His habitual fears of death and eternal damnation increased, and Mrs. Thrale's lack of warmth towards him made matters worse. Dr. Johnson had other reasons, too, for his despondency. Not long before the stroke, his lodger, the apothecary Levitt, had suddenly died after lapsing into a state of speechlessness. Still more disturbing was the memory of the terminal illness of his great friend Dr. Lawrence (Fig. 7). As the result of an apoplexy Lawrence sustained a right hemiplegia and a severe aphasia, and Johnson was in close touch with his friend up to the time of his death 10 weeks before he himself was stricken with a cerebrovascular accident. Indeed in a letter to Dr. Lawrence's daughter Johnson had written: "If we could have again but his mind, and his tongue in his mind, and his right hand, we should not much lament the rest"† (Chapman 802). This particular letter was despatched 10 months before Dr. Lawrence's death or 10 weeks before Johnson sustained his own aphasia.

His depression lifted, for a time at any rate. On 1 July Fanny Burney noted in her diary that she had called on Dr. Johnson and had found him gay and cheerful. On 19 April 1784, she reported that he was amazingly recovered, perfectly good-humoured, comfortable, and smilingly alive to idle chat.

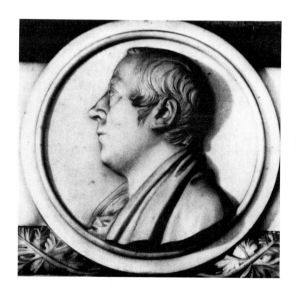

FIG. 7. Dr. Thomas Lawrence. (Courtesy of Canterbury Cathedral and the Royal College of Physicians.)

---

*The only conceivable hint to the contrary was an observation he made during his visit to Paris. He went to watch the royal family at dinner and made a note that "the King fed himself with his left hand *as we*" (my italics).

†That some measure of cerebration was spared is shown in the incident when Lawrence, wanting to be given a dose of laudanum (or "black drops" as was the common term), failed to articulate the necessary words. In his frustration, he took up a pen in his left hand, dipped it into the inkwell, and then scattered the blots upon a sheet of white paper. In this way he made himself understood.

Medical views on aphasia were muddled in Johnson's time and remained so until the end of the eighteenth century. This is illustrated by the treatment which Johnson endured with blisters applied to his head, face, and throat in an effort to stimulate the organs of speech. That his lesion lay in the brain rather than the larynx was not realised. At that time, no clear distinction was recognised between the muttering delirium of mental disease; hysterical affections of speech ranging from dysphonia to mutism; the various types of dysarthria or faulty articulation, central or peripheral in origin; and aphasia proper, that is, an effacement of the faculty of language, spoken and inscribed. Only too often an inability to talk was attributed to a palsy of the tongue, and desperate efforts were made to goad that member into activity. The conception of an incomplete affection of language with faults in speaking, writing, and comprehending spoken or printed words developed belatedly.

As a matter of fact, Dr. Heberden happened to be well ahead of his contemporaries in his thinking. Thus in his *Commentaries on the History and Cure of Diseases*, a work which appeared posthumously in 1802, he wrote: "When a person has been struck on the left side, and has at the same time lost his voice, there is no certainty of his being able to signify his feelings, or his wants, by writing. They ... have sometimes been able to do it, though in a confused manner; and the same person on different days would either write intelligibly or make an illegible scrawl."

This shrewd observation was in advance of current notions of the possible results of an apoplexy. A little later we find him also writing: "The inability to speak is owing sometimes not to the paralytic state of the organs of speech only, but to the utter loss of the knowledge of language and letters which some have quickly regained, and others have recovered by slow degrees, getting the use of the smaller words first, and being frequently unable to find the word they want, and using another for it of a quite different meaning, as if it were a language which they had once known, but by long disuse had almost forgotten. ... One person was forced to take some pains in order to learn again to write, having lost the ideas of all the letters except the initials of his two names."

It is not known exactly when these remarks were made. Heberden died in 1801 at the age of 91, and his writings were not published until a year after his death. Johnson's stroke may well have inspired these perspicacious comments.

Sir Richard Blackmore, royal physician and poet, had in 1725 observed the phenomenon of paraphasia, whereby a patient might unwittingly say one word instead of another, but like his contemporaries he attributed this to a disorder of the tongue. Other eighteenth century writers who made brief reports of similar misuse of words were R. James (1743), Linnaeus (1745), Delius (1757), Morgagni (1769), Spalding (1772), Gesner (1772), Falconer (1787), A. Crichton (1793), and Goethe (1796). None of them realised that the explanation of the fault lay in a cerebral lesion. The conception of aphasia, a disorder of language due to brain damage, did not really materialize until the work of the writers Pinel, Gall, Bouillaud, Auburtin, Broca, Trousseau, and Dax, and, most important of all, Hughlings Jackson.

Johnson's autopathographic account is therefore an important element in the early history of aphasia, worthy of being aligned with the better known personal accounts made by Professor Lordat of Montpellier and Professor Forel of Zürich.

Rarely does a professional writer continue to work after an aphasia, even though language functions are apparently restored. Johnson lived 18 months after his stroke, but although he regained his ability to express himself he was by now a gravely sick man. Nevertheless, his literary output did not cease altogether. As he informed Mrs. Thrale on 19 April 1784 (Chapman 954), his nights were sleepless and he would while the time away by turning Greek epigrams into Latin. Ninety-eight of these were published by Bennet Langton in volume XI of *Works* (1787). During this period Johnson also wrote a dedication to Charles Burney's *Commemoration of Handel*, which appeared in 1785. He intended to write a preface to the collection of the works of John Scott, but this was never completed.

In November 1784 he translated into English verse Horace's ode *Diffugere nives, redeunt, jam gramina campis*. He had also intended to have written an epitaph in Latin verse to David Garrick, but he found himself unequal to the task.

An entry in Johnson's personal diary dated 1 January 1784 contains supplication that he might be relieved of "all such scruples and perplexities" as encumbered and obstructed his mind.

Johnson died on 13 December 1784 from cardiorenal failure. James Wilson performed the necropsy on 15 December 1784, and his manuscript record of the event (Fig. 8) is contained within the library of the Royal College of Physicians. An illustration of Johnson's emphysematous lung (Fig. 9) appeared in Matthew

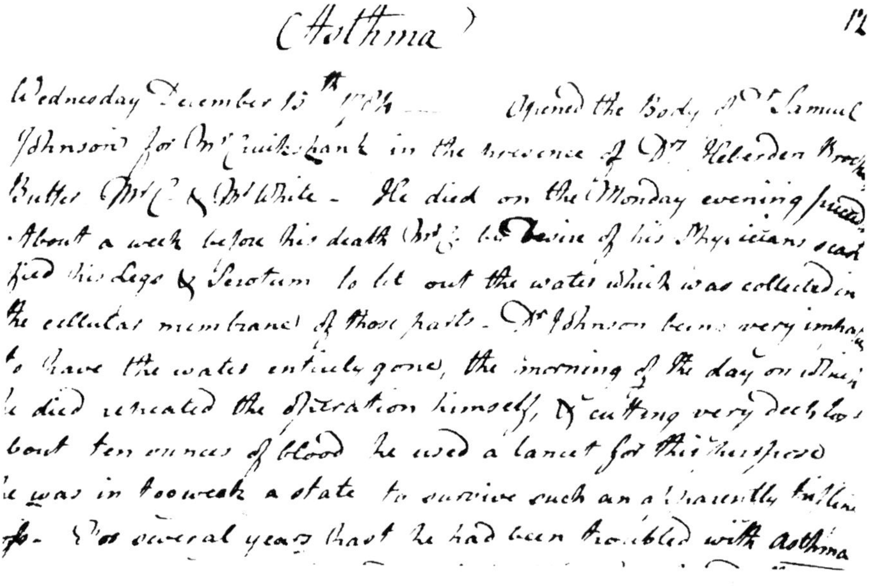
(Asthma) 12

Wednesday December 15th 1784 — Opened the Body of Dr Samuel Johnson for Mr Cruikshank in the presence of Dr Heberden Brocklesby Butter Mr C & Mr White - He died on the Monday evening preceed- About a week before his death Dr [illegible] one of his Physicians scarified his Legs & Scrotum to let out the water which was collected in the cellular membrane of those parts - Dr Johnson being very impatient to have the water entirely gone, the morning of the day on which he died repeated the operation himself, by cutting very deep, lost about ten ounces of blood he used a lancet for this purpose he was in too weak a state to survive such an additionally [illegible] - For several years past he had been troubled with asthma

FIG. 8. Record of Johnson's necropsy. (Courtesy of the Royal College of Physicians.)

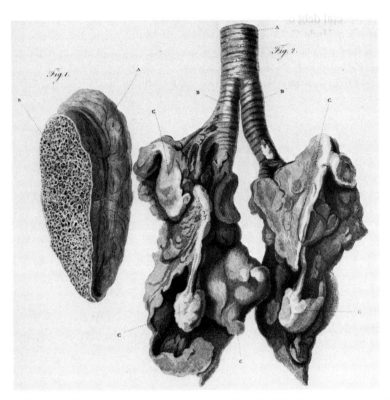

FIG. 9. Drawing of Johnson's emphysematous lung, from Baillie's *Morbid Anatomy* (1793–1799). (Courtesy of the Royal College of Physicians.)

Baillie's *Morbid Anatomy* (1793–1799). The drawings were made by William Clift (1775–1849). Dr. Johnson's right kidney was removed and preserved by the mortuary attendant, Mr. White (subsequently Dr. White). No examination of the brain was made. While stitching up the body, Mr. White pricked his finger with the needle and developed a septic infection.

So perished the gigantic Samuel Johnson, with his anthology of ailments. Let us, in conclusion, turn from further examination of his darker days, and carry away a memory of what he said in a gayer heyday mood:

"If I had no duties, and no reference to futurity, I would spend my life in driving briskly in a postchaise with a pretty woman; but she should be one who would understand me, and would add something to the conversation."

Acknowledgments

For facsimile reproductions of the Johnson letters quoted in the text, I am indebted to the New York Public Library (Berg Collection), the Prime Minister's Library at Chequers, and to Mrs. Donald Hyde in particular. To the last-named I owe an especial debt of gratitude for allowing me to reproduce the copy of Chapman 850 from the Hyde Collection, Somerville, New Jersey. The President of the Royal College of Physicians has been very kind in allowing me to reproduce the manuscript description of the Johnson autopsy. Mr. Payne, the then College librarian, has always been most courteous and helpful in his assistance.